Acknowledgements

Those who need to be acknowledged: Jim Kasmir, Katherine Kasmir, Barb Obermeier, David Cintron, Carol Cintron, Sandy Sowards, Ken Wright, Rafael Tellez, David Buehrens, Tere Buckingham - Davis, Karl Parker, Peter Gillham, Rafa Tellez, Stacy Plasch, Robert Harrison, Darryl Sanford, my best friend Ron, my brother, my mom and dad.

Unread books are glorified paperweights. If you love this book, share your stories and let those interested read directly from it. It is very easy for me to look at someone and quickly detect what is physically wrong with him or her. Some call me intuitive. I have been told that I have the wisdom of an ancient sage, and the formulation ability of a long dead Chinese herbal master. In this book I am passing on those abilities in a form that can be duplicated. If you intend to give this book away as a gift it is a good choice. Our future is in our kids. Kids immediately get the gifts in this book. Be sure to share this book with the under twenty crowd.

Neff/Harry Publishing ©2009 First and Second Cover Design by Gregory Barnett | rocknmotion.com | Second Interior and Third Cover Design by David Buehrens | Fourth Cover Design by Barbara Obermeier Design
First Printing November 2005 | Second Printing January 2006 | Third Printing June 2006
Fourth Printing May 2007 | Fifth Printing March 2008 | Sixth Printing May 2009

Diagnostic Face Reading
and Holistic Healing

by Roger Bezanis

Table of Contents / Sections

There is much acrimony surrounding this book. Big Pharmaceuticals and the medical establishment as we know it are terrified that you will say "ENOUGH." That is why you are reading this book.
-Roger Bezanis

1 Starting Your Adventure

This is **your** book. **You** wanted to read it. In these pages you will find the jewels that will allow you to change your life. These same gifts are there for everyone you know. Unfortunately, some of your friends and family are not where you are in your life, health and consciousness. Of course, sharing this book and all of its gifts is just what you will want to do. When you do, please do not force it down anyone's throat. No one ever likes being force-fed. A rejected book is a useless book. If you badger people with the content of this book you will lose friends. Once the door is closed it tends to remain closed. Ergo, all those you could have helped are lost.

Individuals who read this manuscript need to discover it similar to the way you did. Let them. Share your excitement.

Set an example and live by this book. When those around you see you winning, they will naturally begin to ask what you are doing. Once this occurs, you have an ear and someone who wants to know how they too can heal. Correcting your health slows down your own aging process. Everyone you know will want to know what you did and how you did it.

RULE 1:
There are four kinds of people in regards to this book. Those who have read it, not read it, borrow it and those who receive this book as a gift. The only value this book possesses is to the reader. It must be read. For the borrower, let him or her keep this manuscript for a day or two or when they trade something of equal value. Only then does the "borrower" have an investment in this manuscript. Generally people very seldom place much value in what is borrowed. Learn by heart, until someone reads this book (as you have), it has no value whatsoever.

RULE 2:
If you are asked to answer questions from this book, direct them to the proper page to read. Again, if you want your friends to read this book, hand it to them. Otherwise you will forever be answering questions. You will everlastingly be their crutch. Verbal answers do not stick. But the written word does. That is why we have books. The written word is your answer.

RULE 3:
You are receiving information that is in a different stratum than what you are normally exposed to. The data in these pages is not taught in colleges or part of any medical curriculum. The alternative health community is just now learning this data. Therefore, do not use this book to make someone wrong. Do not make wrong those who cannot see beyond what they know. Do not make wrong your parents, friends or associates. They are all doing the best they can with what they have and know. Kindness will win more battles than all the steel that you can muster. When someone asks to see this book, show it to him or her. Live by example and you will win.

RULE 4:
Do not forget who holds the keys to the Earth's future. It is the young since kids instantly understand and can use this book. Our young have not been fully brainwashed by our media, therefore get this book into their hands. They will save this planet.

"Diagnostic Face Reading and the Holistic Healing" is not like other books you have read. DFRHH is one of the more complicated books that most people will come across. The reason this book is such a challenging read is not because I wrote in language long dead and forgotten, but because I am saying things that are contradictory to what you have been taught. In this book I am giving you concepts that are foreign to what you currently know. This book will fly in the face of everything you have been told in a number of areas, that you think you know very well.

Therefore, considering the sheer "Oh come on," "What exactly did he say?" and the "Now hold on here a minute, that is impossible" factor of this book, it will need to be read multiple times. Test show that three reads per chapter is sufficient for people to really grasp what I am saying. The best way to read this book is one chapter a night and then sleep on it. Then reread the same chapter two more nights in a row. The first reading is for exposure to this new data, in the next nights reading you will start to grasp what I am saying. By the third reading you should be thinking with what I am saying. I want you to have the certainness that I do. That is the purpose of this book.

Realize that I made no mistakes in this book. Nowhere did I say something that I did not mean to say. Whenever I have included something in this book, it is because it works. These findings have been tested for years. Thousands of individuals have validated these results at a rate of better than 95%. Therefore it is very important for you to fully understand what I am saying.

Please understand that you should read this book with a dictionary at hand. When you do run into a word that you do not know the meaning of, you can look it up in your dictionary. If you do this, the book will make sense. To ignore this, I guarantee will leave you with blank spots (or sections) all over this book.

Again, when you find a word that you do not know the meaning of, look it up in a dictionary. If this book is not making sense, look for a word just before that section (that is confusing) that

Roger Bezanis

you do not comprehend. Do not read any further until you comprehend what that word means or the next few paragraphs will be a blank.

**SPECIAL NOTE: Throughout this book I use the word poison. Because of that I am defining it here.
poi·son (poiˊzən)
n.
1. A substance taken internally or applied externally that is injurious to health or dangerous to life.
2. A chemical substance that inhibits another substance or a reaction.

Without understanding, this book is as good as a brick. Understand my words and capture understandings that you and less than 50,000 people on the planet recognize. If you fully appreciate what it is that I have written, you will be able to identify and repair any problem of the body.

2 The Man Eating Machine

We often think that those in charge are "in charge" because they can be trusted. Every day we make investments, life changing decisions, take drugs and signoff on surgeries because "a trained professional" said it was the thing to do for our health or welfare.

We place our trust in our mayors, governors, generals, cabinet members, parliaments, presidents, large firms and government agencies. We do this because we "believe" that these individuals and groups are "interested in" and or "defending" our best interests.

Sadly this is rarely the case. Our "best" or welfare is second to the bottom line. The following story is true and is a matter of public record. It weaves an amazing story that was so appalling, that legendary film maker and actor Clint Eastwood brought it to the screen in the 2008 movie "The Changeling."

On 10 March 1928, Walter Collins (son of Christine Collins) disappeared from Los Angeles California. There had been a number of child abductions and Christine was worried. That afternoon she contacted the Los Angeles Police Department (LAPD) to file a missing persons report. She was told that she could not make a report for 24 hours. This delay cost valuable time and may have ensured that Walter would not be found.

Collins' troubles came at a time when the LAPD did not have a good public reputation. They were known for corruption and extreme strong arm guerilla tactics built around intimidation and violence. The force was "on the take," commonly known as taking bribes. The LAPD was assisting the criminals by turning a blind eye to their nefarious activities. They did so with an outstretched hand to be lined with green cash for their assistance.

To the chagrin of the much maligned LAPD, this new abduction / disappearance grabbed national attention and sympathies. The LAPD was now in the public spotlight, just where it did not want to be found.

Faced with negative publicity and increasing public pressure to solve the case, the LAPD was thrilled when a boy claiming to be Walter Collins was located in DeKalb, Illinois. The boy was brought to Los Angeles for a public and media reunion with Christine Collins. All seemed well, except the boy presented to Christine was not Walter. Christine knew immediately that the boy presented to her as her own flesh and blood, was in fact an imposter.

The reunion was about to go horribly bad. True of self assured (and often delusional) seemingly omnipotent organizations and individuals, Captain J.J. Jones was confident he could navigate even the worst storm.

During the initial meeting Christine Collins loudly claimed that the boy presented to her was not her son. Captain Jones insisted that Christine was wrong and that she should take home "her son" and "try him out for a couple of weeks." Amazingly, Collins capitulated and gave in to the captain's demands. She took the imposter home as the camera's snapped away. Because of this the story seemed to die.

It died in the press, for Captain Jones and the LAPD, but not for Christine Collins. Who would know her son better than she?

Three weeks after the boy was given to Christine to "try out," she had had enough. She marched into Captain Jones office hoping to persuade him to see her point of view.

She did not.

The captain did not budge one bit. He insisted that she was mistaken and that the LAPD and its investigative work were beyond reproach. Christine went home without satisfaction to the imposter claiming to be her son.

Captain Jones was not finished with the missing boy's mother at all. The LAPD dispensed a psychiatrist to convince her that she was misguided due to tremendous stress and other mitigating factors.

He was attempting to undermine Christine's own certainty. This was on a par with trying to convince you, the reader, that your own memories are all hallucinations. If this horrible treatment with the psychiatrist was not so alarmingly true it would be a funny story.

The psychiatrist visited Collins and spewed his psycho babble, flamboyant jargon and expert opinion for the sole purpose of instilling doubt in her own motherly observations. The hope being that she would ideally "fall in line" behind the police and their "line."

If this story hit the papers it would cause a huge embarrassment for the beleaguered police department and its captain. Hit the papers it did.

This awkward attack only hardened Christine's resolve to inflict her will on the wayward – LAPD and their claims that she was wrong about her own son. She gave the story to the newspaper and again approached Captain Jones.

This time she was armed with medical and dental records, height differences as well as compelling circumcision information. The new boy was even shorter than her Walter. Again Jones disallowed her claims and she was deemed a trouble maker.

She was committed to the psychiatric ward at Los Angeles County Hospital under a "Code 12," used for those who were "difficult" or "an inconvenience."

Consider what you have just read. Christine Collins was imprisoned in a psychiatric ward because she was a problem. She was attacking (with just cause) a government agency. So abhorrent was her defiance – that she was silenced in a mental ward. These are the same kinds of tactics later employed by Hitler in Nazi Germany and Stalin in the old Soviet Union.

Hitler had a policy of zero tolerance regarding speaking out against the government. Where did he get this idea? Could such tactics be used today?

Fifteen days after her imprisonment, Jones (to his credit) questioned the imposter and discovered that he was actually a boy named Arthur Hutchins, Jr., a runaway from Illinois who was originally from Iowa. A drifter had given the boy the idea to attempt the ruse of impersonation, due to his resemblance to the missing Walter.

After the interview and a tirade of bad press, Christine was released from her incarceration.

Eventually, it was discovered that Walter Collins had been abducted and murdered by Gordon Northcott as part of the notorious Wineville Chicken Coop Murders, which took place from 1928 to 1930.

The significance of this story is staggering.

A sane individual who had proof that she was being lied to, confronted her accusers and demanded redress. Without inspection of her facts she was savagely rebuked. Collins was labeled "a trouble maker" and locked up without consideration. The legitimacy of her claims did not match the truths that the "powers that be" had determined were true and she was summarily punished.

She was imprisoned for speaking the truth! She was imprisoned for presenting a well constructed contrary/dissenting opinion to "those in charge." How dare her! This story clearly reveals that to governments and large organizations such as Ely Lilly, the FDA, AMA, etc. absolute truth is not important. Your truth is insignificant. The only truth that matters is "their truth." The only truth that matters is "what we say the truth is."

If we make too much noise we are attacked by forces far beyond our ability to cope or conceive. Consider this: in California there exists today the California Welfare and Institutions Code called the 5150. It states that a person can be held against their will for up to 72 hours in a psychiatric ward if there is a complaint against them.
The following is the 5150 code:

Section 5150, Allows a qualified officer or clinician to involuntarily confine a person deemed (or feared) to have a mental disorder that makes them a danger to him or herself, and /others and / or gravely, disabled. A qualified officer, who includes any California peace officer, as well as any specifically designated county clinician, can request the confinement after signing a written declaration. The 5150 hold may be written out on form MH 302, Application for 72 Hour Detention for Evaluation or Treatment.

The state's ability to place a person on an involuntary hold in a psychiatric ward is the only situation outside of law enforcement where your rights and freedoms can be swept away in seconds. With the stroke of a pen and a complaint you can be detained against your will. Many states have a variation of this code.

All it takes is a complaint of irrational behavior for someone to be locked up. Once incarcerated a psychiatrist (who really is crazy) will evaluate the individual and decide if they "need" to stay longer.

Every day we switch on the TV, read newspaper headlines, listen to radio and devour electronic media piped onto our computer screens that tell us what to think. We are told that black is not black and that white is not white. We are told that tobacco does not actually cause cancer. We are told by esteemed government agencies that what we believe to be true is all lies. We are told that we are weak, feeble and that our government will protect and heal us.

The seat of responsibility is a very serious one to hold. Thinking that those who would control or influence our destinies are good benevolent beings is a serious flaw in judgment. Every night our own TV broadcasts propaganda of a nature that is intended to create doubt and duress. Twenty four hours a day our media is driving to make the public docile lambs waiting for slaughter. When the power to inform is subverted and used to maliciously control and abuse, it becomes a crime akin to terrorism.

Every person on Earth must be made aware of the unspeakable nature and magnitude of this crime.

Roger Bezanis

We must be cognizant of the oxymorons of government intelligence, truth in advertising, better life via chemistry, etc. or we are doomed to surgeries, feeding tubes, drugs and an early painful death.

No one is beyond the reach of the government if it finds you to be an annoyance. Never forget the power of the 5150 code and Christine Collins. Beware of the otherworldly power of the IRS. Of course we all know that the IRS is never used to exact revenge, ever. The IRS is just a benevolent and sedate agency with our best interest in mind.

We know this down to our core, because they say so right on TV. Everyone knows that if it is on TV, it must be true.

This problem is not a predicament germane only to the United States. Every government on Earth has studied the lessons learned regarding public control and indoctrination. It is a well known business maxim that control equals income. Under different flags world governments have the same basic intention, which is to survive. The influences of the old Soviet Union, Nazi Germany, the Japanese Empire and charismatic leaders like Jim Jones are microscopically studied for their workability.

Look at Korea, Iraq, Iran, the mediaand the political and mind controlling might of the United States. The only way to rise above such attacks is to willfully band together, speak as one, say no and fight back. One man cannot stand alone and only invites slaughter.

We are the architects of our own doom. If we mindlessly watch TV, which has been proven to be hypnotic – we fall victim to their insidious plan. Poison-pushing advertisers know this and count on its brain washing affects. The sad truth is that those who wish to control us intimately know the power at their disposal. The absolute best way to program the public is mass brainwashing done simultaneously every time we switch on our favorite program or sporting event. Advertisers hate TIVO and other devices like it that block or cut out their messages.

When we begin to think that we are sick or need the next new drug or junk food item, we have lost. When we know advertising slogans as well as our own zip codes, we are automatons. Soon we no longer insist that white is white. No longer do we have the backbone strength to stand up and say that we are being lied to.

Sheep need a herder to make decisions. Cattle walk blindly and obediently to their own bloody end. The milking machine of big business is connected to your wallet and soul as they are being pumped dry. I am sorry but this is the world that you live in. Your finances are siphoned away directed to those in ivory towers. There they sit smoking cigars of human flesh while they line their pockets with ill gotten gain.

Totalitarian states yell to make you subservient and docile. Your thoughts are wrong; you must believe what they tell you. If you fight against them they will deal with you. Be obedient or the consequences will be grave. The men in black suits are waiting to pay you a visit to make you disappear.

That is what to expect if you live in a totalitarian state. What kind of state do YOU live in?

The fate of Christine Collins is not an aberration. The fact that her story seems so isolated is very unusual. How many like her never survived or never escaped psychiatric incarceration?

Tragic as it is, we are each and every one of us Christine Collins. Learn her lesson of defiance. Stand up with all of the free thinkers and protest. This book is a beacon in a night of unspeakable turbulent danger. Right now it is guiding you to the safe harbor where your friends are waiting. Use the life changing power of these pages to protect yourself. I invite you to take responsibility for mankind and help others to awaken on safe and sunny beaches where health is not a privilege and freedom is for everyone!

3 Man's Responsibilities To Man

Like it or not, every one of us has a responsibility to OUR FELLOW MAN. Should man go extinct, it will be a cooperative failure. Collectively burying our heads in the sand while ignoring what is happening around us will make mankind a footnote in Earth's history. You have a huge accountability to your family, friends, you and all of mankind. Being productive and useful, you must survive and survive well.

Living to tell your tale and passing on what you have learned is vital to all of us. Isolation begets death. Every society in history that has isolated itself for an extended period of time has crumbled. A solitary man is no different.

If you are not surviving in good health, you are dying a little bit more every day.

The example **you set** does not go unnoticed by your peers. When you are spied eating a candy bar, you are communicating that candy bars are the things to eat. If you are seen eating a salad, salads are validated. The example you set could very well change someone's life. You never know who will be watching.

When you pull yourself out of the muck, your awareness improves. Imagine a man with a headache. Where is his awareness? On his head! If that same man feels good (no aches or pains) where is his awareness? Answer? Wherever **he** chooses to put it. Sick people are of very little use to anyone as they are trapped being sick. Ailing individuals require vast amounts of attention and are draining on those around them.

Therefore, you have a responsibility to yourself and the planet to be in your best possible health. Excellent health is invaluable and needs to be sought after, respected and cherished.

Simply correcting your health allows you to be more responsible for the world you live in. Your new unfettered attention is then available for placement on problems of a global scale, rather than just on your woes. Good health is your responsibility to pursue, own, and nurture. Be healthy and you begin to take responsibility for all of us.

Your questions are always welcome. I am here for you.

Hippocrates said "Let food be your medicine and medicine be your food."

4 In the Beginning

The greatest single known source of information in the ancient world was the Great Library at Alexandria erected 283 B.C. and destroyed by fire in 47 B.C. The city of Alexandria lies along the coast of Egypt on the Mediterranean Sea. Alexandria was founded in Egypt by the greatest conqueror of the ancient world, Alexander the Great. His successor was Pharaoh Ptolomy II Soter, who founded the Museum or Royal Library of Alexandria in 283 B.C.

The Museum was a shrine of the Muses modeled after the Lyceum of Aristotle in Athens. The Museum or Library was a place of study, which included lecture areas, gardens, a zoo, and shrines for each of the nine muses as well as the Library itself. It has been calculated that between 400,000 and 700,000 scrolls (equal to our books of today) graced these halls at one time. The documents were a multinational mix from Assyria, Greece, Persia, Egypt, India and many other nations. More than 125 scholars lived at the Museum full time to perform research, write, lecture, translate and copy documents. The library was so large it actually had another branch or "daughter" library at the Temple of Serapis (also in Alexandria).

The library held scrolls containing data on the workings of the first mechanical clock, the first vending machine, surgical instruments (like the ones used today) and no doubt the blueprints and technology used to build the pyramids. Because it is gone and has been for centuries, man is still rediscovering lost technology. I am referencing it here, because the data that is contained in this manuscript has existed before. Perhaps it too was contained on a scroll or several. Much of the information on these pages has been hidden, much of it in plain view. But without the right key or context to put it in, the data would make little sense.

In the next two hundred plus pages, what was once a mystery will be explained. The mystery of you will unfold and for the first time make sense. Truth has a way of making sense. Imagine for yourself what would happen if civilization, as you knew it, suddenly disappeared. What would happen if all the people who knew how to fix our technology suddenly were taken from us? What if most of the world was destroyed except a few million individuals? How long might it take us to recover? Imagine further, that all of the plants and manufacturing facilities were gone. No books, no manuals.

What would become of us? When would the next inventor come along and reinvent the electric light bulb? This is the nightmare that would befall the inhabitants of the ancient world in Alexandria one night in 47 B.C. A majority of what was then known was swiftly gone as fire swept through the scrolls of knowledge housed at the Alexandria library.

If such a catastrophic event as mentioned above occurred today, at what future date would we replicate computers or re-harness the atom without someone or something to lead the way? We could dig ourselves out from such a morass, but it would take quite some time, if not centuries. Archeologists are just now discovering that not only was "our present day technology" known in antiquity, it was widely used.

On these pages are the missing puzzle pieces collected and reset in proper order. The "experts" told you this knowledge DID NOT EXIST. They told you that you were stupid. They were wrong. Micro study of anything proves little. Examining an elephant's tail says little about the whole animal. The so-called best minds on the planet love to study the micro aspects of life. This proves nothing. If altering one atom for the better imbalanced the system in general, it is a bad correction. Microscope jockeys only seem to care about what they are myopically looking at. They pray for the day when they will witness matter & antimatter colliding.

This book is devoted to making life simple & livable for anyone. What matters is what the whole body is doing in relationship to the total body's functions.

What I have completed is revolutionary; I have combined seemingly incongruous modalities and practices into useable, tested techniques and data so that you can experience what it is to be in charge of your body and life. I take all the puzzle pieces and lay them out exposing the full, understandable big picture. You will not have to reinvent lost technology. I have spelled it out for you; your job is to test it and see if it is true for you.

I had no intentions of writing this or any book. I honestly had no idea I had anything to say. I had no idea that what I was teaching people was anything different than what others were already preaching. Yet, year after year as the looks of amazement kept swelling in number I realized that what I was saying was unique. When other experts started cultivating my ideas and approaches, I began to get a glimpse that what I was doing was very special.

Teachers, professors and doctors started attending my lectures repeatedly. They all insisted that what I was teaching was quite unusual, so much so that it seemed otherworldly.

My work is your work; I am just presenting it to you in book form, as you must have forgotten it

Roger Bezanis

long ago. You the public demanded that this tome be written and advanced. This is your book. Every technique in this book has been observed and then tested again and again. The empirical data is staggering. The human body **ALWAYS HEALS ITSELF**, unless its owner is actively poisoning it.

Do not lose sight of how simple fixing your health can be. I am not going to have you study your cells under a microscope. Nor will I have you subject yourself to x-rays or experimentation. I am not interested in micro-managing one aspect of health. We are all a collection of circuits and connections. It might be possible to learn something about an elephant by studying its tail, but it would be difficult and not something I am pursuing in this book. True natural medicine, or holistic medicine, treats the body as a whole.

If you cannot obtain 100 high-quality years out of your body, the question becomes, why? This is my total focus: healthy longevity.

It is because of this kind of work and my "no excuses" attitude that has made me a requested lecturer. I never intended to lecture. I constantly refused to lecture, regardless of how inspirational people told me I was. I refused to lecture until I was sure that I had incredible things to articulate.

Thanks to you, I lost the lecture battle almost 10 years ago.

Becoming one of Earth's leading formulators of herbal products was not on my list of things to achieve as a budding adult. Nevertheless, my lab tinkering caught the attention of many when I began sharing my formulas. Honestly, the vast swelling of medical community demand caught me off guard. Wasn't everyone making the same great products? Couldn't formulas similar to mine be gotten everywhere? No, as other formulators did not know how to think outside the box of tradition.

I had to produce my products "en masse" or go broke being a charity worker. All of the observation that came from developing my products became the footnotes that eventually became this book. Testing again and again and noting what I was observing led to the most remarkable discoveries.

Because of my formulas, I was presented with a windfall of time, which has allowed me to give you this astonishing book.

I had to write this book or open up a practice. If I had a practice, I could only see 40 or so people a day. With this book, millions can be helped every minute. This soft cover is not a fad or marketing tool. Without question, it is soon to be your best friend and confidant. I give you this book so that I can help you, even though I am not physically holding your hand.

Because of my integrity, nowhere in this book will I attempt to sell you something. This is not a sales pitch for a number of new improved (fill in the blank). Nowhere in this book is my herbal company listed. This book is self-contained. If you follow what is in this book, you will never need supplements, drugs and surgery.

You are on a collision course with discovery unlike anything that you believed possible. The public loves what is in this book because it all works.

To sum up, this book, like my formulas, is the result of curiosity, a burning drive to make a difference and a sudden avalanche of demand foisted on my shoulders. This book was never going to come out until I was forced to write it. Thank you for demanding it.

Feel free to attend my lectures and classes. There are those who have heard me speak dozens of times and are still getting new data. Use this book to save your life or the life of someone very dear to you.

Nothing for sale here! If you need to be sold the latest "health fad", turn on your T.V. some Sunday morning, or any late night, and watch away.

Here's to a new you!

If people want to read this book they will ask for it. You will not have to ask them. Let them ask you for it. If they do not ask for it you have not interested them in reading it. If you offer to let someone borrow this book without them asking you first, you have jumped the step of him or her reaching for the help this book offers.

5 The Door of Health Swings Both Ways

This book holds no allegiances or alliances with any group. I am not beholden to anything except results and your health. I am not on the payroll of a special interest conglomeration. I have no covert or nefarious agenda. I will not spew the brainwashing rhetoric of pharmaceutical scoundrels or lead you astray. I will never preach doctrine that could encumber your health or essence. The money I spend is not tainted by lies of blood-smeared principals.

I have one purpose, to teaching you:

- How to diagnose via reading the face
- How to diagnose via your fingernails
- How to diagnose via your tongue
- How to diagnose via your hands.
- How to diagnose via your eyebrows

- How to diagnose via your hair
- How to diagnose via symptoms
- How to heal yourself from any malady
- How to decode the world of medical speak
- How to take 100% responsibility for your health
- How to know if your supplements are working
- How to handle addictions
- How to awaken your latent powers of perception
- How to lose weight and keep it off

I do not trust teachers, writers, formulators or speakers that live their lives in ivory towers, never actually experiencing what they talk about. In my opinion, an educator, to be legitimate, had to have studied and worked in his field to be sufficiently conversant, to pass it along. Not only have I walked in your shoes and had all of your problems, I have been worse than you in many ways.

Fortunately, I have lived through it all to tell you about it. Through these pages I am passing along experiences culled from my life that have shaped and saved the lives of many. I have not just lived my subject, I have exhaustively studied and experienced it. I have listened to the so-called experts and whenever I happened upon something promising, I tested it on myself, and then, if successful, on others.

When I could count on a 95% success rate or better, I passed it on. I have since formulated products to support these findings. Today I see my creations achieving a 98% success rate.

When I write about diet, I write from a position of having lived all the options. I know how to recover from knee surgery while walking without a limp or pain, 24 hours after the operation. I know what happens if you drink 240 ounces of water in one day. I have been down to 6% body fat. I know what happens if someone tries to live on B-Complex, etc.

In order to really know anything, you must get down and dirty in the stuff of life and envelop yourself in it, and I have. We have all been conditioned to believe that it takes time to correct long-standing conditions. The fact is, "The door to health swings both ways." Memorize that statement, say it again, and pronounce it out loud, "The door to health swings both ways"!

Whatever has gone wrong with the body CAN BE repaired if given a chance.

Grey hair has corrected itself if caught in the first stages of graying. I know this as I have changed my own hair color. You have heard about people going grey overnight? We all have. It is therefore more than possible to reverse it. What changed overnight can of course reverse.

Advancing this simple postulation to include the entire body, any condition can reverse! The door of health swings both ways!

The misguided world of diseases or chronic health issues would not only have you believe otherwise, they are counting on your confusion. The deception starts with the definition of disease.

Definition of Disease (circa 1850) — From Answers.Com

"A pathological condition of a part, organ, or system of an organism resulting from various causes, such as infection, genetic defect, or environmental stress, and characterized by an identifiable group of signs or symptoms."

TRANSLATION: *Your condition (sickness) is not your responsibility. You had nothing to do with it. To fully understand what was originally meant by the word disease you must understand the word history or derivation.*

WORD HISTORY: Disease; The condition of not being comfortable or not relieved or no freedom from pain. [Middle English disease, from Old French: des-, dis- + aise, ease; see ease] Prefix: dis- not or dissimilar PLUS no ease (experiencing pain). Simply, the word disease is supposed to convey IN THE PRESENCE OF PAIN.

Because the word DISEASE has been so altered and twisted by the medicos for the past 250+ years, I am redefining it and giving it the definition below.

DFRHH Disease definition: "A weakened condition of the body brought on by personal choices and ignorance of the natural laws that govern biology"

Additionally: You are 100% responsible for your condition. Your choices have brought about the condition you are in.

To further make it clear as to what the source of a problem of the body is, I am coining a new word. This word sparks a revolution in viewing sickness and now leads to correct handlings.

EXSURPO: Meaning EXACT-SOURCE-PAIN or exact source of the pain. Derivation: Ex: Latin, exactus = exact + Latin, surgere = source + Latin, poena = Pain.

Henceforth we will say the exsurpo of _____ (pain) is the kidney, liver etc. Being sick requires a total and complete disconnection from you as source of you being sick. You must participate in ignoring **what you did** to cause or aid your illness. This ignorance is required for you to remain sick and thus REMAIN a victim of your **acquired** condition.

Sickness is the result of intelligent life granted freedom of choice, then brainwashed to believe there is no choice. If I did not have firsthand experience, I might agree with, "What is broken stays broken."

If you doubt the above paragraph, it is because the fear mongers have stolen your will to live! Take your life back! The Powers That Be promise little while handing out candy-coated death. They want you ignorant to the fact that the human body is resilient and heals without drugs and surgery.

I will explain this in detail in the chapter "Disease Labels and Who Owns Them"

Your body is not only intelligent, it instantly reacts to stimulus. Do not remain blind to this fact or next you will accept the drug company's lies that your only hope comes in a bottle with a warning label.

You feel bad from a cocktail of chemicals, colorings, dyes and drugs. They affect you on contact and always have.

Big Pharma has invested billions to program you to believe that health improvement takes time: days, weeks, months or is impossible. Imagine what would happen if the current drug-company trained doom-speaking witch doctors started handing people hope rather than promising death within 30 days.

Families would sue!

Today's witch doctors don't dare breathe the possibility of hope and recovery. This is a fascinating dilemma. Doctors, who have no idea how the body heals, try to heal it. The public, ignoring its own intuition, intention and determinism, sit idly by, waiting for the death wagon to arrive.

We are taught to worship our witch doctors in lab coats dispensing their drugs and surgery. Thanks to conditioning we glumly ask for a forecast of survival. If the doctor says anything other than "I don't know" or "Death in 30 days", he gets sued. Survival predictions not realized equal lawsuits. Let us all give a big "Thank you" to the American Bar Association.

You can see the problem: the blind are leading the brainwashed.

Promising death (or a bad outcome) protects the doctor and the drug companies. If you buy into the notion that it takes time to recover, then any therapy appears to work. Why? Because the body is so resilient, even in the face of toxic drugs, it can and often does heal on its own, in spite of the doctor's efforts to kill it off.

My approach is completely different. I know that when the right item (or items) is given to the body, the body starts to correct itself immediately. Pain will dissipate; fever reduces, swelling releases, freedom of movement returns, sleep improves, high blood pressure lowers. The list goes on and on.

As far as supplements go, it is a fact that correctly made supplements point themselves at a target organ, and ALWAYS react on contact with the system. To understand more about this, read the chapter called "Your Body is Smarter than you." Pay special attention to the Energy Balancing Technique.

In a nutshell, your body feels sensation moment to moment as opposed to later. This is a survival mechanism. Imagine what would happen if your body took an hour or so to sense heat or taste.

You could singe your skin or exterminate yourself with spoiled food. The body reacts with everything it comes in contact with right **now**, not a week from **now**. When you smell cigarette smoke and sneeze, it is because your body is rejecting it **now**. Your body needs but a 100th of a second to process that information. You smelled it and then sneezed.

With that in mind, I have successfully tested these intimate universal phenomena hundreds of thousands of times. As a result, I question why supplement companies don't mention the "instant response." Supplements and all foods affect the body every time they are introduced. You are not told of this reaction because supplement and drug companies either have no awareness of the phenomena or are hiding what they know.

At least one pharmaceutical company does know this reaction. In their own commercials they warn woman not to touch or handle their product because of a specific birth defect. What about the rest of the drug companies, do they know too? Do they know or care that they are killing you?

You must demand that all supplement makers produce ingestibles that are so good, they create a known instant, positive response on the body. Why won't all companies be doing this anytime soon?

Because it would require:

- Awareness of the phenomena
- Relearning all that they know
- Reformulating at least 50% of what they currently produce
- No longer copying other formulator's work
- Inventing products that actually do work
- Willingness to accept that 2% of the public will claim to not have a noticeable instant response

Money is the reason we will not see this change until you demand that it takes place. Cigarette sales are falling because you have said enough. One voice is the start of a chorus when another voice is added.

Big business does not like to take chances. Even though the supplement business is puny compared to the drug industry, they still follow the same path of least resistance. I, on the other hand, have no problem rocking the boat. I tell it like it actually is. Immediate results are something that supplement makers do not want to be involved in.

If we do not expect immediate results, we are not upset when they don't come.

Any company promoting this idea of immediate results is putting their hindquarters on the line with every bottle. I admire that.

Take a moment to realize that if you sit and wait long enough, something will always happen. It may have nothing to do with your therapy or treatment, but something will happen. If you can't sleep, wait long enough and you will. Have a sore back? Wait long enough and it won't hurt.

In general, when people feel physically or emotionally better, they rightly or wrongly give credit to the product they have been taking. Conversely, when they feel worse, they again blame the product. You must be asking yourself why I am writing so many paragraphs to make this point.

This is why:

Feeling better or worse has practically nothing to do with the product you are taking, UNLESS FEELING BETTER OR WORSE OCCURED ON CONTACT WITH THAT PRODUCT. Contact = **the moment you touched it.** Yes, I said **the moment you touched it.**

The moment you touch anything, your body NOTICES and changes accordingly, even if only slightly.

If you think that I am saying that you can touch some food or supplement and pain will go away, THAT IS EXACTLY WHAT I AM SAYING.

When you take a supplement and hours go by before you feel better, it was because your body finally adjusted on its own. Perhaps a new substance that you just contacted did the trick. Should you feel worse, it was something you JUST ate, JUST drank, JUST inhaled or JUST splashed on your skin. Something you JUST contacted was the straw that broke the camel's back.

Therefore, if you eat a cookie and feel bad, it was from the cookie, not your job or the yard work. If you pick up a slice of pizza and notice that your low back suddenly hurts, it is your body saying HEY MISTER, PLEASE DON'T FEED ME PIZZA!

Every time you feel bad it is due to something that you just came in contact with that has pushed you over the edge.

But what if you took something and within a few seconds you felt better? **That is to be expected.** The only wild card in all of this is hormones from stress. Stress releases hormones and will stress the liver and give you a symptom. The treatment is the same, find the supplement or food that resets the liver and you will feel improved.

Instant body / condition / symptom improvement is an outrageous and foreign idea for most. There will be those who will read this entire chapter and question what I am writing about. I assure you instant response is not only possible, it happens every day, and you never noticed it.

If all drug companies and supplement makers were held with their feet to the fire until they produced products that created a noticeable balance in the body, we would have a lot of burned feet.

We ignore the violent instant reaction from poison oak, poison ivy, pollen, peanut oil (causing, in some cases, anaphylactic shock and death), ragweed, dry cleaning solvents, the smell of tobacco, ammonia, industrial solvents, perfume, etc.

The poor allergist understands some of this yet even he is in the dark. He toils trying to cover or suppress symptoms. He is aware that some substances make his patients feel poorly, yet he has no idea that all substances have the ability to improve or worsen the system on contact.

When you use a supplement, you should feel improvement now, not later.

Below is how the body actually works

The Reactions
At the moment of contact with any substance the body will:
- Get hotter
- Get colder

- Contract / tighten
- Expand / loosen

- Feel more pain
- Feel less pain

- Accelerate or speed up
- Decelerate or slows down
- Age faster
- Age slower

- Release waste

- Retain waste

- Release water
- Retain water

- Relax
- Become tense
- Oxygenate
- Deoxygenate

- Awaken / more energy
- Sedate / less energy

- No reaction or neutral response
  This occurs when the body is balanced and has the reserves to stay balanced.

In treating yourself you must remember the eleven categories above. If you find yourself taking a supplement that produces no perceivable benefit, ultimately it is a waste of money. You would probably not wash your car every hour. Taking supplements for no reason without defined benefit is akin to such an activity.

6 You and Your Doctor

Hippocrates studied patients over and over; he was fascinated in their stories but especially how they appeared. He trained himself to smell sickness as well as listen for it. He developed a sharpened eye and for him face reading became second nature. Thus he perfected an expert technique that has been lost. If you have ever wondered what "being in practice" meant, ask a doctor. He / she will tell you that what they learned in college, while valuable, was second to what they learned in the field or in practice.

Put yourself in the shoes of Aristotle; he too noticed the look of the ill. He saw dark, gaunt or swollen regions of the face and knew they meant something. He knew enough to ask. Eventually he knew it was a symptom of ill health.

Have you ever noticed what a stroke victim looks like? Aristotle, Hippocrates and I have. You will too. Good doctors care and ask questions.

Throughout history certain individuals have earned our respect and praise. They perform miracles every day and involve themselves in life and death.
They are called doctors.

Many feel their doctors walk on water. Even the worst practitioners of health receive praise and curiosity. Such was the fate of Nazi Doctor Josef Mengele, a mad man and murderer. Hitler's personal doctor, Dr. Theodor Morell, clearly a quack, pumped Germany's WWII Fuhrer full of a cocktail of B-Vitamins and Amphetamines (speed, a stimulant). Then there was the father of modern psychiatry, Wilhelm Wundt, another mad man. Finally, Atlanta dentist turned gunfighter, card shark, Tuberculosis sufferer and friend to Wyatt Earp, Doc Holiday. Not all doctors are serving up good health. It is their own ethic level that will determine their legacy. Witness the twisting road of Dr. Death, Jack Kevorkian, as he is both scorned and hailed.

The human race has placed this profession on a pedestal. When any individual can control the terms of life and death, reverence naturally follows. Is it deserved? You bet it is.

What makes a good doctor?

- Compassion
- Intelligence
- Knowledge of his field
- Ability to listen
- Ability to learn new things
- Little or no ego
- Good bedside manner
- Interested in you and your problems
- Knowledge of new advancements in medicine
- Intuition
- Willing to ask for help
- Understanding that they can always learn
- Willing to say "I don't know" and then find the answer
- Willing to hand off to a more qualified expert

The above description makes a good doctor. How does your doctor stack up? Is he listed above or do the following characteristics seem more accurate?

What Makes a Bad Doctor?

If he is:

- Always right
- Argumentative

- Makes you wrong
- Won't listen to you
- Spends little time with you
- Dispenses drugs without an understanding of what he is dispensing
- Not willing to learn
- Not interested in what you have to say
- Little or no compassion
- Poor bedside manner

If the list above describes your doctor, RUN!

Your doctor should be a partner in your health, not the driver. When a doctor practically foaming at the mouth yells at you, it is often because you ventured into the sacred territory of diagnosis or self-diagnosis.

You need to be encouraged to participate in your own health care. You beyond all doubt have one true friend. This comrade knows everything about you. This companion goes everywhere you go, eats what you eat and has all of your habits. That friend is you.

Who is better qualified to give you a hand than you? You have personally observed yourself 24 hours a day for your entire life. You are over qualified to assist yourself with just a little training. Your doctor can help you get to this level or he can stop you.

Clearly, with a little work and some study, you could be your best ally in securing a healthier future. That is the purpose of this book. To teach you the basic principles of health that school, T.V., advertising, the AMA, FDA and God knows who else never taught you.

You can be healthy regardless of what your doctor, spouse, friend or confidant told you. When you show this book to your doctor, he or she should want to read it. He should be in favor of your reading it. If not, this is a bad sign.

When your health care practitioner is against you educating yourself and insists that his care is all that you need, get a new doctor. Should you be yelled at, belittled or made to doubt the validity of your decisions about your health, again this is red flag; find a new doctor.

You can be better, healthier and stronger and it starts now.

7 The History of Medicine

Much has been said about the rise of Traditional Medicine (also called Allopathic medicine) at the expense of Natural Medicine. This chapter brushes aside all the bias and rumor and just gives you the facts regarding who did what and when it occurred. Many of the players you will have heard of. You will probably be shocked to find out why your health care choices are so limited today. The demise of Natural Medicine was no accident. It was a well-crafted and devious plan.

As you read this chapter you will begin to understand how deep health care corruption really runs.

Why is it that natural medicine was assigned the new name of alternative medicine after 1900?

The history to be covered in this chapter includes:

7995-2995 BC, Ayurvedic Medicine appears in the mountains of Tibet

2630-2611 BC, Imhotep treats patients in the Third Dynasty of Egypt

Circa 2400 BC, Acupuncture and Chinese texts outline the use of herbs

1500 BC, Egyptian physicians write down techniques for the healing of the Pharaohs

1200 BC, soldiers are treated for wounds during the siege of Troy

400 BC, Hippocrates forms the first school of medicine; Naturopathic medicine is practiced

55 AD, Dioscorides documents herbal formulas for the Europeans

159, Galen invents new procedures and the instruments to perform surgical work

500-1400, the Dark Ages, no known advances in medicine survived this period

1200, Unani Medicine begins being practiced in the Middle East

1801, Homeopathic medicine is created

1810, with a mail order medical certificate, Jenner creates the Smallpox vaccine

1814, Germany starts issuing medical degrees

1841-1866, various forms of anesthesia started to be put in use

1847, the American Medical Association groundwork is put in place

1848, Samuel Weiss was fired for requiring surgeons to wash their hands

1867, Joseph Lister champions antiseptic surgical practices

1869, Pasteur creates Pasteurization and, with Koch, develops many vaccines

1880-1900, German psych-trained doctors begin taking positions of power in major American medical colleges

1906, the FDA is created with the Federal Food and Drug Act

1907, the AMA investigates medical colleges of the United States and Canada

1908, the AMA allows the Carnegie Foundation to investigate medical schools for them

1910, the Flexner Report on Medical Education in the United States and Canada is released

1910-1940, Carnegie, Rockefeller, Kellogg, Ford and others start paying off (bribing) medical schools that will implement new drug therapies (created by companies they support), while doing away with the current natural curriculums. Non-approved medical schools are forced to close at a mad rate due to a SUDDEN lack of funding and students. The country drops from 160 medical schools to 80 almost overnight. AMA membership soars, as all allopathic doctors must join to practice.

1915 to present day, Drug Company profits soar, as more drugs are created to combat the new diseases described and named by the AMA. All new drugs receive the blessings from the FDA and follow a diagnosis from the AMA. The world is starting to be drugged.

The Practice Of Medicine/An Unabridged Timeline

Ayurvedic Medicine 7995 to 2995 BC: This is considered the oldest form of healthcare in the world. It was born in the mountains of Tibet in what is now known as present day India. Passed down verbally for generations, in approximately 2500 BC, it was written down in Sanskrit (recognized as the world's oldest surviving language) on stone and clay tablets. These tablets are known as the Vedas; they are the oldest written knowledge found on Earth. Often called the "Mother of healing", Ayurveda spread to China and advanced through much of the then known world. It influenced Hippocrates in Greece and became known throughout the Middle East as Unani Medicine.

Current Ayurveda is drawn from three later sources, primarily the Caraka Samhita (approximately 1500 BC), the Ashtang Hrdyam (approximately 500 AD) and Sushrut Samhita (300-400 AD). These works are considered classics as they describe the basic principles and theories from which Ayurveda has evolved. They also contain large amounts of clinical data on the management of a multitude of diseases.

2630-2611 BC Imhotep: Egyptian physician to King Djoser (third dynasty) is believed to be the first physician in recorded history. He is credited with diagnosing & treating at least 200 diseases; many diseases of the abdomen and bladder, a dozen of the rectum, 30 of the eyes, and almost 20 skin, hair, nail and tongue problems. He's credited with treating tuberculosis, liver / gallstone problems, colon issues, appendicitis, kidney problems, diabetes, gout and arthritis problems. He performed surgery and even practiced some dentistry. Imhotep extracted herbal medicines from plants and knew the position and function of the vital organs as well as understanding the circulation of the blood system.

China circa 2400 BC: their first medical texts were laid down, documenting the use of herbs and diagramming the structure of the body, including meridians and organ function. Many believe that for thousands of years Ayurvedic and Chinese Medicine, which included acupuncture, were the only types of medicine being practiced on earth.

1500 BC: Ancient Egyptian physicians, in the court of the Pharaohs, understood the body and documented these findings in papyrus documents still being unearthed today. Machaon and his brother Polidarius treated soldiers at the battle of Troy, circa 1200 BC, for arrow wounds. Together they saved many lives on the battlefield.

460-377 BC: Hippocrates was born on the island of Cos, Greece. He laid down the "Hippocratic Oath" (the pledge that doctors take today). He became known as the Father of medicine and was regarded as the greatest physician of his time. Hippocrates said "Let food be your medicine and medicine be your food."

Circa 400 BC: Naturopathic Medicine is first noted with the rise of the Hippocratic School of Medicine. Hippocrates preached "The healing power of nature" or "Vis Medicatrix Naturae" and the use of hydrotherapy and hygienics. The style of medicine being practiced was called "Eclectics", as were the doctors, since they used whatever means necessary to heal the patient.

Circa 55 AD: Dioscorides (Greek) compiled written formulas and herbs that were often direct forebears of what has been used for the last 1,000 years. His formulas and approach were largely unchanged in Western pharmacopeias until the twentieth century.

131 AD: Galen (Greek) studied at the historic medical school in Alexandria, Egypt. By the age of 28, he was saving the lives of gladiators. He was a pioneer in surgery and is credited with inventing most of the medical instruments used today. Galen favored the beliefs of Hippocrates and called on the healing power of nature to balance the body. He observed and noted symptoms and often treated with opposites, i.e. if a man appeared to have a fever, he treated it with something cold, if a man appeared to have a cold, he would be treated with heat. People who were weak were given hard physical exercise to build up their muscles. Those who had breathing problems due to bronchial issues were given singing exercises. He was a prolific writer and was still influencing doctors 1,000 years after his death.

1200: Unani Medicine, the framework of which is based on the teachings of Hippocrates. Unani was the culmination and the convergence of the works of Galen (131-210 AD), Islamic physicians Al-Razi, (Iran, 850-925 AD), Ibn Sina (Persia, 980-1037 AD), Al Zahravi (present day Spain) and the surgeon Ibn Nafis (Syria, 1210-1288 AD). Unani medicine has been practiced all over the Middle East and is considered the best of the medicines of Egypt, Syria, Iraq, Persia, India, China and other Middle East and far East countries.

500-1450 Middle Ages of Medicine: this period was basically a standstill. The use of bloodletting for curing illness was prominent. For lesser problems, leeches were used. Astrology started to influence medicine. No major advancements were made.

1801, Homeopathy appeared: In 1801 Samuel Hahnemann, a German physician, created Homeopathy (from Greek Homois=similar + Greek Pathos= suffering, Homeopathy = similar suffering). He codified the earlier suppositions of Hippocrates. After repeated direct success in applying his principals, he created Homeopathy. The label of Homeopathy would stick in 1902.
1810 Edward Jenner (1749-1823): in 1790 he purchased a medical certificate from St. Andrews University (a standard practice until 1814). After many troubling failures he finally developed a vaccine for Smallpox in 1810.

1814: Germany invents the "Degree" to show a level of proficiency and graduation from college.

1848 Samuel Weiss: A surgeon at the University of Vienna Medical School. Weiss noted that doctors routinely went directly from the morgue (handling the dead), to birthing wards delivering babies. When this practice was followed more than 50% of the infants died. He concluded that there was an element being carried from the dead to the infants that resulted in their premature deaths. He required surgeons to wash their hands before surgery. Due to the believed silliness of his supposition, he was fired.

1867 Joseph Lister (1827-1912): He literally cleans up surgery. He was the man who finally convinced the field of medicine that washing hands between surgeries is vital. Lister is known as the "Father of Antiseptic Surgery." "Ward fever deaths", caused by the un-cleanliness of surgeons and hospitals, fell from 12% to 1%. Lister insisted that all wounds had to be thoroughly cleaned and covered with a dressing soaked in Carbolic acid. As a result, his patient's mortality rate ran less than 2%.

Circa 1869 Louis Pasteur (1822-1893): Developed the "Germ Theory," that a weakened immune system can be attacked by germs that cause illness. He developed Pasteurization to kill bacteria. He collaborated with Dr. Robert Koch who had a detailed understanding of the human body (that Pasteur lacked) to develop numerous vaccines.

Due to the rapid expansion of the population across North America, good medicine had a very difficult time keeping up. Except on the settled east coast, standard or routine medicine was not being practiced in America. The new west was not a good place to be sick. Not that home remedies did not work, but it was the Snake Oil con man that was the problem. The lack of plentiful well educated Naturopaths and Homeopaths left America in the dire need of experts.

Early 1800s: powerful drugs came into recreational use all over the world. At this time in history Opium addiction was common in China, Europe, England and the United States. In these places more opium was consumed than beer.

1842 Dr. Crawford Williamson Long: On March 30, 1842 made the first use of ether to remove two tumors from a patient's neck. He used ether in minor surgery as early as 1841. Dr. Long eventually published his findings in The Southern Medical and Surgical Journal in 1848.

1843 Dr. Alexander Wood of Edinburgh: He loaded syringes with morphine and injected them in patients prior to surgery. This use gave far better results than oral administration. Wood found that injection was three times more effective than any other delivery method of killing pain. **1844 Dentist Horace Wells of Hartford, Connecticut:** He promoted nitrous oxide anesthesia to the Boston medical community but there was little interest. Unfortunately, in demonstration after demonstration, he received poor responses from colleagues and the public.

1846 Dr. Charles Jackson: He tutored Dr. William T.G. Morton in the use of nitrous oxide. During the next five years the American Dental Association adopted its use. Morton began secret experiments with ether. On September 30th, 1846, at his Boston office, he painlessly removed a tooth from a city worker.

1847: The future American Medical Association (AMA) was formed with one doctor as its sole member. The fledgling American Medical Association was incorporated in 1897.

1847: James Young Simpson first tested chloroform on himself on November 4, 1847. It created a very powerful narcotic effect and was known to cause death quickly when misused. The first fatality was a 15-year-old girl called Hannah Greener, who died on January 28, 1848.

1850 through 1899: Because the AMA was struggling to get members, there needed to be a way to drive up membership and thus drive up income.

1850-1866: the use of anesthesia started to become more common but the Civil War interrupted its progress and actually caused its use to slow until after the war. Nevertheless, those who did experience anesthesia appreciated the results.

1860-1865 American Civil War: doctors used unorthodox medicines and procedures often made up on the spot. For pain, they sparingly used medicines such as morphine, nitrous oxide, ether and chloroform. The normal treatment of a severely infected wound was amputation. As harsh as amputation was, it saved more lives than it took. Due to lack of supplies, common surgery was still being performed on patients who were given only alcohol and opium.

1875-1930: German physicians and psychologists / psychiatrists start moving from German universities to positions of prestige within major universities in the United States. The leader of this movement was Wilhelm Wundt (1832-1920), German physiologist and psychologist, generally acknowledged as the founder of experimental psychology.

1875: Wilhelm Wundt takes a position at the University of Leipzig, and sets up the first German psychological lab. Simultaneously, William James, a student of Wundt, set up a similar lab in America. Wundt's students found a pipeline directly into university positions in the United States. Most of these Wundt graduates went on to become eminent psychologists in the United States. It is widely accepted that the covert work of prestigious wealthy individuals living in America made all of this possible.

PROGRESSION OF NATURAL MEDICINE TO ALLOPATHIC MEDICINE AND SURGERY

Unity with the body	Natural Medicine	Homeopathy	Allopathic Medicine
Spirituality Prayer Breathing Exercise Fasting Water fasts Fruit fasts Vegetable fasts Laying on of hands Massage	Enemas Use of herbs Ayurvedic Medicine Oriental Medicine Acupuncture Iridiology Unani Medicine Naturopathy Osteopathy Chiropractic Colonics	Discovery that like substances can heal in the body in small amounts Vaccinations Drugs are used for the first time	Doctors are taught to cut open the body and remove defective parts. Microscopy and cellular study allows man to attempt to reverse engineer the body issues at a cellular level.
Food used to align the body and spirit.	Surgery pioneered.	Surgery used more extensively.	Use of powerful drugs genetically reprogram the body changing function.

8 Crimes against the Soul of Man

In the last chapter we met Wilhelm Wundt. This one individual was responsible for the beginnings of the German / European attitude that man was an animal. A soulless being has no rights, can be owned and experimented on. Ask any lab rat how he feels about that. Without a soul a man and his brain can be (and has been) sliced up like a Christmas Turkey. Thinking begets consciousness and the presence of a soul was what Wundt wanted to separate from man. He knew there was no soul inherent or connected to man. His own writings and later actions prove it.

Wilhelm Wundt wrote the following in "Lectures on Human and Animal Psychology."

"The old metaphysical prejudice that man "always thinks," has not yet entirely disappeared. I myself am inclined to hold that man really thinks very little and very seldom. Many an action, which looks like a manifestation of intelligence, most surely originates in association.

The Wundt Effect

Wundt was in the right place at the right time to change the course of psychological history and medical history. His students were plentiful and hungry for positions of power. The following is a list of Wundt's students who filled positions opened for them by very powerful and influential people. The wealthy industrialists that facilitated this drastic change are well known to you. A handful of men determined the way in which medicine would be practiced in the Americas. They attempted to predestine your medical future.

To overthrow any institution you must seize power at the top. The following list illustrates how a few of Wundt's students did just that.

James Mckeen Cattell was the first Professor of Psychology in the world (University of Pennsylvania, 1887). He studied in Leipzig under Wundt in 1882 and was appointed a fellow at John Hopkins University. He also lectured at Bryn Mawr, 1887; was the Professor of Psychology, University of Pennsylvania, 1888; head of the Department of Psychology and Philosophy at Columbia University from 1891-1905. He was the President of the American Psychological Association in 1895.

Edward Bradford Titchener, receiving his degree from Leipzig in 1892 was then appointed Assistant Professor of Psychology at Cornell University in the same year. He was made head of the psych laboratory that was founded the year before by Frank Angell, another Leipzig graduate. He went on to become the editor of studies from the Department of Psychology of Cornell University (1894-1927), American Editor, Mind (1894-1917) and Editor of the American Journal of Psychology (1895-1927).

Hugo Munsterberg moved from Germany to the United States to serve as the professor of psychology (1892-1916). He became the Director of the Harvard psychological laboratory in 1905.

G. Stanley Hall (1844-1924) pioneered American psychology in its early years. Hall taught briefly at Harvard before assuming a position at John Hopkins University in 1881. In 1887, Hall founded the American Journal of Psychology. He also served as the first President of the American Psychological Association in 1892 and was re-elected shortly before his death in 1924.

Lightner Witmer transferred to Leipzig University in Germany to study under Wilhelm Wundt. He obtained his Ph.D. in 1892, from Leipzig and then moved to Philadelphia to head an experimental laboratory at the University of Pennsylvania. Witmer established the world's first psychological clinic in 1896.

Charles Hubbard Judd completed his Ph.D. in 1896 under Wilhelm Wundt at Leipzig at only 23 years old. He later taught at the University of Cincinnati, Yale University, and finally the University of Chicago, where he was appointed as the Director of Education from 1909 until his retirement in 1938.

John D. Rockefeller, Andrew Carnegie, Will Keith Kellogg and **Henry Ford** became more and more interested in the German model of medicine. They independently decided to support the integration of German and American medicine. These multimillionaires and their vision would soon reshape the way medicine was practiced in America. Thanks to the efforts of the men listed above, foundations and groups like the FDA and AMA would flourish. I will be writing more on this topic of the FDA and AMA in later chapters.

Greed Takes Over

Prior to 1910, medicine in America was a melting pot of therapies. Doctors were good, but consistency was not the same when compared to the rigid doctors of Europe and Germany. The American doctor often had little training and used old time (yet effective) home remedies.

Homeopathy and Naturopathy were gaining more and more popularity. It worked and it was readily available in large cities. Yet, there was no formal medical degree as there was in Germany (first issued in 1814). Medical credentials could be purchased through the mail in America, while they were "earned" in Germany. It was clear that a large number of doctors received far less than adequate training.

Homeopathic doctors were flourishing in 1900. 100 homeopathic hospitals existed. Popularity of homeopathy in all classes of society soared. There were 22 homeopathic schools and over 1,000 homeopathic pharmacies.

But the AMA had no jurisdiction over homeopaths. Fighting for recognition and its very survival, in 1907, the AMA formed a committee to study American Medicine as it was being taught. The Council on Medical Education was formed with the intent to offer up reforms for medical education.

Surely a publicly made study would drive up membership and gain much needed repute for the organization. It was not to be as the committee ran out of money in 1908. This came to the attention of Andrew Carnegie, who created the Carnegie Foundation in 1905 to support such ventures. Realizing the benefits and buffers of an organization versus private donation, John D.

Rockefeller started his foundation in 1911.

Independently they decided to alter the landscape of American medicine forever.

Understanding the woes of the AMA, the Carnegie Foundation dispatched Henry S. Pritchett, President of the Carnegie Foundation, and Abraham Flexner. Flexner was educated at the University of Berlin and at Johns Hopkins University. At the Carnegie Foundation he was a researcher. Flexner had a gift for assimilating large amounts of information and then forming it into an understandable format for readers. Via the Carnegie Foundation, Flexner spotted an opportunity to alter and thus control post-graduate education in the United States. Flexner and Pritchett were to meet with the AMA. Pritchett was instructed to make an offer of help that the AMA could not refuse.

The plan was to take complete control of the AMA study and thus control of their findings.

Pritchett was instructed to:

- Offer to absorb the previous cost of the AMA study

- Offer to take over the rest of the study for the AMA and therefore absorb any future costs. He had a directive from Carnegie to offer any amount of money it took to get the AMA to let Pritchett and Flexner finish off the study and compile the findings. Acceptance of this gift was the first step in a master plot to take over and change medicine in America. The cost of taking over the work was only $10,000!

The story goes, on a cold day, December 8, 1908, it took less than an hour and the deal was struck. Flexner would compile an exhaustive study of over 160 medical schools in America. Based on his findings he would recommend which schools should be shut down and which should be approached to improve their conditions.

This was the first nail in the coffin of natural medicine. The "Flexner Report" was a clever mix of truth and subtle deceptions. It painted a gloomy picture of natural medicine. Flexner's copious report "Medical Education in the United States and Canada" (1910) was disseminated to the public in droves and did much to change public opinion. Soon pharmacology courses would be standard curriculum in new research departments at all qualified medical schools. Schools that gained the Flexner seal, of approval would receive huge amounts of grant money.

Ultimately, the decision as to who should and should not receive money went right to the top of the Rockefeller Foundation, Carnegie Foundation and others. These groups were anxiously signing grant checks. Homeopathy had been practiced in the United States since 1801, yet most Homeopathic schools were shut down. No chiropractic schools received any money. Osteopathic schools complied with Flexner's edicts and did get money. Soon thereafter, the Osteopathic

Medical Doctor was created.

Expected AMA membership soared off the charts as doctors rushed in panic to protect their livelihood. In 1910, 1 billion dollars in grant checks found homes at favored universities. Those willing to play the new Flexner game were flourishing and paid very well.

Over the next 15 years, Flexner toured North America visiting, reforming and bestowing checks on schools that met his standards. In 1913 alone, the Rockefeller foundation gave away another 80 million dollars in grants. Not a small amount of money considering that the total gross budget for all US medical schools in 1920 was only $12 million.

It paid to be on the right side of the fence. Not all the money came from the R&C (Rockefeller and Carnegie) Foundations. The Henry Ford Foundation, Kellogg Foundation (Kellogg Cereal Fame) and the Macy Foundation contributed mightily as well. Nevertheless, R&C were the most prolific givers in this arena.

To be on the receiving end of this money a college had to affiliate itself with a "recognized" teaching hospital. All professors had to be full time instructors and not see patients to supplement their incomes. This was used against Homeopathy as the instructors at the smaller institutions with smaller enrollments had to practice to make ends meet. Not to mention that now finding a "recognized" hospital affiliation for a Homeopathic college would be impossible.

Agents friendly to the AMA and R&C now managed recognized hospitals. For a short while they were rewarded (with grants) for toeing the new line. This further closed the doors of "non- approved" colleges from surviving. Without the funds to attract faculty and pay for new equipment, Chiropractic, Naturopathic, Homeopathic and Osteopathic colleges were nearly dead.

The schools that survived were those who would accept the yoke of the Rockefeller-Carnegie and their new Allopathic (drug based) curriculum. If it were not for newly formed and aggressive alumni organizations with private investments we would no longer have natural medicine.

The term allopathy was coined in 1842 by Hahnemann to designate the usual practice of medicine (allo = other + pathy = therapy, or use of drugs) as opposed to homeopathy (use of like substances).

In 1906 the FDA came into existence with the passage of the Federal Food and Drug Act. This act / law made it a crime for a processed consumable to be sold without an FDA approval. The FDA later partnered with the AMA to control the flow of drugs. Today, drugs approved by the FDA are those that can be isolated through chemical reaction (laboratory process). This of course excludes all natural substances such as herbs and herbal formulas as they do not go through lab processing. The chemical process renders drugs patentable as they are created in a laboratory and not in nature. The FDA does recognize Homeopathy due to its limited laboratory processing.

The only processing that herbal formulas receive is via cold pressing into capsules or tablets, hardly a dense chemical- laden laboratory process. Because of that, the dried leaves, roots, twigs, flowers and barks used in these mixtures are still viable and healing to the body. Therefore, the FDA does not recognize herbals as their lack of processing precludes them. The FDA is only interested in chemicals, drugs and big money. Herbal formulas are small potatoes compared to the remarkably lucrative drug industry.

In essence, this aspect of the FDA charter forever closes the door on herbal formulas being recognized by our Food and Drug Administration. Unless the FDA changes its charter, no one will ever see an herbal formula receive FDA approval.

Connecting the Dots!

Those of you who love a good conspiracy theory will love this. This is not a theory. The Rockefeller's, Carnegie's, Ford's, Kellogg's and Macy have conspired to run an influential agency (the AMA) from 1908 until circa 1920. This is due to the Flexner report "Medical Education in the United States and Canada" (1910). With that report, sweeping policies were affected that changed the practice of medicine.

Is there any reason to believe that these "moguls" ever relinquished control?
Is there a direct link from the FDA to the AMA?

It is well known that the AMA names the problem (disease). The FDA approves the drug for the disease and takes an 800 million payoff from the lucky pharmaceutical company who will make the drug. Who controls the FDA? We know who controls the AMA.

Are trillion dollar families such as the aforementioned and the Rothschild's (bankers in France and England) still calling the shots for health care worldwide? Can it be possible that they are acting as puppeteers over world governments?

If you were handed pseudo government power and could manage the flow of trillions of dollars in drug sales a year, would you relinquish control? There are many who believe that the FDA is a government agency under private control.

Using the Rockefeller Effect to Beat Them Back

The reason the tactics of this chapter were so effective in changing medicine was due to the strategy of "Getting them while they're young." Doctors had to be educated at the foundation root student level if they were going to be of any use. The brainwashing rhetoric had to be beaten in hard with no other option given. This profound incessant indoctrination led us to the insanity of what is called "modern medicine."

If you want to change this planet, get this book into the hands of kids. Yes, I have explained face reading to 10-17 year olds and they instantly get the simplicity and ease of the technique. Since face reading is so simple, anyone can do it. Yet the other gifts of this book are even deeper and again our future is riding on us doing something about it.

Kids instantly get what I write and say. Why? Because their un-brainwashed minds instantly recognize truth. This book is bursting at the seams with easily understood and tested truths.

Get this book to your nieces and nephews. I have often said that giving this book away is a bad idea. When it comes to kids, give it away. Give lots of them away. Purchase dozens of them for donation to elementary and high schools. Find out where I am lecturing next and bring your sons, daughters and their friends.

For you under 20 year olds reading this book, **you can change the world**. Yes, all of you young / pre adults can transform the humankind. Like it or not, you and your friends are going to run this planet. I am appealing to you to do something about the creeping crud that is overwhelming society today. Get all of your friends to read every page of this book. Have your high schools invite me to spend three hours presenting all of the truth contained herein. Do a book report and present it to your class. Use your high school budget to purchase this book for your school library. On these pages are the kinds of Earth shaking truths that can change mega-business and man's future forever.

If you don't do it, you are condoning the poisoning of your friends. They will become sick.

It all starts with you! I cannot do it alone. I need your help, as I cannot be everywhere. We have to do this together. The world needs you and me standing together shoulder-to-shoulder marching forward. I am counting on you.

9 Murder for Money—Psychiatric Crimes and Liver Function

In his book "Why Does Television Grovel Before Psychiatry?" Professor of Psychiatry Emeritus, Dr. Thomas Szasz states:

"From entertainment to news, television is enthralled, awe-struck and dazzled by the mysteries of virtually anything that smacks of psychiatry or psychology." The statistics and

statements poured out on major talk shows, morning news and magazine shows by these "experts," "present as scientific 'fact' what might well be only a scientific fiction."

You have a target on your back and are being hunted by rabid dogs intent on sucking the life out of your body and soul. The rabid dogs are the American Psychiatric Association (APA), World Health Organization (WHO) and Big Pharmaceuticals (I.E. Ely Lilly, Pfizer, AstraZeneca, Bayer Corporation, GlaxoSmithKline, Schering Sales Corporation, TAP Pharmaceuticals) and others like them.

Their devices for promotion and indoctrination are the TV and all media outlets! Every day we invite these pariahs into our homes and eat dinner with them.

Later Dr. Szasz adds:

"On television, everything can now be a psychiatric 'illness' as long as there are psychiatrists willing to 'diagnose' and 'treat' it... [they] invariably label the behaviors as 'illnesses' which are therefore uncontrollable and comparable to alcoholism or drug addiction. Child molesters and murderers are thus depicted as poor patients who are not responsible for their 'sick' behavior."

Psychiatry seeks to reach the largest public possible for the most financial gain possible. This demonic "branch of medicine" sees man as a sickness. Man is to be controlled like mice in a habitat for observation. Somehow through privilege, breeding or insanity, psychiatrists believe they have risen above mankind and therefore should be his caretaker.

The major nations of the planet have a backbone made up of so called psychiatric medicine and agenda. Not since Nazi Germany has the commingling of psychiatry and government plans been so pervasive.

Since the 1950s, world governments have radically attempted to control and direct their populaces by use of psychiatry and its drugs. An awake and questioning public is a danger from the legislative process. These ruling cowards seek perverted and covert control under the guise of world health care.

The following is directly taken from the "Depression and Bipolar Support Alliance." This group is a non-profit organization with full time lobbyisst in Washington pushing their agenda.

According to them:

*The **Depression and Bipolar Support Alliance** (DBSA) is the leading patient-directed national organization focusing on the most prevalent mental illnesses.*

__DBSA__ interacts and works with alliances in the mental health community such as the Mental Health Liaison Group (MHLG).

(POISONS) Medications for Depression and Bipolar Disorder

Your HCP might prescribe one or more medications to treat your symptoms. These may include:

Mood stabilizers, Antidepressants and Antipsychotics

Notice the 3 categories of "help" above are d r u g s—d r u g s and of course more toxic d r u g s.

DSBA is well known for its love of children and fighting their problems with medication. The reason why children are being targeted is because they must be absorbed into the "system" early or psychiatry risks losing a potential patient.

The following is again from their website:

Depression and bipolar disorder (also known as manic depression) are both highly treatable medical illnesses.

The above statement is patently false. Medical illness includes colds, pneumonia, cancer and items that are known and described entities like appendicitis. Psychiatric "illness" cannot be tested for. There is no blood test, just the opinion of the observer which is filtered through his emotions and personal experiences. The old saying "opinions are like assholes, everyone's got one" is applicable here.

(The DBSA website continues)

Unfortunately many people do not get the help they need because of misunderstanding the issues surrounding the illnesses or the fear associated with stigma. The following information can help you learn more about the signs and symptoms of mood disorders so that you can get the help you need for yourself or a loved one.

The following proves the notes in bold above. While reading the list of symptoms for depression below, ask these five questions:

1) Why is the condition or "state" of normal not described?

2) Why do they ignore the role of diet and lifestyle?

3) Is life supposed to be without ups and downs?

4) Are we normal only in a comatose drugged state?

5) Why are drugs being used to crush creativity?

DBSA Signs and symptoms of depression
- *Prolonged sadness or unexplained crying spells*

- *Significant changes in appetite and sleep patterns*
- *Irritability, anger, worry, agitation, anxiety*
- *Pessimism, indifference*
- *Loss of energy, persistent lethargy*
- *Feelings of guilt, worthlessness*
- *Inability to concentrate, indecisiveness*
- *Inability to take pleasure in former interests, social withdrawal*
- *Unexplained aches and pains*
- *Recurring thoughts of death or suicide*

The medical model teaches that disease can be isolated in a laboratory setting and diffused via interaction with antibodies that can replicate in the human body.

So called psychiatric disorders such as "Bipolar disorder" and "depression" are akin to fairy dust as they do not appear anywhere to be diffused. Depression is not found in a beaker or seen under a microscope only drugs are. Therefore with nothing to treat psychiatrists with the help of Big Pharma and the AMA are criminally treating opinions with drugs.

(DBSA website) Signs and symptoms of bipolar disorder
- *Increased physical and mental activity and energy*
- *Heightened mood, exaggerated optimism and self-confidence*
- *Excessive irritability, aggressive behavior*
- *Decreased need for sleep without experiencing fatigue*
- *Grandiose delusions, inflated sense of self-importance*
- *Racing speech, racing thoughts, flight of ideas*
- *Impulsiveness, poor judgment, distractibility*
- *Reckless behavior*
- *In the most severe cases, delusions and hallucination*

(DSBA) Symptoms of depression - the "lows" of bipolar disorder
- *Prolonged sadness or unexplained crying spells*
- *Significant changes in appetite and sleep patterns*
- *Irritability, anger, worry, agitation, anxiety*
- *Pessimism, indifference*
- *Loss of energy, persistent lethargy*
- *Feelings of guilt, worthlessness*
- *Inability to concentrate, indecisiveness*
- *Inability to take pleasure in former interests, social withdrawal*
- *Unexplained aches and pains*
- *Recurring thoughts of death or suicide*

Psychiatry and psych drugs are now intended via marketing to appear benevolent. This could not be further from the truth. Psych drugs are positioned to sooth and cradle life in a bosom of safety. The above list if read by the unsuspecting seems harmless and inviting. With regard to that it is hard for these people to stay off these drugs.

The sole intent of the AMA, World Health Organization and Big Pharma is to ensure that everyone is on at least one psych drug. Ideally they would like the people of Earth on a clutch of their poisons.

The coupling of government with Big Pharma is an ominous and dangerous duo. Humans have ups and downs because that is part of being human. It is part of the autonomic nervous system and is an indicator of the health of the individual. Having a bad mood is no different than getting hot.

The heat index of the body indicates how the machine is running. If something stresses the body on a structural level the heat rises. Should the body receive a chemical or some shock that created a hormonal release heat may be the result depending on liver load. These hormones arrive at the liver for detoxification but should they fail to be processed by an overburdened liver all manner of havoc may ensue.

The response is that the body gets hot and we then misidentify the chemical overload and take a drug to cool us off. This is akin to a child asking for water and his mother instead giving him a cup of sand.

Whenever we have emotional stress of any type the key is not to drug and block it. We must understand the reaction as a cry from the body for help. The oldest records of emotional stress come to us from China 4000 year ago. What was noted then is still accurate today.

The Chinese stated "The liver and emotions are linked!"

In simple terms the liver must detoxify all that we come in contact with. Today it is overloaded with more work than two livers could keep up with. Because of this we notice tendencies towards lack of sleep, bad moods, aches and pains, moodiness etc.

The Chinese gave us one of the oldest statements about liver function to persist through history unchanged. The statement mentioned above has not changed in over 4000 years. Again they said "The liver and emotions are linked." The Chinese found that emotions were colored by the good or bad function of the liver.

This statement persists yet the true nature of the liver including the proper care of it was not readily translated from Chinese to English.

The Chinese court physician to the emperor had a tremendous task helping his highness stay in top physical form. If the emperor was "off" it could become a very bad day for anyone coming in contact with the sovereign leader of China. This is why keeping his emotions in check was so important. A bad 24 hours full of heated emotions would not only impact the life of the physician but all of China.

It was based on this challenge that the epiphany that "The liver and emotions are linked" was first postulated and proved. Even 4000 years ago it was clear that oil coated the liver and made it inoperable. This factor and many more impacted and forced the liver "off line" into a realm of quiet desperation as the body tired to cope. Even today the first signals from the liver indicating stress are heated emotions and poor judgment.

Summarizing 4000 years ago Chinese biologists, herbal formulators and nutritionists made note of hundreds of substances that offended the liver.

They also noted and categorized the responses when toxicity was affecting the liver. Much of this sage wisdom has not made its way into English.

The liver is the emperor of our body. Like 4000 years ago it is a matter of life and death to keep the emperor happy and healthy. Today our lives are very different than they were 4000 years ago and our liver is far more taxed. Therefore balanced emotions are harder to come by and still very pro-survival to strive for. In the present day just as 4000 years ago these chemical and food based foes quickly heat up the liver and the emotions.

This should be of paramount concern to anyone wishing to achieve emotional balance in life. I have spent ten years working on this data and the best way to heal the liver. Milk Thistle is a commonly used herb that is touted to "protect the liver" or "is a liver protector." Shockingly or perhaps not so shockingly the masses are completely wrong with their blind use of milk thistle.

If one understands the simple rule of cause and effect they too would establish what is not only good for the liver but the whole body.

I am a formulator, researcher, educator, author, lecturer and one who is driven by the guiding light of results. I thereby am perplexed by those who cannot think outside the box and do not use results as their yardstick. When I developed my own liver formula I was stymied by conflicting data indicating gaping holes in commonly held "everyone knows" beliefs and the facts. Trusting milk thistle, I tested it and tested it and the results were horrible when they should have been golden. People became worse with its use, not better.

So perplexing was this enigma that it took me weeks before I would believe my initial confusing and disturbing results. How could I be sickening people by following the centuries old rules and beliefs regarding the healing of the liver?

In my world it does not matter what something is "supposed to do" the only thing that matters is what it actually does. The mystery revolving around the vaunted herb milk thistle and the actual nature and function of the liver was very taxing.

Routinely formulators copy other formulators thus propagating the same robotic misguided mistakes. "Monkey see monkey do" may be good enough for primates but among humans it is senseless, appalling and damaging. I was learning this first hand.

Habits die hard as does the false data and false beliefs accompanying blatant inaccuracies even in the face of overwhelming logic.

I then made several mixes some with milk thistle and some without. Those without milk thistle worked and those with it failed. This one ingredient milk thistle consistently exacerbated liver symptoms at any dosage.

Milk thistle is the most commonly recommended and deeply respected herb on the planet for healing the liver. History has given us 4000 years of references all clearly stating that milk thistle is a liver protector.

Interestingly the Chinese were not using milk thistle yet they identified it as a "liver protector." Clearly this statement is a warning prohibiting milk thistle use. Protecting the liver which protects the body is akin to supply ships trying to protect battle ships and destroyers.

Milk thistle directly interferes with the purpose, action and activity of the liver. The liver must protect the body 24 hours a day, seven days a week, including weekends holidays, ground hog day and leap year.

The liver is the body's protector and must be active 24 hours a day. It is the Army, Navy, Air Force, Special Forces and Marines of the body. It is first on the scene when anything enters the body; it works the hardest and is the last to leave.

The liver is not without defenses as it is the only organ in the body with the power to regenerate Not quite as advanced as Terminator 2'cyborg the T-1000 played by Robert Patrick or Kristanna Loken's T-X of Terminator 3, yet the human liver is very affective and almost superhuman in its repair ability. Up to 25% of the liver can be removed and it will still grow back.

The liver cannot rest for even a moment or we start to become ill.

When the liver is running correctly liver symptoms calm and dissipate to an unperceivable level. If liver interference is present for an extended period of time the body starts to deteriorate and die. The simple action of monitoring urine pH demonstrates just how important the liver is to life in the human body. Healthy urine pH should fall between the levels of 6.8-8.0.

The body does not have a voice yet it must communicate with us. It does this with sensation. The liver signals us with a variety of symptoms that without a trained eye or expert understanding would go unnoticed. The last thing we should ever do is "treat" these sensations with a pain killer, antidepressant, antipsychotic or "mood stabilizer."

Classic liver symptoms are:

- Bad moods or depression
- Irritated eyes
- Red eyes
- Fuzzy vision
- Poor memory
- Poor mental focus
- Inconsistent / poor energy
- Head aches
- Poor sleep
- Itchy skin
- Dry skin
- Skin broken out
- Irritated skin
- Burning skin
- Tingling skin
- Fibromyalgia
- Shallow breathing
- Emphysema
- Lung tumors
- Lung cancer
- Poor lung function
- Poor digestion
- Right elbow pain, soreness or stiffness
- Right shoulder pain, soreness or stiffness
- Right side neck pain, soreness or stiffness
- Right pectoral pain, soreness or stiffness
- Right scapula (shoulder blade) pain, soreness or stiffness
- Right bicep pain, soreness or stiffness
- Right triceps pain, soreness or stiffness

- Right deltoid pain, soreness or stiffness
- Right upper back pain, soreness or stiffness
- Burning tongue
- Burning (inner) mouth
- Lung issues and congestion
- Sinus issues or congestion
- Congested nose / sinuses
- Intense or extreme emotional responses
- Addictions

The liver and kidneys are the hub / keystones of the body's immune system and survival net. When encountering a substance the body swifts it away to the liver for processing. The number of symptoms the body experiences is in direct proportion to the level of toxins in receives. When the load is insatiable on the liver; symptoms will fully display (see the list above). Being very clear when our body comes in contact with any substance via the skin, lungs, eyes or mouth; that material it is rapidly contained and sent to the liver. Think of the liver as a washing machine and processing plant.

All material absorbed via the above routes are sent to the liver which is a sponge-like hepa filter. Once this matter arrives at the liver it is inspected whereby it will be used, stored and or disposed in quick fashion. This is how the liver operates under optimal conditions.

When liver load is overwhelming, as it often is in as much as 90% of the public, the liver becomes a besieged spectator as the body seems to melt down with toxins.

The liver becomes toxic due to drugs, food preservatives, processed oils, fluoridated water, colorings, dyes, white sugar, caffeine, alcohol, man-made foods and environmental hazards.

A common and misnamed problem of the liver is swelling which is the same thing as inflammation. Hepatitis means the same thing as a swollen liver does. Even though Hepatitis means that the liver is swollen or inflamed the word Hepatitis is alarming. It creates worry and mystery as to what it is Hepatitis is. It sounds as though the "hepa monster" has gotten you or some such thing. Perhaps you caught a germ! Hepatitis is never caught and it is not scary but the word is intimidating.

Even if you know what it is, it sounds far worse than what it actually is, as the word Hepatitis does not describe the condition. Again, hepatitis is just a swollen irritated liver.

I surveyed 100 people I asked them:

1) Do you know what hepatitis is?

2) Do you know what a swollen liver is?
3) Which sounds worse?
4) Do you think you could treat Hepatitis by yourself?
5) Do you think you could treat a swollen liver by yourself?

28% Knew what hepatitis meant
98% Knew what a swollen liver was
85% Thought that hepatitis sounded worse than a swollen liver
54% Felt they could fix or treat a swollen liver on their own.
2%   Felt they could fix or treat Hepatitis on their own.
40% Didn't think they could fix or treat either of them
6%   Didn't know how to answer

The June 2001 issue of the "Townsend Newsletter for Doctors and Patients" recommends the herb bupleurum for all three forms of Hepatitis. They also recommend its use for liver cancer, cirrhosis, Epstein Barr, chronic fatigue, tumor growth, Leukemia and alcoholism.

It is a Chinese herb that resets or turns on the liver. Hepatitis is created due to liver overload and congestion as its workload is far above its ability to cope with the job at hand.

Review the list of liver friendly foods listed later in this chapter and you will have a leg up.

It does not matter whether you have been told that you are suffering from bi-polar, OCD, ADHD, ADD, depression, anxiety, mania or Hoingy Boingly disease (<<just a made up disease like the rest) they are just names for issues that are solved by cleaning up the system and turning on the liver.

The so called foods and substances to be avoided are:

• All processed oils (they coat and choke off the liver)
• MSG, as it preserves the body and is a known carcinogen
• Oil based supplements as they are often rancid
• Hot spicy cooked food
• Salt, as it keeps the body from utilizing water
• Sugar, as it suppresses the immune system by 95% and up to 8 hours
• Sodium, as it acts just as salt but also acts as a preservative to the body
• Caffeine, as it is a diuretic and robs the body of fluid
• Dairy products, as they congest the body and constipate the colon
• All breads, as they convert to sugar
• Tylenol, as it destroys the liver
• Pain killers, as they block liver function

- Drugs, as they poison the body and break it down
- Fluoride, as it attacks the liver and is a carcinogen
- Alcohol, as it rots the liver and poisons the body
- Steroids, as they shrivel the liver
- All sodas, as they are loaded with poisons

The liver is healed with the following foods: Blueberries, carrots, oranges, tangerines, grapefruit, lemons, limes, onion, garlic, broccoli, asparagus, red cabbage, cauliflower, green beans, tomatoes, bell peppers, romaine lettuce, apples, beets, arugula, avocado, blackberries, raspberries, ginger, radishes and strawberries.

When eating foods found on that list it is best to eat them raw otherwise you greatly decrease their life changing benefits.

The herbs that heal the liver are bupleurum, gentian root, hyssop, cayenne, astragulus, bilberry root, dandelion root, orange, tangerine, irish moss, yellow dock, sarsaparilla, safflower herb, grapefruit fiber, lime fiber, red clover, peony root, lemon fiber, garlic, ginger root, lemon verbena, thyme, goldenseal and marshmallow root.

Large amounts of spicy cooked foods are especially bad for the liver as they heat it via chemical reaction. To the human body heat applied via cooked food is the same as heat from a fever. In either case the body thinks that it is fighting an infection.

This chapter examines liver function, psychiatric crimes, psychiatric drugs, psychiatric abuses and herbs and foods that heal the liver. To a psychiatrist body function is an enigma. They are trying to treat a time tested liver problem caused by toxic overload with drugs that add to the toxic overload.

Psychiatrists have no notion of liver function thus no clue what they are doing. The crime known as psychiatry knows nothing about body function. This wayward group only acknowledges the liver as an organ, certainly not the center of emotions.

Psychiatrists based on their actions and own literature do not recognize that man has a soul. Amazing when you consider that psychiatry means the study or healing of the soul.

Webster's defines psych this way;

Main Entry: **psych-**
Variant(s): or psycho-
Function: *combining form*
Etymology: Greek, from psyche breath, principle of life, life, soul, from *psychein* to breathe; akin to Sanskrit *babhasti* he blows

From Medicinenet.com
iatry: Suffix meaning medical treatment. From the Greek "iatreia" meaning healing which came from "iatros" meaning treatment (or physician). Psychiatry is literally the medical treatment of the psyche.

When you consider the above definitions it becomes painfully obvious just how true the statement is that psychiatry does not recognize the soul. Why else would they cut up the brain, shock the brain and deaden the brain with suicide causing drugs?

Psychiatric crimes:
- Frontal lobotomies
- Frontal leucotomy (ice pick surgery)
- Gamma knife surgery
- Shock treatment
- Drugging

The history of psychiatry is an appalling excursion into debauchery and torment. Psychiatry is sadly misguided in their efforts and costs hundreds of lives every year.

Most of us agree that man has a soul, sprit or élan' vital. Even the atheist admits that the body is animated with energy. A casual look at the esoteric aspects of the body reveals a very interesting story indeed.

Below we will examine the nature of man with regard to the body, spirit, soul and élan vital or life force.

Is personality a function of the:
- Soul
- Body

Is charisma a function of the:
- Soul
- Body

Are the memories of your life a function of the:
- Soul
- Body

Is creativity and creative thought a function of the:
- Soul
- Body

Is intelligence a function of the:

- Soul
- Body

Are emotions a function of the:
- Soul
- Body

Is honesty a function of the:
- Soul
- Body

What part of you do some people believe could live forever:
- Soul
- Body

Most people acknowledge that the answers to the above questions all have the same answer, the soul. Yet psychiatry ignores this.

If you are an atheist this is all a moot point. But for the rest of us it is obvious that we are a soul. For psychiatry we are just a piece of meat. Otherwise why does this profession assign all of mans difficulties to the brain? Are you your body or are you, you. Are you your brain that will one day die or are you an immortal sprit or energy? Psychiatry insists that chemicals in the brain make you unstable and in need of their "help." They insist that you (as a spirit) are flesh only. Therefore they offer solutions that affect only the flesh.

Psychiatry probably thinks that your eyes decide what to watch on cable TV or that your hands drive your car. For the psychiatrist since the mouth is attached to the head and it makes noise and since the brain is not far away, then you must be your brain. Silly is it not?

Most people have never thought about what the soul is. Nevertheless it is clear that it is not a piece of meat or a body part.

Since you are a spirit or energy where is the spirit found in relationship to the body? Is part of the body? Is it around the body? The answer to this riddle is simple. The sprit or soul can be found around or in the body. Because it is not anchored to any specific part of the body its location will change. It is safe to say, that if there is a living breathing body nearby, there is a soul somewhere very close to it.

Since the soul can move, this explains the out of body experience.

To recap psychiatry believes that you are your body. This is similar to thinking that the actors being watched on your TV are actually in the TV itself. If you have ever looked you have noticed that John Travolta, Brad Pitt, Dakota Fanning, Josh Hartnett, Will Smith, Scarlett Johansson, Justin Long and the actors from Saturday Night Live are not across the room hiding behind your TV screen.

The brain is a nerve center that opens and closes the eyes and computes optimum solutions to the physical strain of daily life. Our brain is a high output computer that can handle a remarkable amount of tasks. All it needs is a body that is healthy enough to support its activities.

Savagely slicing up the brain with operations such as the frontal lobotomy or the new bloodless Gamma Knife surgery (surgery via focused radiation beam) is still butchery.

Such is the history of psychiatry. The reason psychiatry insists that you are a piece of meat is because then they can administer drugs and surgery. These arenas are huge money making ventures. If you buy into the concepts offered by this profession you have agreed to be a slave to their mindset and procedures.

Psychiatry is invalid for four basic reasons:
• They deny you as a spirit or soul
• They insist that you are your brain
• They do not recognize that the liver plays a huge role in emotional intensity
• They therefore do not understand that a toxic liver increases emotional intensity

Since psychiatry does not recognize the soul, they therefore deny the existence of God. Further the insidious aspect of psychiatric drugging of emotions is tantamount to pouring gasoline on a fire to put it out. Science has proved as did the Chinese 4000 years ago that a toxic liver is the result of all antidepressants and psych drugs. They actually put the user asleep. These drugs often result in suicide and other questionable deaths.

Why do emotions get worse with the use of psychiatric drugs?

The reason why is simple the liver must now work harder to get your attention. Emotions actually get far worse as the liver is further beaten up. Since the liver communicates to us via increased emotional response, deadening it with drugs is the wrong thing to do. The result is it must increase the intensity of its emotional output to get your attention. Therefore, your emotions get more and more dramatic.

Drugs ingested increases the load on the liver pushing it further into the muck.

Remember the first symptom the liver gives us when it goes "off line" is feeling of unease or upset about random happenings or life. Suddenly small problems become elephants. If you see a doctor who is psych drug friendly and you bring your elephant in tow you may end up on drugs or worse.

Roger Bezanis

More and more data is being uncovered everyday demonstrating that man is still being damaged by psychiatry. The horrors of psychiatry are so heinous that it is amazing that the medical field recognizes these madmen as doctors and not as criminals. For some time it was believed that "shock" treatment was a thing of the past. Sadly it is not. What used to be called Electroshock or Electroshock Treatment (EST) is now usually called "Electro-Convulsive Therapy", often abbreviate ECT.

The term is misleading, because ECT is not a form of therapy, despite the claims of its supporters. ECT causes brain damage, memory loss, and diminished intelligence.

An article in the March 25, 1993 *New England Journal of Medicine* (page 839) says: "ELECTROCONVULSIVE therapy is widely used to treat certain psychiatric disorders, particularly major depression".

The March 26, 1990 issue of *Newsweek* magazine reported that "electroconvulsive therapy (ECT)...is enjoying resurgence. ...An estimated 30,000 to 50,000 Americans now receive shock therapy each year." (p. 44). Other recent estimates say the numbers skyrocketing to more than 100,000 ECT's per year.

In his textbook *Psychiatry for Medical Students*, published in 1984, Robert J. Waldinger, M.D., said "ECT's mechanism of action is not known. As with other somatic therapies; in psychiatry we do not know the mechanism by which ECT exerts its therapeutic effects". (pp.120 & 389).

Psychiatrists claim unhappiness or so-called depression is sometimes caused by unknown biological abnormalities in the brain. They say by some unknown mode of action ECT cures these unknown biological abnormalities.

There is no good evidence for these claims. Other than by causing mental disorientation and memory loss, ECT does not help eliminate the unhappy feeling called depression.

This is true even though currently unhappiness or "depression" is the only "condition" for which ECT is a recognized "therapy". Indeed, rather than eliminating depression, the memory loss and lost mental ability caused by ECT has caused some subjected to ECT so much anguish they have committed suicide after receiving the "treatment".

ECT consists of electricity being passed through the brain with a force of 70 to 400 volts and amperage of from 200 milliamperes to 1.6 amperes (1600 milliamperes).

The electric shock is administered for as little as a fraction of, to as long as several seconds. The electrodes are placed on each side of the head at about the temples, or sometimes on the front and back of one side of the head so the electricity will pass through just the left or right side of the brain (which is called "unilateral" ECT).

Some psychiatrists falsely claim ECT consists of a very small amount of electricity being passed through the brain. In fact, the 70 to 400 volts and 200 to 1600 milliamperes used in ECT are quite powerful.

The power applied in ECT is typically as great as that found in the wall sockets in your home. It could kill the "patient" if the current were not limited to the head.

The electricity in ECT is so powerful it can burn the skin on the head where the electrodes are placed. Because of this, psychiatrists use electrode jelly, also called conductive gel to prevent skin burns from the electricity.

The electricity going through the brain causes seizures so powerful; the so-called patients receiving this so-called therapy have broken their own bones during the seizures. To prevent this muscle paralyzing drugs are administered immediately before the so-called treatment. Of course the worst part of ECT is brain damage not broken bones. Do not let yourself, your family or friends be subjected to this or the insanity of psychiatry. It is horrific to consider that psych drugs can be administered in many school systems without parental consent.

Speak to your school administrators to DISCOVER "their attitudes" and then DECLARE YOUR OPPOSITION to their policies. Make your wishes known for how your child will be treated. If you don't stand up and say NO, you may be RUN OVER by the barbaric powers covertly operating under your nose.

It does not matter whether you have been told that you are suffering from bi-polar, OCD, ADHD, ADD, depression, anxiety, mania or Hoingy Boingly disease (just a made up disease like the rest) they are just names for issues that are solved by cleaning up the system via diet and detoxification and by resetting the liver.

Do not treat a liver condition with drugs that ultimately make the condition worse. Use nature to help you as the answers are in the kitchen and in what you put in your mouth.

Under no circumstance should your liver be protected with milk thistle or any substance. Not even a swollen liver (hepatitis) is a reason to protect the liver. So called experts who enforce milk thistle for the improvement of and healing of hepatitis are misinformed.

The liver capacity to alter chemicals, produce food and police the system of waste is not infinite. When you feel the symptoms mentioned earlier in this chapter it means that our liver is overwhelmed right now. Like a typist that can handle 60 pages a day; when it is given 70, 80, 90 or more pages a day it to falls behind in its work. That typist may feel a little taxed.

When considering this simple response it is criminal that psychiatry, in its German beginnings over 100 years ago, seized this emotional response and assigned it to the brain.

See your chiropractor and get regular adjustments. A colon hydro-therapist can be your best friend as colonics have a direct and marked affect on the liver.

Learn face reading and your liver symptoms by rote so that you can foresee liver issues years in advance of actual problems. In this way you are being proactive with your health. This is the best approach to maintaining your vitality.

Do not let yourself be placed on psych meds as they will destroy you. Re-read the previous chapter as many times as needed to ensure that this data is burned into your memory and ready for easy use.

I am here to help if you need me.

Your friend,
Roger Bezanis

10 All About the Liver

You have read that the liver and emotions are linked. What does that statement mean? It means that 4000 years ago in China the physicians to the emperor started noticing strange behaviors emanating from "His Highness."

He would get emotional, i.e. angry, sad, depressed, nervous, edgy, fearful, paranoid, etc., after coming in contact with different substances. Shakespeare, Francis Bacon, Jean-Baptiste Poquelin (Moliere) and other dramatists knew of this relationship, as did medicine of the 14th century.

With that in mind, look at the definition below of melancholy. It is very revealing as this emotion was directly tied to the liver and the gallbladder function. The exact location of the gallbladder can be found attached to the right underside of the liver. It produces bile, which is a digestive aid and stool softener.

1mel·an·choly
Pronunciation: me-in-kä-lï
Function: noun

Inflected From(S): plural mel·an·chol·ies

Etymology: Middle English malencolie, from Anglo-French, from Late Latin melancholia, from Greek, from melan- + cholï bile — more at GALL

Date: 14th century
1 a: an abnormal state attributed to an excess of black bile and characterized by irascibility or depression B: BLACK BILE C: MELANCOLIA 2 a: depression of spirits: DEJECTION B: a pensive mood

It was believed that when the gallbladder produced too much bile, depression would follow. We now know that the liver regulates all emotions, not just depression. We have also mapped out the direct relationship to substances ingested and our liver function and therefore moods. It is further observed that, as his immune system goes, mans' emotions follow.

4000 years ago in China the Emperors physicians started to fully appreciate how delicate the liver was. They noted that the liver's (the center for detoxification for the human body) ability to do its job was directly impacted by the food or chemicals the emperor ate or absorbed.

Cleansing the body of impurities is the liver's job. Based on the construction of the body, the liver, via one of its channels (colon, lungs, skin or mouth), comes in contact with every substance the body contacts first. This means the liver is the hub of your body. All roads lead to the liver.

Keeping the liver clean and free of waste was of paramount importance to these physicians, as the emperor's mood would not only affect all of China, but their lives directly. If he was in a foul mood, he could have had them removed from his circle of court physicians or even beheaded.

Either way you would certainly lose status (headless or jobless) by being disciplined. To simplify and add clarity, the body, being perfect, has several built in alarms that we are supposed to react to.

Such as:

Hunger = Eat
Thirsty = Drink
Tired = Sleep
Pain = Bad / Avoid

The above four points are accepted and non-arguable. The following five points have been neglected:

Itchy skin   = Liver
Watery eyes   = Liver
Emotional stress   = Liver
All bad moods   = Liver
Coughing   = Liver

When the Emperor's physicians gave him certain mood enhancing drugs, his mood would alter, but when he came down from the drugs, he was worse off than before. Therefore, what was happening? The physicians had inadvertently increased the load on the liver. Yes, the drugs initially made the emperor feel better (as he was somewhat sedated). All the while his liver was working overtime to break down the substance to drive it from the body. They found that the best way to control his mood was by being sure that the emperor had a healthy, fully-functioning liver. Healthy liver function with no drugs was paramount to keeping the emperor in the pink. His diet was the key. Water, seasonal fruit and herbs (food) were the best approach. Waste not processed by the liver dispenses into the system. Escaped waste lodges in the fatty tissue, connective, tissue or muscle tissue. There it will stay until such time that the liver can process the waste.

When we get moody, it is the liver signaling us that it needs help. The irritant can be hormonal; yes, testosterone and estrogen can cause liver overwhelm. Therefore, menopause and your period are especially brutal on the liver and, as a consequence, your emotions. But, it is all a liver issue. Improve liver function and you will feel better.

The true source of fear demands a special note. It is believed by many that "fear" is controlled or regulated by the kidneys. This is not true or the Chinese would not have written "liver and emotions are linked." This belief is derived from the observation that terrified people often lose control of their bladder. Therefore, it is easy to conclude that fear equals fluid release and is directly caused by "fear" hitting the kidneys.

The correct sequence is fear-stimuli cause the body to release a hormone or chemicals. The liver must quickly address this substance but fails in the attempt. In response, the liver goes into crisis mode and attempts to flush the substance from the system and releases water to the kidneys. If you recall, the liver is the "washing machine" of the body. The Released fluid rapidly hits the kidneys. The kidney as directed by the liver flushes the fluid and the person, in "fear", urinates.

Please correct anyone who you discover has this common misconception.

Weight Loss and the Liver

Weight loss has been a mystery since man became physically and socially aware. The liver must wash the body free of waste. When the liver is impaired or running slow, it will not be able to flush waste out of the system. Efficient liver function is paramount to wash toxins and fat from the structure of the body.

Steroids and the Liver

Steroids suppress the immune system yet are given for poison ivy and poison oak. These two irritants cause the body to itch and swell. The reason why is because your body has been attacked by an acid irritant. Treating it, your practitioner will tell you that you must take steroids to prevent this inflammatory response.

Please understand that your liver regulates your skin. When you have stumbled onto poison ivy or oak your body is fighting an irritating poison. The last thing anyone should ever do is turn off the immune system when there is an immune system challenge.

Therefore, do-not-take-steroids-ever. Understand that your immune system is under siege (via your liver) and support it with liver herbs, water and citrus.

Steroids will keep you sick longer as your liver will not be functioning.

Support your liver. Do not shut it down.

Mad Men in White Coats

One has to then ask, why did psychiatry start giving people psychiatric drugs for liver issues? The answer is simple yet complex.

Every field of endeavor on the planet is trying to help everyone all the time. That being said, psychiatrists had an intention to help. But, by not knowing structure and function of the body, they only added to the problem and made things worse and worse.

The problem with psychiatry started with its roots. The term "psychiatry" literally means the "doctor of the soul," coming from the Greek, "psych" meaning soul, and "iatros" meaning doctor.

This term acknowledged a fundamental truth:

"That man has a soul."

Man was not a piece of meat that could not think, he was a spiritual being. Johann Christian Reil (1759-1813) coined the term psychiatry in the West in 1808. Reil clearly recognized that the soul was what animated the body. He called it the "Vital Force" that separated living organisms from inanimate objects.

But in his own work, while championing the "Vital Force" (which we could call the soul), he also called for the dissecting of the body to better understand the vital force. This immediately creates a problem as he had just combined the soul and the body into one mechanism: a piece of meat.

In the following statement, he inadvertently created a stage where the future dissection of the body would be acceptable.

Reil wrote:
"It would be advantageous for theoretical and practical medicine if we could analyze the different kinds of degrees of organization, if we could reduce their most complex tissues to their most simple elements and if we were able to, we would then be able, more happily, to analyze many phenomena and to reduce them more accurately to their principles."

Reil's rambling and effusive observation may very well have been misunderstood and taken to mean that man was an animal and therefore without a soul.

He concludes with:
"Follow them (the systems) from the original most elemental organ to the most complex animal organs."

All of this came to a head in 1811, two years before his death, as a professorship of "psychiatric therapy" was established in Leipzig, Germany. A similar chair in Berlin followed this. That same year, 1811, the first laboratory opened up designed to study the human mind via dissection of the brain. This idea is as ludicrous as dissecting a TV to look for the actors.

Germany spun out of control as it was involved in a political chess game that would affect every class of people in Europe. Germany needed to control larger masses to be successful. If experts (there is that word again) claimed it so, it would be accepted as true.

This need for control was part and parcel behind these oddball observations and postulations:

Psychiatry As A Political Tool

Psychiatrist C.T. Groddeck, 1850, psychiatrist, awarded a doctorate for his dissertation entitled: "The Democratic Disease - A New Form of Insanity." In Groddeck's view, every democratically inclined person was insane.

Psychiatrist C.J. Wretholm (Groddeck's colleague) 1854, "discovered" the still shocking "Sermon Disease". Wretholm believed that anyone who enjoyed church was disturbed or insane.

Psychiatrist P. J. Mobius, circa 1854, extensively lectured in Germany and in Europe on the "Psychological feeble-mindedness of woman."

Psychiatrist Adolph Hoppe chimed in with his contribution to mental disorders with "Political and reformatory insanity." Therefore: All political reformers were insane.
Psychiatrist Adolph Hoppe later added the politically damning and World War I stimulating "French mental illness" for those born in France, as he considered France cursed.

The above observations while primitive and laughable by today's standards are not laughable at all. They are horrifying. These ideas were believed and acted upon.

Otto Von Bismarck (World War I Chancellor) used these twisted ideas as justification to start World War I. Hitler had the groundwork laid for WWII with the rest of these works and many more. Germany, being racially pure, had as its divine right to purify and direct the people of Earth.

Kind of like a global policeman. Sound familiar?

Anytime one group sees itself as senior / smarter / closer to God or more righteous than another, war follows. The masses will pay the ultimate price. Every war fought in history had this idea at its core.

These observations / hypotheses served as a useful tool to squash dissidents to the military and political opponents. With a mental program explaining that man was indeed an animal (a twist on Reil's work), Bismarck - the leader of Germany – did indeed use this "science" as a cause for a justifiable war.

No doubt, Wilhelm Wundt (1832 – 1920), the future father of psychology, read Reil's papers. Later Wundt would theorize that man was an animal and that all thought was brought about from the result of chemical reactions in the brain. Today, Wundt is still highly revered in the field of psychiatry.

It was one of Wundt's students, Emil Kraepelin, who became known as the "Father of Psychiatry."

He believed that mental symptoms were hereditary and he supported the sterilization of certain "mentally ill", so defective genes could not be passed on. Ernst Rudin was a student of Kraepelin, and he was a rabid eugenicist. His racial theories were sold to Hitler. The resulting "Master Plan" for a pure Aryan race was created. Hitler was often correctly described as the "most evil man in Nazi Germany."

The Chinese Liver vs. the Psychiatric Brain

PROBLEM: Ragged emotions

1993 BC - China , Chinese doctors conclude:
- The liver is the center of body detoxification
- The liver modifies emotions
- The brain is a nerve center
- The spirit is not housed in the body

Result - Fix the liver and emotions will balance

1854 - Leipzig Germany, Psychiatry concludes:

- Man has no sprit
- Man is an animal
- The brain is a nerve center
- Slicing and medicating the brain disconnects emotional response

Result - Fix emotions by dissection and drugs

Because the Chinese saw the problem as a simple organic problem of waste management, it was straightforward to solve with liver support. Both groups saw the same thing. Psychiatry even had the benefit of the earlier Chinese work. They, in essence, ignored it.

4000 years ago the Chinese saw a chemical overload of the LIVER with a resulting symptom of heightened emotions. They discovered it was easy to "cool" the emotions by addressing the liver.

2120 years later Psychiatry saw a chemical overload of the BRAIN. Read on to find out what the psychs did besides help to start world wars.

In 1897, German legislator Julius Lenzmann attacked the psychiatric community in a speech on January of that year. In part, he said, "Most, if not all of the doctors of the insane are extremely nervous individuals. I have knowledge of the trials where all of the participants were of the opinion that the only insane one was the doctor." Lenzmann saw the writing on the wall but was ignored.

Thanks to that blind eye and all the ones before his, unspeakable atrocities would follow. Soon to come were brain experiments, including medications (or poisons) such as calomel (a colorless, tasteless compound, $Hg2Cl2$), which was originally used as a purgative and insecticide. Also used were leather gags, hand mitts, straightjackets, restraining chairs, solitary confinement; electro shock, insulin shock; frontal lobotomy and ice pick surgery.

You have been introduced to the players from the beginning. The players from Germany and France are all on the play list, but what was happening in America? We now jump across the pond and into North America. Meet John Fulton of Yale, Egas Moniz of Portugal and Walter

Freeman, an American psychiatrist. They all met in 1935 while attending a neurological conference in London. Imagine the stories they must have had to share!

Fulton completely removed the two frontal lobes from a pair of chimpanzees, a "Lobectomy." The procedure had radically altered their chimpanzees' behavior. Fulton could no longer generate experimental forms of neurosis in the animals. They were seemingly proofed against agitation.

The maniacal symposium droned on and on. Finally the discussion about the significance of the frontal lobe removal arrived. The assembled company hedged gently around the delicate issue that Fulton's chimpanzees raised. Eventually, Egas Moniz asked the question that Freeman had wanted to ask. "If frontal lobe removal prevents the development of experimental neurosis in animals, and eliminates undesirable behavior, would it be possible to relieve anxiety states in man by surgical means?"

A year later, Moniz attempted this butchery on a female patient and eventually several more. By 1945, Freeman developed the Ice Pick or Transorbital Leukotomy, a slash across both frontal brain lobes using an ice pick. The pick is shoved up through the top of the left and right eye sockets. The surgeon then uses a sweeping motion to destroy the two frontal lobes. The Transorbital Leukotomy replaced or pushed aside the Lobotomy.

Psychosurgery was on its way. By 1955, Psychosurgery was common, as were the drugs to combat mental disorders such as Thorazine, the precursor to psych drugs including Prozac, Zanax, Zoloft, Paxil and Haldol.

Eventually, brain operations were banned. But, amazingly, shock treatment never fully was and it is still practiced today. The new brain surgery is completed with the Gamma Knife / Radiosurgery (emotion altering brain surgery done with radiation).

Complaints against psychiatry are not new. In 1882, reports on psychiatric treatment methods, which were sadistic, had prominent German individuals such as the parliament, journalists and scientists, protesting. One statesman said, "One of the most pronounced problems with psychiatry had been its inability to recognize what the problem actually is with the mentally ill."

However, psychiatry did not disappear. I hope you are outraged reading this. You may be able to prevent psychiatry's next victim if you speak up. Psychiatry in the United States has the backing of the government and is expanding the same way it did in Germany. There was a time when the psychs were on the run. Since the mid 1990's, they have been gaining strength. We must fight, and fight hard. Drugs do not belong in schools. Columbine and Virginia Tech did not have to happen. Psychiatry remains one of the most evil tortures known to man.

You thought electro shock and insulin shock have been banned?

Roger Bezanis

In 1993, Dr. Steven Rasmussen became the first U.S. physician to treat OCD with a surgical tool known as the gamma knife, which focuses 210 gamma-ray beams into a single point. A tiny hole is burned in the brain creating irreversible damage. The brain is still ripped apart with less mess. Patients are left violently and grotesquely damaged. Yet they *are* meek, manageable, quiet and docile. Patients may be docile and quiet, however they are still angry and suicide is very common.

I have successfully aided individuals diagnosed with OCD to become normal by just repairing their liver. Anyone can do this. It is not just I; we can all make a difference when we decide that we can.

Again slicing up the brain to improve emotions is akin to cutting open the TV to look for the actors. Now wouldn't it be safer to just clean up the diet and then the liver? The answer is yes and, over the last 16 years, I have helped thousands of people get off their psych drugs, thousands more to not get started on them, and thousands more to feel good every day without drugs or dangerous surgeries. Toxins and emotions are a liver problem.

Every day the AMA (American Medical Association) working in concert with the APA (American Psychiatric Association) invents new names / diseases for behavior that is either normal or fixable with nutrition, herbs and vitamins.

Sweaty palms are now a disease called Palmer Hyper Hydrosis. Post Partum Depression didn't exist 20 years ago. RLS (restless leg syndrome) wiggled on to the radar five years ago. All of these reactions are now diseases. Not to mention ADD, ADHD and more. Imagine crowded AMA / APA conference rooms full of executives "brainstorming" the newest malady to **sell** to the public.

Thanks to our dedicated and hardworking AMA / APA we have a never-ending reason to drug ourselves. These labels with peer and employer pressure force people to seek out Psychiatry, which means they will be buying drugs and stimulating the economy. They will also be dying a little more every day.

Remember the absolute roots of psychiatry can be found earlier in this book, in the sections on Phrenology and Physiognomy.

When you treat your body like it is whole, complete and perfect, it heals. If you believe that bad moods are calls for Prozac or a Prozac deficiency you have been brainwashed. Treat the proper organ the correct way and begin to love life again. A headache is not an aspirin or pain killer deficiency. Remove the offending poisons and the body always heals.

You can choose to be healthy. So can your friends and family. Anyone who is on the fence about psychiatry or psychiatric drugs needs to read this chapter; you may save their life.

11 The Liver and Your Skin

Earlier in this book and again in the last few pages, I have indicated that the liver monitors or regulates the skin of the body. What is often forgotten is how delicate this relationship happens to be.

Anything that gets on the skin immediately affects the liver. Taking a shower or a bath is actually a simple technique for washing of the liver. When you rise in the morning, you are washing your liver and jump-starting your immune system. If you have insomnia (a liver issue) and take a shower prior to bed, you usually sleep better. Why? You have drawn toxins out of your liver that might have kept you awake.Hepatitis is a swelling of the liver. It is believed that the dirty inkwells of tattoo artists cause numerous cases of hepatitis B and C every year. This is not true in a direct sense. There is no question that tattoos and hepatitis are linked. There is no question that the inkwells of many tattoo artists have Hepatitis in the mix.

Yet the equation is backward. One does not get Hepatitis from inkwells, as it cannot be passed from one person to another. What does happen is that tattoo ink is a strong poison and brings on a swollen liver. Then those who come back again and again for their next tattoo fix leave Hepatitis markers in the inkwells of the artist.

Those with tattoos have a 75% higher chance of contracting hepatitis than those without tattoos. The more tattoos one gets, the higher the probability that Hepatitis will be contracted.

The problem, while obvious, is usually ignored. The ink is a poison and it is directly applied in a very dense fashion to the skin. In essence, you are indirectly attacking your liver with tattoos.

Another very interesting aspect of tattooing and liver function is that the liver fades or eats your tattoos. The liver is constantly eroding the dye of the tattoo. If given enough time the liver will remove tattoos completely.

Remember the last time you accidentally smeared permanent marker on your hand? The color faded even without washing. The color was not rubbing off or "wearing off"; it was being absorbed into your body.

Most people believe that washing was what removed the stain from their fingers after an episode of "oops, I got that all over my hand." Washing did help. But a huge part of what happened was your skin absorbed the foreign matter and (hopefully) sent it to your liver for processing. As for tattoo ink, this is the simplicity of why they fade. Again, with the right formula or herbs and diet (or some combination of the same) tattoos can and will eventually become a faded memory.

Migraines

Migraine headaches like all headaches are a product of liver overwhelm. The odd element of the migraine headache is that it does not act a run of the mill headache. Normal headaches are not affected by usual liver supplements or foods. Why don't Migraines react like other headaches and easily resolve?

General run of the mill headaches respond to good liver formulas, water, food, vitamins, rest and various combinations of the above. The answers as to what makes Migraines so different come from their traits.

Traits of a Migrane

Sensitivity to light (liver issue)

Sensitivity to sound (kidney issue)

Throbbing pain in the head (liver issue)

Head pain may be localized or involve the entire skull (liver issue)

Can be accompanied by nausea (liver issue)

Odors can make them worse (liver issue)

Blurry vision is common (liver issue)

Foods can make them worse (liver issue)

May last for several hours

Equilibrium problems can occur (kidney issue)

Another interesting and telling fact about migraine headaches is that they will affect women at a rate of four (4) to one (1) over men.

The above pieces of data are all very telling and start to paint a picture of what is at the heart of debilitating problem.

How can migraine headaches affect more woman than men? What could be pushing these statistics?

There are factors that affect many women but not men as the list below will illustrate. Women due to advertising, culture and thousands of years of conditioning have become a test plate for the latest musings of the "woman recreationist mind." If men were required to adapt to the habits and requirements that we impose on women, there would be revolt of a global proportion.

The following list delineates what separates men from women. Keep in mind that much of this list is self-imposed.

In the 21st century women participate in the following:

Makeup

Earrings

Nose rings (95% more women have this than men)

Tongue rings (97% more women have this over men)

Acrylic Nails

Nail polish

Nail cleaning and preparation chemicals like acetone

Birth control pills

Contraceptive jells

IUD's

Hair colorings / dyes

Perfume

Tampons

Panty Liners

Perm solutions

Implants

Face lifts

Botox

Cleaning solvents (some women clean with these far more than men)

High heels

Moisturizers for the face

Cleansers for the face

Moisturizers for the body

Cleansers for the body

Douches

Fertility drugs

Hysterectomies

Tubal ligation

Nylons

Bras

Eating disorders (reported only) affect women by upwards of a 7 to 1 clip over men

More

During the bygone days, there was a time when Lysol (popular bathroom and house cleaning solution) was used as a douche. As you might have guessed, some women died from this practice.

Considering the list above, every item on this catalog has the potential to be toxic to the human body. Many of them are <u>very</u> toxic to the body.

The items and habits above can block the system interfering with liver and kidney function. They all have the potential to cause system wide irritation. When you study human function as I have, this conclusion is apparent.

Tremendous liver and kidney-overwhelm causes migraines. The solution is reduce as many of these irritants as possible and then support liver and kidney function via diet and supplements.

Otherwise woman's' wellbeing will be affected on a daily basis and wreak further migraine issues.

Migraine culprits or facilitators are in the above list without fail. The sooner we can address these problems and start eliminating them, the sooner we will be able to not only address migraines in women but better health for women up and down the line. A mystery remains as such until the light of observation is shown directly on it. Then the pieces fall together as they do above. Assay yourself against this list and see if, at the moments of your worst pain there was something that "set it off." Now imagine that all of these factors or a good portion of them are attacking the immune system of our challenged young woman

Therefore, the recipe for handling migraines would be to return function to the liver and kidneys with various herbal formulas, herbs and foods while eliminating as much of the above list as possible.

The foods that activate the liver and kidneys can be found earlier in this book. Please look them up and employ as many as possible.

12 Showering and the Liver

You know that the liver regulates the skin. One of the easiest ways to affect change in the liver is to take a hot shower! Why? Because the skin is part of our excretory system thus taking a shower opens up these channels and aids the liver.

This is also why taking a hot shower to start the day is so vital. Simply, this activity jump-starts the immune system by activating your liver and kidneys. The kidneys are activated with your shower water as well via water absorption.

The results on sleep can be seen the first night.

Taking a hot shower before bed insures better sleep as insomnia is just due to an overworked liver. The same process that activated the liver in the morning helps to calm down the system at night.

Dry skin brushing is another way to insure better liver function.

The practice of dry skin brushing is very old and dates back thousands of years. But when employed in a daily routine is very beneficial. The ability of the skin to excrete toxins is of paramount importance for good health.

It is a fact that skin brushing is one of the optimal ways of TURNING ON the immune, endocrine system and all the glands of the body very quickly. In addition, at the same time, it triggers an increased physical and mental well being as the liver that regulates the skin is now very active.

The Benefits of Dry Skin Brushing

Dry skin brushing helps the body to shed dead skin cells, which helps to improve skin texture and cell renewal.

Skin Brushing encourages the body's discharge of metabolic wastes, which greatly aids the lymphatic drainage of the entire body. When the body rids itself of toxins, it is able to run more efficiently in all areas.

Brushing also helps to tighten the skin because it increases the flow of blood. Increasing the circulation to the skin can also help lessen the appearance of cellulite.

Dry skin brushing stimulates the lymph system to drain toxic matter into the correct channels, thereby purifying the entire system. This enables the lymph to perform its house-cleaning duties by keeping the blood and other vital tissues detoxified.

Skin brushing may help with muscle tone, and a more even distribution of fat deposits.

Because of direct liver function improvement, skin brushing aids the nervous system by resetting the connection to the skin via the liver.

(Note: using a good strong brush in the shower is very beneficial in cleansing the liver via the skin)

Waste cannot persist in a body teaming with circulation. Help your body improve circulation by removing its waste with skin brushing. Try it and find out for yourself.

Final note, the skin can be brushed wet (via shower or bath). If it is done in a wet environment, it must be brushed harder using something that is semi-stiff, such as a loofah sponge. Exfoliate can be used but must was completely off. If you have been paying attention, you will agree that the fewer chemicals used for the cleansing of the body the better. Remember, soap is manmade and therefore has little place on the body for any length of time. Soap does have its place as a disinfectant and abrasive scrub, but a little goes a long way.

13 The Liver and Oil

Even before man learned to write, the importance of oil was well understood. Without question, oil has been sought after, hoarded and fought over long before recorded history. Archeologists and scholars agree that in man's vast panorama of existence, he has had many obsessions, from fire to microchips but none more consuming than oil.

Even though much of the early record has been submerged, lost, buried, burned, or forgotten oil has left its indelible stain. Oils of all types have been coveted at one time or another. Olive oil may have been the first vegetable processed where the end result was a valued lubricant.

The Yom Kippur story from the Torah is a celebration of oil and its importance. People will die for oil and have throughout earth's history.

World War II was fought over oil. The Germans and Japanese didn't have it, and needed it to expand. Expansion based on a national thirst for oil was what started and ended the bloodiest war on record. Regardless of what we are being told, we are now in the Middle East for the same reason.

The "black gold" has been used as a food, lubricant and fuel. It has been used for the anointing of kings, protecting warriors, an additive in the manufacturing process and in medicines. How important is oil to religion? The word Messiah literally means "the anointed one." The name Christ comes from the Greek, khristos, "the anointed one," a literal translation of the word mashiach.

Translation: "**Our savior is the one anointed with oil**!" Oil has been given a lofty place in the story of man.

Oil in the body is very mysterious. During youth we do not want it (oily skin). Aging, we cannot get enough of it as our skin has "dried out." The obsession grows as we hydrate, moisturize, slather, soak and paint on masks.

Cosmetic companies indoctrinate us into the belief that the body is too stupid to run itself. The right question would be, is oily skin the cause of blackheads, pimples and skin disorders, or is it something else?

Television, radio, newspapers and the Internet tell us that, to be healthy, we must override our body's natural oils with all manner of creams, salves and washes.

By the age of five we morph into little automatons that suddenly NEED to run right out and purchase the next new and greatest thing! Advertisers understand this and now target huge parts of their budgets at pre-teens. Begging, pleading and cajoling leads to pestered parent purchases.

Our shopping mantra is:

"TV, radio, internet and newspapers do not lie... Buy!! Buy!! Buy!!

"Ignore the body"

"Science knows best"

"What is new IS better"

"Own it first"

Our oil obsession, like the shopping mantra, is deeply rooted in our psyche.
Do humans really need **TO ADD** oil to their diet? The answer is **NO**. Read on.

Anatomy 101: The liver is a chambered organ that filters much like the air filter found on your car. Everything you ingest quickly arrives at the liver for processing. Without processing, your body would be swimming in poisons. Remember the liver is the lynch pin of your immune system.

Hepatologists have long studied the oil and liver function quandary and unflinchingly acknowledge that the risk for damaging the liver is extreme when oil is ingested. Understand that all oils coat your liver, leaving it inoperable for hours immediately after ingestion. Warnings about the dangers of oils on liver function are not new, just ignored.

The "inhale and exhale" of the liver must be steady and constant. It must (much like your lungs) take in and then release, take in and then release. Like a sponge, it wipes up and rinses out, until it gets congested or immobilized. Sucking air out of a brick is of little use, as is a tired, overworked, oil-coated liver.

The body has no defense for processed oil. None! It can only try to release it into the bowel. Have you ever noticed an oily stool? Oil is the last element to leave the stomach. It floats in the stomach as it floats on water. Does that mean there is no human use for oil at all? Under strict supervision, while utilizing a detoxifying sauna program, exercise, and proper vitamins, oil creates untold benefits. This type of program is the finest approach to detox that has ever been found and is now offered around the world. Under these conditions oil has a purpose and aids the tissues to release waste. Unquestionably, using this approach with supervision creates amazing results.

But the random taking of oil supplements can be very irritating and potentially damaging if done willy-nilly. Remember, the liver is the hub of your immune system and cannot go offline or be slowed.

Today, many women take Evening Primrose (EP) oil to help with menopausal symptoms.

It is commonly used to relieve hot flashes, neck pain, shoulder pain, sleeplessness, poor concentration, low energy and bad moods. In an oil preparation it is useless. Those who take EP routinely notice that moods and other symptoms actually get worse with its use.

Why? Because processed oil is the carrier or delivery system for EP.

EP in a dry form is very beneficial to the body. After sixteen years of investigation and years of personal firsthand experience, this fact has been borne over and over again.

When the body does need some oil, how should it get it? The body distills all the usable oil it needs from our fresh fruit and vegetables. Have you heard of orange oil or avocado oil? Oil is so prevalent on earth that it is a component in all-organic life.

Yet, once we process the oil out of its original whole source, it becomes useless to the body.

Roger Bezanis

Here is the rule to follow:

- *Never, ever, use oil supplements unless under supervision as part of a detox program.*
- *Derive your oil intake from whole food alone and then it is 100% bio-available to the body.*

The following is a list of problems that can occur with the use of processed oil:
(This includes cold processed olive oil):

Looking or feeling bloated
Gassy digestion
Gallstones
Hepatitis- like symptoms
Itchy eyes
Burning eyes
Watery eyes
Itchy Skin
Tingling skin
Poor concentration
Poor moods (anger, depression, etc.)
Hot flashes
Right side neck pain or stiffness
Right pectoral muscle pain or stiffness
Right deltoid muscle pain or stiffness
(round part of the shoulder)

Right rotator cuff pain or stiffness (inside of the round part of shoulder)
Right scapula pain or stiffness (large flat bone behind your shoulder)
Right elbow pain
Low energy between 9 PM (night) and 3 PM (afternoon)
Fuzzy vision
Headaches
Congestion (nose, sinuses or chest)
Fidgety
Restless
Hot tempered
Confusion
Sleeplessness

Again, if your body does not derive its oil under its own power, through its own processes, the body cannot use it.

Avoid these foods:

Popcorn
Butter
Margarine
All nuts processed and raw
All seeds processed and raw
Mayonnaise
All oils (in bottles)
Fish oils (in capsules)

Oil supplements (in any form)
Vitamin E-oil supplements (except dry vitamin E)
Salad dressings (pour off the excess oil and you should be fine)
Sardines
Cheese

If the worst thing you eat is a little salad dressing, so be it. Remember, if you eat a salad dressing that separates in the bottle, pour off the excess oil, as it adds nothing to taste and is only filler.

You can regulate your health with the information found in this book. It is up to you to use it.

14 Behind the Medicine Cabinet

Transgressions and crimes from WW I have been buried for almost 100 years. Surprisingly, details from this long dead conflict are still influencing our lives today. One very well known company was a huge player in both world wars. It is still a huge player today. This mystery company is not one you would associate with death, yet it has had a direct hand in the deaths of millions.

- The company that invented Aspirin in 1899

- Produced Mustard gas for Germany in WW I

- Developed Heroin in 1898, used as a pain killer

- Developed Tabum, a nerve gas used in WWI

- Developed Chlorine gas, used in WWI

The company was Bayer and Co.

With war looming in the future, a decision was made in 1925 to consolidate Germany's industrial might "under-one" banner. Brokered by Hermann Schmitz (who would 20 years later be convicted of war crimes at Nuremberg) a mega merger was about to take place. Hermann married the following companies: Bayer (the Aspirin folks), Badische, Anilin, Hoechst, Agfa, BASF, Hoechst, Griesheim-Elektron and Weiler-Ter-Meer. These chemical / drug companies would form one of the largest drug dye and chemical conglomerates known to man. The new company was christened I.G. Farben (full name, Interessen Gemeinschaft Farenindustrie Aktiengesellschaft).

I.G. Farben's purpose was to make war possible for the Nazis and Hitler. In 1948 Schmitz was convicted of war crimes and sentenced to two (2) years in prison. It has been suggested that if Standard Oil, Ford Motor Company and Dow Chemical had not sold to I.G. Farben and the Nazis, WWII could never have been launched. Since Hermann Schmitz was a convenient fall guy, Ford Motor, Standard Oil and Dow Chemical were never brought up on charges.

I.G. Farbetn supplied the following to the Nazis:

- 100% of the Zyklon B gas chamber gas
- 95% of all poison gases used in gas chambers
- 84% of the explosives used by all German armed forces
- 100% of the synthetic rubber used by the German armed forces
- 70% of the gunpowder used by all German armed forces
- 46% of the German aviation fuel

- 90% of the plastics used by the German armed forces
- 95% of the nickel used to make weapons
- 100% of the lubricating oil used by the German armed forces

Farben also operated Auschwitz, labor camps, used slave labor and conducted human experiments with Joseph Mengele. The list of atrocities committed by Farben is long and gruesome. The 1945 Potsdam Agreement called for the breakup of I.G Farben. It wasn't until 1951 that it changed its name and resumed business as Farbenfabriken Bay AG. In 1972 the name was again shortened to Bay AG. The post World War II Bayer is built on the ashes of millions of Jews, gypsies, dissidents, the racially impure and Russians. Bayer's roots are forever firmly planted in the manufacture of death from two world wars.

There have been more recent transgressions in the drug world but to list them here just becomes redundant. Do more investigative reading by looking up the history of Prozac and Ritalin on the Internet. These stories are tragic. Please note that the practice of Allopathy, the use of drugs to treat illness, supports drug companies who make and sell drugs, which in turn directly supports the FDA.

How does the FDA operate? They take payments from drug companies who want to introduce new drugs to market. The payment for the FDA to rubberstamp a new drug is 800 million dollars. The check should hopefully include any applicable lab testing guaranteeing the drug's safety. Often this step is brushed aside: witness the unexplained "new drug deaths" every year. The cost to bring drugs to market in the United States is astronomically high. This is where the patent process comes into play. Patents ensure seven (7) years of product copy protection before generics can be introduced. Example, first there was Viagra, now there is Levitra, Cialis etc. All exist for erectile dysfunction (ED). The first drug to market for ED was Viagra.

After the FDA signs off on your product, you are free to advertise and sell your new drug for the full 7 years without competition. A new drug, if marginally successful will pull in over 1 billion dollars a year.

Hippocrates said "Let food be your medicine and medicine be your food."

Hippocrates did not say, "Swallow dangerous chemical poisons and hope for the best."

WHAT IS IN YOUR MEDICINE CABINET?

15 The Sanctity of Women

It is a genetic predisposition for both sexes to seek approval. The difference being that some men have capitalized on this and make it their business to expect and exploit the trait.
- Author Roger Bezanis

One gender of human is not better than then other. Yet one gender has inflicted its will on the other since the beginning of time. If mankind is to survive that must change.

Earth is populated with two genders of humans, men and women. Much of human history is dominated by the male sex as they scribed the dusty pages of our historic texts. Warriors seem to make for interesting reading and many people just adore ingesting tales of blood and guts. Examine today's list of action heroes / action stars and our taste for violence becomes devastatingly obvious.

It is not that women have not made history, it is that they have been ignored by the writers of history. Namely their husbands and jealous boyfriends.

Yet without question the future of Earth is in and has always been in the hands of women. Women rear the young and mold every mind and body that walks the planet. This sentient fact holds true not only in the world of Homo sapiens but the animal world as well. It is the role of the lioness to rear the cubs. Monkeys, apes and bears follow the same pattern along with elephants and other species.

Yes the male and female roles are defined but neither role is any less important than the other.

Life on Earth has not been equal among the two sexes. But due to religious upbringing, historic patterns, genetic coding or some other heretofore not mentioned answer, women have remained in support of men.

Due to that role or affliction, women have often been treated as possessions not people. In some parts of the world women still hold a very low standing. Prior to 1850, women were seen as assets, not citizens. Until 1920 women did not have the right to vote in the United States. The historic record is littered with the egregious treatment of women. It is sad that it is necessary to have to state that, "Women are not second class citizens."

When you consider the importance of women to the advancement and rearing of mankind, we must examine just who women are.

Some women have demanded world awareness and humankind has been better for it. Witness the emergence of Hillary Clinton and Sarah Palin. Some will point out that Palin was initially the focus of jokes and ridicule but she has survived. Memo to those keeping score: it takes a big person with a lot of horse power to create that kind of stir and such stinging ridicule. Let's face it, when the world news, Saturday Night Live and standup comics are deriding you on world stage, you must be a threat to someone.

If we glance at the history of Earth, women have consistently changed the planet and been its leaders.

Roger Bezanis

Consider these women:

Mother Theresa	Helen of Troy	Cleopatra
Margaret Thatcher	Joan of Arc	Amelia Earhart
Harriet Tubman	Katherine Hepburn	Indira Gandhi
Eleanor Roosevelt	Sally Ride	Cora Aquino
Golda Meir	Oprah Winfrey	Eva Peron
Princess Diana	Queen Nefertiti	Annie Oakley
Billie Jean King	Danielle Steele	Dororthy Parker
Meryl Streep	J.K. Rowling	Queen Hatshepsut
Queen Elizabeth	Mary Queen of Scots	(recognized as an Egyptian King)

The women listed above are / were all exceptional leaders. They either lead or set the standards the world has attempted or is attempting to emulate.

There is an obvious fact that we as a society routinely neglect to place enough importance on. Women carry the responsibility of the future of mankind on their shoulders. The womb must be regarded as the most sacred place on the planet. Every soul births from this holy place. If it is not faultless, clean and powerful, new generations of humankind will get weaker and weaker.

Ask yourself how many movements you are aware of that champion the perfection of the woman and her womb. It is so obvious that this is important it is almost silly. But just like gravity, if we ignore it, we become a statistic caused by ignorance and neglect.

One of my favorite authors, Shonda Parker, has written several books, all pushing for a pre-pregnancy detoxification. Later in this chapter you will discover that I am recommending a regiment far deeper.

Let's further reflect on the importance of women.

In marriages that have fallen apart, it is often women who are revered most by the prodigy. This is not a slander of men at all. It is just a fact derived from empirical evidence. It is also of note that Mothers' Day celebrations are almost as old as recorded history.

The history of Mothers' Day is centuries old and dates back to the ancient Greeks, who held festivities to honor Rhea, the mother of the gods. Early Christians also celebrated the Mother's festival on the fourth Sunday of Lent to honor Mary, the mother of Christ.

Interestingly, Mothers' Day was made inclusive of all mothers thanks to the work of a religious order. They named it Mothering Sunday. The English colonists settling in America discontinued the tradition of Mothering Sunday.

In 1872 Julia Ward Howe organized a day for mothers dedicated to peace. It marks the beginnings of our present day Mothers' Day.

In 1907, Anna M. Jarvis (1864-1948), a Philadelphia schoolteacher, began a movement to set up a national Mothers' Day in honor of her mother, Ann Maria Reeves Jarvis. The first Mother's Day observance was a church service honoring Anna's mother. Anna handed out her mother's favorite flowers, the white incarnations, on the occasion as they represent sweetness, purity, and patience.

She then solicited the help of hundreds of legislators and prominent businessmen to create a special day to honor all mothers. Anna's hard work finally paid off in 1914, when President Woodrow Wilson proclaimed the second Sunday in May as a national holiday in honor of mothers.

How important are mothers? In the United States Mothers' Day preceded Fathers' Day (1956) by 42 years. On the timeline of human history, Mothers' Day occurred circa 2000 years before Fathers' Day.

What an amazing dichotomy. The history of man demonstrates a true appreciation of mothers and women, yet the United States has been slow to catch on. The U.S. is the most celebrated country on Earth today, yet many Americans still see women as "eye candy." Revisit Sara Palin, like her or not. There are many people who only remember her for her fashionable eyewear. On several fronts we revere women but unless a woman demands respect with billions behind her such as Oprah Winfrey, we remain mum regarding their true contributions.

My words are not meant to foster uprisings in the home or world conflict. They are all a preamble to the concepts, truths and ideas that now follow.

Why the title of this chapter is called the SANCTITY of women will soon become obvious. Because what we do to women, we consequently pass down to future generations of mankind. If we poison women, we doom mankind.

There is nothing more pious than the care and nurturing of women.

Does this mean that women should be carted around in a wheel barrow or carried by strong men on a golden pillow? No. Of course if anyone, man or woman, can ethically garner that kind of treatment, I want the formula.

We all deserve to be healthy yet it all starts in the womb. Obesity and addictions are now known to start in the womb based on what a woman eats or "takes" during pregnancy.

This fact has been sighted in the book "The Zone" by Dr. Barry Sears and is often reported by the BBC. On Friday, 30 March, 2001, in the United Kingdom, the BBC reported "Obesity starts in the womb" and quoted Professor George Davey Smith, of the University of Bristol. He told a meeting of leading obesity experts that obesity and the nutrition of the mother during pregnancy play a significant part in child development.

He later stated "If the mother is poorly nourished when pregnant their children could be obese in later life."

Womb created health conditions are a vast subject and need to be copiously studied with bank rolls of billions before anyone will really take notice. This chapter is devoted to some of this amazing data.

Mother to womb passed health conditions are not an obvious fact and because of that they are often overlooked. During pregnancy the baby and the mother share the same food supply. What the mother eats, the baby ultimately ingests.

Mothers that smoke during pregnancy are smoking for the baby as nicotine and all of its carcinogens circulate throughout the system via the blood supply. The entire chemical history of the mother is passed on to her unborn child. If she has toxins lodged in her fat, she passes them to the baby as these chemicals decompose and enters into the blood supply.

Sugar intoxication and addiction starts in the womb with almost every birth. What mother eats is passed to the growing life she is carrying. Sugar not only races your heart but the heart of your unborn child. If it is in your body it is in your blood stream and eventually in your breast milk.

Chemical Calories

A diet of "Big Macs and fries" ensure that the infant is getting a shocking amount of sugar, salt, sodium, colorings, dyes, yeasts, preservatives and other chemicals.

The above list does not include chemicals fed to cattle via their food supply to increase the beef yield per animal. Agricultural chemicals are sowed into the plants that are fed to cattle, slowing metabolism. The result is a bigger slower animal with reduced organ function. When humans at any age ingest these chemicals via beef or non-organic produce, in essence we too are being "fattened for slaughter."

We have knowledge of the dangers of sugar, salt and sodium, but chemical calories may be even more pervasive and body altering. You do not have to be a scientist to see the differences in adolescents and teenagers today. They are often taller, fatter, balder and bustier than 30 years ago, all attributable to chemical additives in the food supply.

Author Dr. Paula Baillie-Hamilton writes volumes on the subject of "chemical calories". She estimates that each of us carries between 300-500 industrial chemicals in our bodies at any one time.

Dr. Baillie-Hamilton also explains that livestock fattening chemicals damage our natural appetite "switch", which tells us when to stop eating. This in turn overwhelms the body causing added fat storage. The solution to healing most health conditions can be found in "chemical calories" and other chemicals which "lurk in every bite of food we eat, every sip of liquid we drink and in the very air we breathe".

From Ruth SoRelle, M.P.H., September 2008 "Childhood obesity may start in the womb."

High-fat diet

Researchers from BCM, the University of Utah Health Sciences in Salt Lake and the Oregon National Primate Research Center teamed up to study what happens to offspring of non-human primate mothers fed a diet consisting of 35% fat. This group was compared with a group that ate a diet that consisted of only 13% fat.

The offspring from the 35% fat diet had non-alcoholic fatty liver disease (comparable to that found in obese human youngsters). In fact, their triglycerides (one form of fat measured in blood) were three times higher than those of the normal offspring.

In some cases, the mothers on the high-fat diet did not become obese themselves but their offspring suffered the same ill effects as those of moms who did become obese.

We are a society of addicts. The fact that this sounds completely impossible does not dilute the reality that it is 100% true. We were weaned on sugar via cereals and bread that converts to 100% white death sugar. Baby formulas are marbled in sugar.

We as a society must make it our duty to ensure that women are strong and healthy. Repairing the race of man has been the goal of many. If mankind is to remain on earth, we must make it our business to purify and heal women or mankind will become a dusty footnote in Earth's history.

From folk song to rambunctious rap music, it is commonly communicated that we live in "a man's world." On the most part women and men are hotwired to please each other. It is a genetic predisposition for both sexes to seek approval. The difference being that some men have capitalized on this and make it their business to expect and exploit the trait.

Consider all that we do in an effort to beautify women. From hot rollers to implants and tattoos, a woman is a canvas to be decorated. Throughout the world it is common to inflict trauma on women of incredible magnitude all in an effort to please their mate.

This longing or desire to be desired is so ingrained that women compete amongst themselves to see who can be more beautiful or alluring.

Due to jealousy and unexpressed rivalry some women even find it hard to be true friends with other women.

The following list comprises much of what women endure to be women.

Make up	Make up remover
Hair colorings	Eyeliner
Eyebrow liner	Lip liner
Lipstick	Mascara
Permanent lip liner, eyeliner, eyebrows & lipstick	Ear piercings (linked to heart disease)
Crash Diets	Nail polish
Acrylic nails	Birth control pills
Contraceptive gels	Contraceptive injections (still in its infancy stage)
Morning after pill	Eating Disorders (a female dominated problem)
IUDs	Tubal ligations
Infertility drugs	Perm solutions
Tampons	Douches
Implants	Face lifts
Men...(Oops)	Botox
High hees (Very bad, just ask a Chiropractor)	Hysterectomies (660,000 performed in 2007)
Moisturizers	Nylons
Panty liners with scents	Bras
Nose, lip, nipple, tongue, belly button, vaginal and eyebrow piercings	Mifepristone (or Mifeprex similar to the morning after pill)
Cleaning Solutions (many women clean more than men)	Eating Disorders (a female dominated problem) More:

The Mutiliation of Women

We have sold women the idea that they must be of a certain shape to be accepted as beautiful. That is patently false as all women are beautiful. In the United States our parades are based on the beauty queen, cheer leader and pin up girl. Since the beginning of time every society has an agreed upon standard as to what the majority considers beautiful.

But the standards are different everywhere from country to country and often region to region in the same country.

It does not matter what the beautification items are. Some societies demand drooping earlobes, the appearance of an extended neck, a tiny waist, tattoos, large breasts, no breasts, painted nails, "plate like" lips or a large frame for birthing. The message is the same. Ascend to this level of beauty or be thought of as a less than a perfect woman.

All of these standards are agreed upon. They are accepted as they are weaved into the fabric of our trained likes and dislikes. Wanting "plate like" lips is no different than wanting the Cubs to win the World Series. The desire is a result of upbringing, tradition, experience and social interaction.

We grasp these values even before we discover our ability to speak. These lessons are communicated visually. We watch who in our society gains respect and who gets attention. This is a survival mechanism. The newborn always allies him or herself with the one in power. To do otherwise is to risk getting less than stellar treatment from those who offer nourishment, comfort and safety.

What the mother thinks and does it transferred to the baby, toddler and young adult. This was passed down from her mother and from her mother before her. All of this is programming done on a day to day, minute by minute basis.

Through education we must change these long ago programmed reactions to societal pressures. By doing so we return the power of choice and the ability to think and perceive to the individual. It all starts with mothers. Of course fathers have an impactful role in the rearing and conditioning of offspring, but it is our mothers who carry the lion share of the load.

To not be aware of the impact that we have on our offspring is akin to ignoring gravity yet again. It almost becomes a group or mob hypnotic trance as we are stumbling around like functioning automatons.

Again remember these standards are not set in stone. They even morph from one decade to another as tastes changed. Interestingly, we tend to emulate those in the public eye such as Babe Ruth, John Wayne, James Dean, Marilyn Monroe, John F. Kennedy, Twiggy (beanpole skinny in the 60's), John Travolta, Farah Fawcett, Princess Diana, Ronald Regan, Michael Jordan, Dale Earnhardt Jr., Sara Palin, Oprah Winfrey, and now Barak Obama.

In much of the world we have our beauty pageants and runway models. Here in the good old USA we export our little trouble maker, the infamous Barbie Doll.

The bottom line is money. Marketers pay attention to who is in the public eye. They then package and sell us that image. In order for change to take place we must first identify that we are being marketed to and then become bigger than the message.

The only way to survive such an onslaught of "image sales," is to set your own image standards. Reinventing who you are is a personal quest, not one that should be left to the boys on Wall Street in their advertising board meetings.

Successful marketing to our worst demon, "self doubt" has changed the landscape of the cosmetic business and fostered plastic surgery. Now the attitude is, if you cannot hide it under makeup "go under the knife."

Some women are in such abject terror about having gained weight they will not venture outside to be seen. It would be wrong to just blame our parents, boyfriends and husbands for conveying these hurtful life changing messages. Teachers, instructors and even employers can add to this mental mayhem.

Why are these individuals and groups so rabid about pushing their views on the so called weaker sex? Again the answer is marketing and therefore money. These individuals and even you are buried under dynamic pressure telling you to buy or die.

Today and for the foreseeable future, these ads will be aimed at younger and younger audiences. This is pure marketing genius using movies, TV shows and cartoons to sell the latest craze to unsuspecting and little influential buyers. What parent can dodge 100% of the appeals by a little boy or girl who is determined to have the latest gizmo?

The best way to influence minds is to get them while they are young. Certain plastic toys are icons of childhood and alter our perceptions of beauty. Yes I am focusing on Barbie Millicent Roberts (her full name) yet again.

Barbie is forever smiling and never talks back. Barbie is not human but to a little girl she has a voice, personality and is completely perfect. In the mind of every young girl playing with her, Barbie is not only human, Barbie is that girl.

If innocent little Barbie was a real woman she would have measurements of 39DD-18-33. Consequently it should not be surprising that the female sex has the highest incidents of anorexia and bulimia.

What a horrible stress to inflict on anyone. How can a woman live up to the standards of a fictional, plastic, card board boxed figure from Mattel? Notice how fixated the children of the 60's, 70's and 80's are on breasts. The aforementioned 40 year time span marks the height of Barbie's popularity. Today Barbie is still not dead.

Barbie was born in March 1959. Take a trip down memory lane, remember how perfect Barbie was? Remember that she is always smiling? If it is a good day, she is smiling. If you drop her on her head, she is still smiling. She is clearly well adjusted as plastic goes.

It is conceivable that part of the rise of psychiatry between 1970 and 1990 was directly due to Barbie, as former little girls are still attempting to have "Barbie smiles."

Striving for perfection is one thing. Striving for inhuman plastic perfection is quite another.

Not surprisingly some studies say that women are victims of psychiatry at a clip of 5 to 1 over men. Many women are still trying to gain that Barbie smile and perfect hair.

Am I blaming Barbie alone? No, it is the contamination of all of these factors commingling with our insecurities that make us all potentially dominated objects. Today marketing is so affective that with a little push people can be made to buy or do almost anything.

If we combined 10 years of world cosmetic sales the total would stand between 500-850 billion dollars. Without question women are powerful consumers. This is the impact that marketing slash brainwashing has on womankind. If womankind and therefore mankind are to survive we must be heady to this brainwashing blitz. But it does not end with marketing for marketing sake. Certain groups seek to control women and abuse them.

The Diagnostic & Statistical Manual of Psychiatric Disorders (DSM) does not define what so called normal behavior is; therefore according to them we are all sick! They want every woman to believe that their only salvation lay in a bottle of tablets called Prozac or something equally as dangerous.

How convenient is it that they will not and cannot define what normal behavior is. If no one is normal everyone needs help of some sort. This help is given in the guise of drugs and in extreme, hospitalization and surgery such as shock treatment.

If normal behavior was spelled out, three things would happen:

1) People would be able to self correct (not everyone would be sick)
2) Psychiatric drugs sale would plummet into an ashcan.
3) Funding for psychiatric facilities and shock treatment would disappear.

It is no stretch to say that psychiatrists think that every human is mentally ill in one way or the other. They think that we are all sick and should be at the very least on a drug. This kind of thinking is so prevalent in our society that we do not bat an eye when we hear such news about a star or associate going the shrink route.

Remember that image and self esteem destroying ad campaigns aimed at women are so

Roger Bezanis

successful, women become easy targets for psych drugs and psych treatments. This further pollutes the future of mankind. If a woman is poisoned, her womb is poisoned and her child is born poisoned.

TO SUMMARIZE

- We have conditioned women to be great consumers by convincing them that they are inadequate and small.

- Advertisers attempts to instill insecurities and fear whenever possible. It is very effective.

- We have trained both sexes to always want whatever is HOT / NEW / DIFFERENT, all because advertising says that it is.

- Marketing has brainwashed women (and to some degree men) to believe that they are less than whole. With this end achieved they can then steer our purchases.

- Women are fantastic traders on the cosmetic and beauty market. Yet they are consuming products where the long term effects are not known.

- The onus of safety regarding what we ingest is woefully lacking at the government level and is therefore on the back of the consumer.

- The Federal Trade Commission will never restrict the use of fear and insecurities to sell products. Therefore you have to be aware of what you are being sold and by whom.

- The next time you hear or see an ad for any product you must tell yourself over and over again "I am being marketed to." "They are trying to sell me something."

- Creating your self-image is vital if you are to remain autonomous from the marketing that seeks to control you. You must develop your own style as an individual.

For those of you who know Jessica Simpson and her younger sister, Ashley, Ashley was a maverick and complete individual.

She was quoted in the September 2008 issue of Marie Claire "Everyone is made differently, and that's what makes us beautiful and unique. I want girls to look in the mirror and feel confident."

Sometime after the article came out she got a Rhinoplasty (nose job). Ashley was cute and quirky in her dress and manner. She is now assembly line, cookie cutter cute like so many others. Her individuality is gone.

Again remind yourself that you are being marketed to. The next time you hear or see an ad for any product you must tell yourself over and over again "I am being marketed to."

WHAT IS IN YOUR FOOD? IS IT HARMFUL?

If you do not have a degree in commercial chemistry and are not receiving regular peer reviews of technical data from pharmaceutical companies you are not alone. To be an expert on pharmaceutical poisons and American Medical Association (AMA) recommended surgeries is impossible unless you are in the insane boardrooms that create such flotsam and jetsam.

If we recognize that no one needs surgery unless it is a life saving procedure or drugs unless it is antibiotics, we are heading in the right direction. Unfortunately we are the minority which is why this tome is so vital. We must spread the word to all men and women to make these words known.

Our milk, beef and poultry supply is pumped full of hormones. Long term affects are completely unknown. We are now seeing more bald young men with reduced sex drive at an early age. Viagra sales to the under 30 crowd is remarkably high.

Is anyone testing to prove the connection? Not on your life as that study would threaten a billion dollar industry.

Baldness is even occurring in high school boys. While adolescent breast size is exploding into uncharted territory, young girls are entering puberty earlier and earlier all because of a hormone rich food supply. Again the long term affects are unknown.

We are striving to be lean yet many of us are trying to live on McDonald's. These two incongruities are without parallel and laughable in scope. Asking anyone to be thin while trying to live on Jack in The Box, McDonald's or any fast food is like hoping to find ice in a fire.

Thanks to this backwards logic, one out of three adolescents is obese! Soon that number will be 9 out of 10. How can we let this happen? Remember the answer is brainwashing. We are conditioned to accept whatever we encounter in the mass media with little fuss. Studies have proven that TV is mind-numbing and hypnotic. As a result we tend to accept anything broadcast over the airwaves. The British Sky News published a study done by the Children's Society on 2, February 2009 explaining that excessive TV watching causes mental illness. Quote "The more a child is exposed to the media, the more materialistic she becomes; the worse she relates to her parents and the worse her mental health." On the other hand this could just be another attempt to prepare to sell drugs to a new crowd of MySpace addicted American Idol fans.

Roger Bezanis

Media ensures that image is our focus and on a nearly impossible to obtain golden ring. Our health needs are buried under electronic media implanted circuits demanding that we accept their chaotic toxic spew.

So called "eating disorders" are far more commonplace than anyone would like to believe. The depth of emotions and drive for acceptance accompanying the causes of these aberrations explain the intense turmoil experienced by those who practice their hellishness.

We are surrounded by those immersed in body image torment every day. Women are bombarded with messages that communicate "you are worthless unless you_____." Turn on the TV and count how many ads in an hour are aimed solely at undermining female self esteem.

Thin is not only "IN," it is the only way. How else could Lap Band or stomach stapling (gastric bypass surgery) have gained prominence so quickly? This is why bulimia and its sister anorexia are on a fast quiet rise.

Drug pushers such as Ely Lily and others have received the green light by the FDA to create drugs to solve these issues. It will not be long before the AMA will approve protocols for correcting eating disorders via brain surgery. We are seemingly at the mercy of big business unless we say no!

Drugs are not the answer but discipline, self esteem, understanding, support groups and diet education are. The next time you hear or see an ad for any product you must tell yourself over and over again "I am being marketed to."

Men rarely report Anorexia and Bulimia, but I was both. These two issues seem harmless and that is their charm or attraction. They are life destroying.

I copiously chronicle my journey to safety in the final chapters of this book. Once someone (male of female) knows what I did, they can walk in my footsteps and become whole again.

The last several paragraphs have given you the blueprint being used by drug companies, government agencies and other nefarious organizations to control both men and women. Succeeding on a daily basis they are weakening all of us. The more women are attacked and drugged the weaker mankind becomes.

Even if we ignore the danger women face and only consider the dangers that both sexes share it is still a scary proposition. Regardless of what we are doing as a public for our health sugar, caffeine, sodium, salt, colors, dyes, preservatives etc are breaking down our system every day.

Many argue with the sage statement that "we are what we eat." Without question this statement is 100% true. Putting ice cream in gives us cottage cheese results. Blaming the companies that make garbage food does not work.

If you buy your own groceries, are not hospitalized or on a feeding tube, then you can control what you eat. We are conditioned to think that we should be able to eat junk food! I just had a conversation with a woman who espoused those very words.

She said that if I followed your guidelines laid out in The Hidden Keys to Weight Loss I would of course lose weight and feel great. But if I strayed from your plan I would gain 10 pounds rapidly. I offer "Oh, I see, it would be kind of like putting your hand in a garbage disposal and hitting the on button. You would expect damage right." She agreed and said your plan is a lifetime plan. I told her exactly as being healthy is for a lifetime.

Women's health will remain just an insipid concern unless we group our voices and raze the heavens. We must demand grandiose transformation or the working order of things will eventually kill us all. In this battle idleness equates death.

What kind of a low point in society have we reached when we readily accept side effects such as infertility, death, blindness, loss of hearing, loss of bladder control, high blood pressure and stroke? The captain of the pharmaceutical ship is insane so we must mutiny or sacrifice more lives.

Regardless of our station in life we can and should jump into a lifeboat and escape to live another day.

How can we be so blind and ineffective? For the most part we are doing it to ourselves.

Most of us have fond memories of PB&J sandwiches? Many good parents lovingly smeared peanut butter and jelly on what would rapidly convert to sugar, namely bread. Simple chemistry proves just how silent and biologically chaotic this common digestive delight actually is. Mom fed you and me a cocktail of sugar layered with sugar.

Think about your favorite foods. Many of those foods quickly metabolize into sugar within minutes of ingestion. All breads, pasta, rice, crackers, cereals, cookies, cakes and flour based products morph into sugar quickly in the body.

Advertisers and food manufactures intimately understand our knee jerk responses to sugar in all of its forms and with malice and forethought nefariously use it against us. They know that our will power is whittled by our day to day stresses. They know we seek comfort in our "sugar time bomb" laden foods. These poisons are polluting all of us from mother's womb to the grave.

The purveyors of this gunk belly laugh all the way to the bank knowing that we do not have the will power to really change. We do not have to eat candy bars to be sick. If we just eat breads and crackers we still lose. Sugar is our loud mouth neighbor so ear piercing in his assaults that we no longer take notice of him. Still he screams but we are numb to his impact until years later when we are broken and sick.

A healthy person has no truck with the mechanical insulin pump yet today kidney health is in such sharp decline they are in astonishingly epidemic use. Is this what you want for your life?

If not, we must band together and break our chains of national nutritional bondage. To remain on the road we are on, we are guaranteed to become an eventual obese, feeble, hairless and near sightless society of wheel chair bound invalids.

Only a personal plan of action can aid you in taking the necessary strides to improve your health. If you are to survive in a healthy manner and not fall prey to continued degenerative physical conditions you must police yourself by yourself.

You as a woman have a responsibility to every woman you know to aid her to understand or remind her of the same lessons that you encountering here. This chapter is not intended to make you wrong. It is simply to alert you that women and children are the number one target of every psych drugs maker on the planet.

Your worth is calculated by the dollars you invest in these toxins. The more you spend on these "dead end" answers, the sicker it is possible to get. I know you are aware of this but unless you speak up to everyone not as fortunate as you, we will all suffer. Hand your friends this book or get them a copy. We must stand up and fight while we still can. You may be long past birthing age nonetheless, you are a visible example to all you come in contact with.

Understand this: the answers to health grow in the ground. Eating Gods candy fruit and vegetables, you will eventually repair your condition. This is not some hoopla designed to sell you something. Read my chapters "A Diet for a New Century" and "The Hidden Keys to Weight Loss" I lay out the self healing tenants that will mend you for a lifetime.

God's self healing Florence Nightingale of survival is fresh fruit and vegetables. Make no mistake, there is no comparison to a diet of fresh earth friendly food versus the same produce that is cooked and degenerated. Fresh veggies and fruit can save your life. Cooked / frozen / canned veggies and fruit are nearly devoid of nutrition. With all this in mind, how can you prepare a nutritious meal and have a life too?

The deck is stacked against anyone who attempts to lead a healthy life as their own friends and families attack their positive changes. Those who should be jumping up and down for joy over your changes are actually uncomfortable.

Your changes are making them feel insecure. That is a tragedy. We must earnestly root for each other.

Your weight alterations can make others feel insecure. It is sad to think that even though we root for our friends to escape the single life and find a mate that we are actually jealous. The same is unfortunately true when it comes to body modification. We all talk about transforming our bodies but God forbid anyone actually does it.

Please, please, please be aware of these tendencies and fight against your demons that want to attack. Earnestly support your friends and avoid knee jerk criticism and we will all be better for it.

Now examining the added stresses and issues that are only germane to women; it is easy to see that it is much harder to make changes. Yet they must be made.

I implore, beg and insist that you read and adopt lessons from my chapter "A Diet for a New Century." It is loaded with easy to use healthy recipes and correct ways to look at food. If you took nothing away from this book other than this chapter, "The Hidden Keys to Weight Loss" and its companion "A Diet for a New Century" you would be a new and healthier person.

A of mankind is up against the razors edge of big business that is propagating industrial poisoning. Never has this fact been clearer. Look at the list of products that   are germane just to women. The bull's eye on womankind's back is huge.

Women are at risk for food "like" and "life style" poisoning by more than 40 to 1 over men. Again review the list earlier in this chapter and you will agree. When you study the list that separates women from men it feels like the fissure between the sexes is the size of the Grand Canyon.

With this abundantly clear table we cannot lose sight of the fact that women are far more likely to breakdown due to these stresses. Therefore it is vital to do everything possible to improve your health.

All people have three basic problems: a sluggish colon, fragile kidneys and a weakened liver. The liver and kidneys are the lynch pins of the immune systems and must be kept in pristine order to maintain stress free health.

Whether declining health is caused by diet, pollution, cosmetics, surgery or bad luck the solution is the same; detox, dietary change, less surgery and avoidance of self imposed poisons. To be at your best, it should be of paramount importance to do a full cellular detox at least once a year. There are many herbal formulas for this. If you study the chapter "Holistic Detoxification" I make it very easy to do.

But the same results can be achieved via:

Dietary change
Exercise
Colon Hydrotherapy

Roger Bezanis

Monitored sauna treatments
Building a toxic free home environment and work place

A deep cellular detox is the easiest approach to take considering the busy schedule that so many women face. Without question the positive results from these changes can be staggering.

1) Improved energy
2) Better skin
3) Weight loss
4) Warmer sunnier moods
5) Constipation eliminated
6) Restful sleep
7) Easier / lighter periods
8) Thicker fuller hair
9) Slowed aging
10) Cancers reversed
11) Tumor turnaround
12) Enhanced memory
13) Menopausal symptoms eliminated
14) Diabetes symptoms vanish
15) Herpes outbreak remission
16) Deeper / fuller orgasms
17) Improved sexual function
18) Reactivated libido
19) Powerful self esteem
20) Recovered cognitive function
21) A superior outlook on life
22) Balanced hormone function
23) Youthful fertility
24) Rapid tissue repair

Dietary change is vital but it is the hardest step to take. This is a further reason to do a detox first since once on a cleanse it is much easier to make nutritional changes. To fully regain and maintain one's health at any age, inner body washing (detox) is a major key.

As stated before the future of mankind is growing in a womb near you. Is it a clean healthy womb? Is it full of tobacco, alcohol, plastic residue? Mankind should not be bathing in a near cesspool of waste.

You my female readers, are vital not only to yourself but to this planet.

No one ever wants to feel helpless or out of control. We talk about "planning our future,"

"Controlling our destiny," etc. Now is the time to do it. Mankind does have a choice and can make his future. Unaware of the game that we are immersed in, our future is a roll of the dice.

I implore you to open your eyes wide and pay attention. If you do not know the rules of the game you are playing or worse do not know you are playing a game misfortune will follow you.

Be well,
Roger Bezanis

16 Who Protects You From Who Protects You?

An ode to P.D. Eastman's, "Are You My Mother?"

Imagine that you are strolling in a field admiring the grass. Imagine also that every blade was beyond your expectations of beauty. Each strand is an inescapable sliver of emerald green. You are thoroughly intoxicated with nature down to your core. Every organ of your body is humming "Mother Nature's song".

Of course you are drenched in incredible relaxation. The cool breeze teasing your skin and the sun warming your back make this a wonderful day.

Your rolling field of green goes on for miles. The sound of geese can be heard in the distance as they wing their way home. Your little dog Chip is at your side taking a nap. There is nothing to worry about as the day could not be grander.

Widening your field of vision you notice that you are among sunflowers and the tender exquisiteness of soft soothing dandelions. What could be better than to be one with nature? Soon blue birds take roost in the surrounding trees of green and rich bark. What a stunning portrait of sanctuary. Nature is enveloping your being while serving and protecting your every need.

Actually the above was all a charade to make you think you are safe. You are not in a field at all! You are being watched and targeted by men in pinstriped business suits and smoking cigars. Chomp, chomp, chomp they chew their cigars dissecting your interests and motives! They know the address of your living room, couch, bed or your favorite easy chair where you sit reading these words.

There is no breeze, that's the fan! You are under a microscope of those looking for a way to pry your will and money away from you.

If someone knocks on your door trying to sell you "The next great health miracle," I did not send them.

You might be getting the idea that someone is trying to control you or "do you in." If you are not certain about this, just look around at the newspapers or turn on the TV.

Now that I have your attention, the question is why would anyone want to harm or undermine you? Who is trying to do you in? Who are these nefarious individuals in pinstripe suits who are smoking cigars and have bad greasy hair?

The list is lengthy and includes fast food makers, among others.

Think back. How many times a day are you told to eat something hot, juicy, new, improved, cheesier, spicier, bigger, better, thicker, meatier or more satisfying?

Maybe you have heard that you can be sexier, hairier, skinnier, more muscled, happier, less depressed, more awake, more sleepy, busier, more relaxed or healthier. All of these promises or claims come from a company trying to sell you something.

Thinking that companies who sell wares for your so called "health" have a clue, your best interests at heart or are reputable, is a leap of tremendous faith. Beware of all of those free offers as free offers are NEVER free.

They have no interest in you, just your money.

None of the above is even remotely bad unless the item sold will damage you by its use.

Laws are set up to protect the purveyors of products and services. Once you are damaged by a product or service, you have to PROVE the product or service is dangerous or caused the damage. Witness cigarettes. We know better, they know bette. Yet they continue to be sold.

As unpopular as this subject is, the same holds true for alcohol. Only a few of us do not drink. Yet if alcohol was put before the FDA today for approval, it would be denied and labeled a solvent not fit for human consumption.

This fact is well known and accepted. Yet we still drink. Why? Is it peer pressure, social habit, history or money?

The answer is all of the above. In the United States the alcohol industry is a billion dollar a year industry. Worldwide, it will one day be a trillion dollar a year industry.

The Food and Drug Administration (FDA) is a government agency that requires 800 million dollars per product for it to receive the FDA rubber stamp of approval.

Those 800 million dollars ensures that a 7 year patent is issued to allow the new product freedom from competition so that the paying company can recoup its investment.

The patent does not guarantee that the product is safe, just that it is not overtly deadly. The FDA does not require proof of research only that "research" was done. That is a loop hole big enough to park a yacht in.

Amazingly, the FDA is not republican or democrat, it just IS.

How did we become such helpless pawns in all of this?

1) We trust the FDA to protect us. Protection is a byproduct of what they do. But, they are not out to protect us. They are out to make money. They are out to stay in business and monitor the inflow of ingestibles to the American public.

   They are there strictly to record each product and take a huge fee for their 7 year patent protection. Each country on Earth has its version of the FDA.

2) The FTC or Federal Trade Commission (another government agency) monitors the visual media, print media, radio, internet (they are struggling to control this medium) and voice transmissions.

The FTC is not out for you either. They take fees or money based on violating its laws or edicts. When a product or service has enough complaints, then the FTC acts and levies fines. Remember the fines levied against radio personalities over the last several years?

If the FDA and the FTC is not out to protect you, then surely the insurance companies are there to protect you right?

Not exactly. Insurance companies work with the AMA (American Medical Association), who sells drugs and surgery. If you recall drugs, and surgery, for the most part, are either dangerous or very dangerous.

Just like in P.D. Eastman's little bird in "Are You My Mother?" perhaps you feel a tad confused. Where to turn for safety next? Ah yes, then, it is your doctor who is your protector!

Doctors always protect us! Yes it is the doctor that we need to see!

There is only one problem: our health care system only pays the doctor if you are sick and receiving treatment. His choices are influenced by what drugs the pharmaceutical companies give him to test. The kickback that he receives from those companies for selling their drugs may influence him as well.

About those drugs. How come he never tests them on himself? Do you think he knows something? Do you think that he read the "side effects" panel and thought better of it? Does he ever test them on himself? Your doctor seldom if ever takes the drugs he is given to test. That is what you are for. You are his guinea pig.

His motives are just like yours. He goes to work and intends to make a living. Your doctor is under pressure to pay his bills just like everyone else. He is only paid if you are sick and taking drugs. If all of his patients are healthy, well, you can see the problem there.

Sure your doctor wants you to be healthy. But he or she only makes money when you are sick. In some parts of the world the doctor is only paid if you are healthy.

Do you have a house payment or rent? How about a car payment? Perhaps you have kids that cost a fortune to keep fed and in clothes. Maybe you have extra money and have toys that require cash to maintain. Some people have boats, fishing rods, cars, skis, bowling balls and other expensive pastimes and hobbies.

Your doctors have the same pressures and responsibilities that you do.

Are doctors bad people? No.

Are they consumers with debts just like you? Yes.

Do they need income? Yes.

Do they make money or receive payment from your insurance on every visit? Yes.

Does insurance determine the type of care you will receive based on what they will "cover"? Yes...

Your doctor is really your insurance company. Again, your doctor is really your insurance company. Are they looking out for you? Yes! That must be it! The insurance companies are looking out for you!

Perhaps you are aware of the AIG Insurance scandal. I guess the answer is no. But there is someone looking out for you and that is you.

Your insurance tells your doctor what to do to treat your problems. He in turn does what he is told or insurance does not pay him.

You body mechanic is your doctor. Most of the time, he is restricted in the type of service or treatment that he can give you. This again is all based on what the insurance company will cover.

Your life and your doctor's procedures are dictated by what insurance covers. Based on his needs, he needs you to comply with his recommendation for surgery and drugs or insurance does not pay him. Your doctor uses drugs and surgery because that is what he is trained in and because he wants to get paid.

Insurance is your doctor. The practitioner standing before you in your doctor's office is just the representative from the insurance company. Sure he went to medical school, but under the "insurance system" he is a medically trained insurance representative.

See a doctor and get an insurance-covered drug or insurance-sanctioned surgery.

See a plumber and get plumbing done. See a florist and buy flowers. It is all very simple.

If you are not looking out for you then it is time to start.

You are the only one who can look out for you. If you become broken it is your responsibility to repair yourself. If you are wronged it is entirely your province as you now know what you are up against.

The authorities are undermanned and are not proactive in their service. Police only pick up broken pieces but are bad at preventing tragedy. Laws are designed to enforce the people's wrath on wrong doers and by default offer a little discouragement to those inclined to commit new crimes.

They prosecute poor behavior but not prevent it. Laws are first-rate at bringing to court wrong doers but putting lives back together is beyond their scope. Laws do nothing at all to heal the harmed or maimed. **What exactly does any of this have to do with you?**

You are, to a greater or lesser degree, part of a machine. This machine is active and churning out its products even if you have not noticed that you are part of it.

You are surrounded by numerous entities that are vying to get you to see their point of view. Every day you are bombarded with data and brain washing tactics that work and work well.

All brain washing is achieved by means of delivering the same message again and again under duress. You may reject the idea that you have ever been under duress and brain washed.

Perhaps that is true.

Consider this... Have you ever watched TV when you were dead tired and more susceptible to suggestion? Ever watched TV when you were tipsy, drunk or medicated?

Have you ever watched TV when you were so mad that you could spit? Ever viewed it while in an intense emotional state? You see, you have had ample opportunity to be brain washed. You have even participated in the plan. Take a moment and think about some of the product jingles that bounce around in your consciousness.

Those little songs and sayings are the result of brain washing.

You must recognize that it is up to you to protect yourself. Any other attitude or relationship with yourself makes you a victim. To a greater or lesser degree, if you ignore this you will remain sick and confused.

You can manage your body and your choices. As a result, you can manage your health. Just kick out those who think they are in charge and take your life back.

Be healthy, be awake!!

Take care of yourself. I am here to help if you need me. It is my honor to direct you to being a stronger and more powerful you.

The future of Earth and mankind is in your hands. It is up to you to know who you are. This is your planet. Take it back before it is too late.

Your friend,
Roger Bezanis

17 Genesis of the Liver and Kidneys

Seconds after the moment of our conception, the first systems to go on line are our waste retrieval and removal systems. Call it a full-blown 24 hour a day / emergency filtering and processing system. All life, no matter how big or small is dependent on this exchange. No advanced organism can exist in a filthy environment of its own making. Some organisms live on the waste of other organisms. But waste deriving from the same organism is dangerous to that organism.

This is not limited to life inside the body. These rules extend to every aspect of life on planet earth.

If you have ever found yourself standing in front of a construction site, watching as a building was being built or razed, there was the obligatory dumpster waiting to be filled. Sure this big long metal thing may have been an eye sore, but it had a very important purpose. What is the job of a dumpster? Its sole purpose is to collect waste for removal from the site. Waste of any size impedes production at every level of existence.

Garbage tends to be acidic and erodes the healthy tissue or organic life. There is a poem that many learned in grammar school that has also been performed in song. It was burned into my memory in my teens. It makes an indelible point about garbage, clearly illustrating the dangers of garbage and why our personal waste removal system is so important.

Circa 1970, Shel Silverstein penned this immortal poem:

Sarah Cynthia Sylvia Stout

Oh Sarah Cynthia Sylvia Stout
Would not take the garbage out!
She'd scrub the dishes and scrape the pans,
Cook the yams and spice the hams,
And though her parents would scream and shout,
She simply would not take the garbage out.

And so it piled up to the ceilings:
Coffee grounds, potato peelings,
Brown bananas, rotten peas,
Chunks of sour cottage cheese.

It filled the can it covered the floor,
It cracked the window and blocked the door
With bacon rinds and chicken bones,

Drippy ends of ice cream cones,
Prune pits, peach pits, orange peel,

Goopy clumps of cold oatmeal,
Pizza crust and withered greens,
Soggy beans and tangerines,
Peanut butter, caked and dry,
Curdled milk and crusts of pie,

Moldy melons, dried-up mustard,

Eggshells mixed with lemon custard,
Cold French fries and rancid meat,
Yellow lumps of cream of wheat.

At last the garbage reached so high
That finally it touched the sky.
And all the neighbors moved away,
And none of her friends would come to play.

And finally said Sarah Cynthia Sylvia Stout,
"Ok, I'll take the garbage out!"

But then, of course, it was too late...
The garbage reached across the state,
It slithered from New York to the golden gate.

And there, in the garbage she did hate,
Poor Sarah met an awful fate,
That I cannot right now relate,
Because, the hour is much too late.

But children, remember Sarah Cynthia Sylvia Stout
And always take the garbage out!

As painful as the above poem may have been, you now hopefully have a much better appreciation for dumpsters and those who fill them. Imagine that there were no garbage men. The Black Plague of the middle ages was made worse by the unclean conditions of Europe at the time. It was common to defecate in the streets and wade through ankle deep household waste dumped from the windows above. These conditions contributed to the unbelievable survival rate of the plague-carrying flea-ridden rats. At the same time, as you know, the rats carried the fleas that passed the plague via bites to humans.

How does this relate to our body? You would not want garbage collecting in your house; the human body (and all organisms) is no different.

The first systems to go on line at conception follow the sequence below.

Conception

Blood or energy flow is established.

Simultaneously the liver and kidneys go on line.

Blastula / First – Second – Third Cell Divisions

Zygote

Embryo

Fetus

Birth

As the body develops, two organs (liver / kidneys) process our waste and safely excrete it. When you consider that all food before it can be used is also passed to the liver for processing, you get the full picture. Without these two vital organs on line quickly, the human body (like any organism) would perish. The result is that, either the liver or kidneys regulate every function of our bodies. It is therefore imperative to keep these two filters up / running and happy.

Even today all life in the human body is dependent on the liver and kidneys.

NOW HOLD ONTO YOUR SEAT... ARE YOU HOLDING? HOLD TIGHTER!

Every malady of the body can be traced back to one of these two major organs.

How to think with what the Liver regulates

The liver regulates the skin of every organ of our body (including the skin itself). To your liver there is no difference between the skin of your pancreas or leg. To the body, anything that coats anything is skin and is under the watchful eye of the liver. The liver also regulates ALL hollow organs.

Therefore your lungs, sinuses, nasal cavities, colon, intestines, uterus and mouth are under the domain of the liver. Your liver regulates the skin of your mouth, tongue and gums. This also extends down to the hollow of your ears, throat (or esophagus), into your stomach. Yet your kidneys regulate your equilibrium.

Your kidneys regulate all organs NOT hollow. This list includes all muscles, the brain, tendons, ligaments, cartilage and the heart (to name a few), all regulated by your kidneys.

This means that a cancer (just an evil word for toxic mass) that shows up on the outside (or inside) of any organ (this includes melanoma) is at its source, a liver problem. Treating any problem such as "surface cancer" as a liver problem solves the problem.

On the other hand "deep tissue cancer" is at its source a kidney problem. If you address each problem correctly, your results will be excellent every time.

You might ask, "Should I work on both the kidneys and liver at the same time"? The answer is of course, yes. You can never make a mistake doing liver support and kidney support at the same time.

To capsulate, the liver and kidney dominate the function of the entire body head to toe. As a result, if you made it your job to help turn on your liver and kidneys and then keep them running, you would be very wise.

With the above data really understood, all of your health choices / health repair choices become uncomplicated. All you have to do is understand your symptoms and they will dictate your actions. With a little practice and attention, this does become trouble-free.

How to think with what the Kidneys regulate

The kidneys are solely responsible for all fluids of your body. They regulate blood pressure, the fluid of the eye, blood, saliva, your sweat, your tears and urine. They also regulate all the fluids made by the other organs and their movements in the body, including bile.

The fluid in your system transports waste from its current location to the processing point for its final handling. Your kidneys must process lactic acid (the result of physical exertion or muscle stress) that is found in the muscle. When it is present to any degree the muscle affected will feel tired, sore and stiff. Muscle cannot fully repair until this fluid is removed after you work out.

If you have ever worked out and felt the "burn", what has taken place was a slight tearing of the muscle. Lactic acid produced by muscle activity is present at the point of the torn muscle. The muscle, if this activity is repeated over a period of days or weeks, grows back larger. Thus we have bodybuilding.

Uric Acid can be found all over the body, as it is a byproduct of destroyed cells. Uric acid is like spent uranium from nuclear fission in the body. Anywhere uric acid is lying stagnant; there will be irritation and some swelling. When allopathic medicine notices sore joints, they call it arthritis. It is just unmoving uric acid creating the pain and swelling. Gout is a severe form of the same phenomena.

These symptoms are the telling signs of weak kidneys. The medical profession does not understand this relationship at all. They want you to purchase drugs to suppress your systems. If you also listen to the ads for drugs, they warn of kidney problems associated with their use. Amazing!

Two Rules/Facts

1) The kidneys process Uric Acid. This acid can be found anywhere in the body but it harbors in the joints. Once there it causes irritation and pain. A large percentage of diagnosed arthritis is actually due to kidney overload, as weak kidneys will have trouble sweeping the joints free

of uric acid. The irritation this acid causes is called "arthritis" which can be reversed without trouble.

2) The kidneys process Lactic Acid. This acid can be found in the muscle after physical activity of any kind. Once generated, uric acid causes irritation and pain. Sore aching muscles are actually due to kidney overload and lack of processing power. Weak kidneys will have trouble sweeping the body free of lactic acid and uric acid.

The moment you are labeled with "has arthritis" and you agree with it, finding the true answer becomes an unlikely prospect. Your medical doctor is unaware of this data. Later in this book you will learn how to test the origins of your arthritis-like symptoms.

Remember, unless your doctor is your partner in your health, he is your advisory. Doctors who insist what is right regardless of what is right must be let go. If your doctor insists that you have arthritis and he will not consider other possibilities (such as he is wrong), get a new doctor.

Arthritis is just a symptom of weak kidneys. I have corrected thousands with extreme symptoms; yours should be no more challenging. Turn on your kidneys and turn off your pain.

It was these kinds of observations that led the Chinese to call the kidneys, "The Master Organ", in large part because of the massive job they undertake. The heart has a job this large and the kidneys too regulate it. The heart may pump the blood but the kidneys monitor it and then keep us healthy moment to moment.

Remember, your kidneys need you to understand them to best survive.

18 Understanding Your Body Clock

Many modalities and traditions recognize the function of the human internal body clock. The existence of this invisible apparatus is not argued by anyone except the uniformed. Yet not everyone knows when and what the body is repairing throughout the day. Few people realize that every organ of the body has a repair or maintenance period. Think of it like the days before cable TV when TV signed off at 1:00 am. Suddenly, all programming would cease (except on the local station which might be playing an old black and white). First, you would see a waving American Flag (in the U.S.) and listen to an instrumental of the Star Spangled Banner. Then you would get a second or two of snow. Finally, the "Test Pattern Indian Chief" would then dominate your TV screen until morning, when programming would resume. You would also be serenaded with a continuous tone (like a hearing test tone). For all those in the dark about what a test pattern Indian is, go to Google and type in "test patterns" and look at the images.

The purpose of this time period was to do technical adjustments for the next day's broadcasts.

In the dark days when there were only 13 local channels, life was rough.

Likewise, each day, whether you like it or not, your body will try to repair the damage done to it from the previous days, weeks, months, years and tens of years. During these cycles you may feel tired, worn out, sluggish, irritable, foggy, etc. If you do, your body is trying to repair major damage and the feelings you have are caused by the energy expended in the repair process.

These are all classic liver symptoms, which I will cover later in this book.

You are about to read the body clock table that has been foreshadowed in the previous paragraphs. More than likely you have never been exposed to this before. It involves the times of the day that your internal organs repair themselves. It is a common question to ask what influences these times. Is it the sun, moon, stars, habits?

All biological organisms are subject to the same natural phenomena from one species to another, from the largest to the smallest. There are no exceptions.

For example, Idaho farmers know that if potatoes are planted in a waxing (lighted area increasing) moon they will take root and grow. This has been verified by science when they took potatoes indoors to the labs. They discovered it did not matter if the potatoes were exposed to the moon or kept in a dark room, they would only grow correctly when they were planted during a waxing moon. In the early Chinese texts, it is said that we should rise with the sun and sleep when the sun sets. Another example of this is in the aquatic world where there is a changing of the guard at sunset as nocturnal animals take over the great reefs as day turns to night.

Man has been trying to beat this natural law and reshape his life. He has attempted to manipulate nature by ignoring it. It is a very unsuccessful thing to do, trying to fool Mother Nature.

A single man can get used to a reverse schedule of sleeping in the daytime. It will play havoc on the body for weeks or months if it is adhered to. The worst possible schedule is the one that is constantly in flux (day sleeping, night sleeping, day sleeping, etc.). Third shift can be difficult to adjust to as well. While your body clock will continue to run the same program, it may slowly alter.

Mankind is not immune or above mutation. In just two generations we have seen the usual robust head of hair replaced by the shaved head. What is driving these phenomena? Is it cool to be bald or is there something else at work? Just as girls are experiencing adolescence at an earlier and earlier age, humans are going bald as a group. The same force that is making young girls full figured and busty at an earlier and earlier age is mutating all of mankind. I will cover this later in these pages. Mutation is a result of powerful forces pushing life to adapt or succumb. These forces can occur due to climatory change (ice age, etc) or directly due to man's changing habits. As a result, if all males suddenly became solely nocturnal it might only be two or three generations before males would have better night vision than females.

Burning the candle at both ends and "second shift work" will take its toll on the individual attempting to live such a lifestyle. Like it or not nature is inflicting forces on all of us that we are only partially aware of. The tides that crash on our shores drive nature and the planet, and will continue to affect us regardless of how we fight it. When we sleep as nature does at sunset and then rise with the sun, we will be healthier and survive better. Nature does not care about our schedules but it will influence us whether we like it or not. The spud and plankton cannot fight with universal forces they can only react to them.

"If man is not affected in-some-way by the Moon he is the only thing on Earth that isn't", (Robert Millikan, 1868-1953, U.S. physicist and 1923 Nobel Prize winner). This, of course, explains why you feel so badly when you are off your schedule, are up all night or pull a shift 48 hours long. To make this chart work for you, apply it exactly by the clock as your body is going to follow the tides as all life has for millions of years.

"Every Cause has its Effect; every Effect has its Cause; everything happens according to Law; Chance is but a name for Law not recognized; there are many planes of causation, but nothing escapes the Law."
— *The Kybalion, 4th Principal of the Hermetic Principles*

"Everything flows, out and in; everything has its tides; all things rise and fall; the pendulum-swing manifests in everything; the measure of the swing to the right is the measure of the swing to the left; rhythm compensates."
— *The Kybalion, 5th Principal of the Hermetic Principles*

The following table is a hybrid of my earlier works. It is now possible to chart what your body will be experiencing at anytime of the day. If more data is uncovered, this chart will morph again.

The repair times of your body:

a) Lungs / Eyes / Liver / Descending colon	3 a.m. - 5 a.m.
b) Intestines / Lungs / Eyes / Liver	5 a.m. - 7 a.m.
c) Stomach / Lungs / Respiratory System / Liver	7 a.m. - 9 a.m.
d) Spleen / Heart / Kidneys / Liver	9 a.m. - 11 a.m.
e) Heart / Kidneys / Liver	11 a.m. - 1 p.m.
f) Heart / Adrenal Glands / Liver / Kidneys	1 p.m. - 3 p.m.
g) Bladder / Reproductive System / Kidneys / Liver	3 p.m. - 5 p.m.

h) Kidneys / Joints / Muscle / Reproductive System / Liver	5 p.m. - 7 p.m.
I) Pancreas / Circulatory & Endocrine System / Kidneys / Liver	7 p.m. - 9 p.m.
j) Circulatory System / Endocrine System / Kidneys / Liver	9 p.m. - 11 p.m.
k) Gallbladder / Liver / Kidneys / Ascending colon	11 p.m. - 1 a.m.
l) Liver / Kidneys / Transverse colon	1 a.m. - 3 a.m.

This list is the result of years of research and is complete. You will notice that the liver and kidneys play a role in every function of the body. Consequently all repair of the body can be modified by this knowledge. With this table you can forecast what issues you will have at various times of the day. How you use this data will dictate how good you feel. You will also know what organs and systems have been causing your health issues

There are exact phenomena that take place when the body is in the repair mode. I will address each of these points one at a time.

Morning symptoms 3-9 a.m.

Coughing
Sneezing
Runny nose
Itching skin
Itching scalp
Itching throat

Itching inner ear
Watery eyes / burning eyes / itchy eyes
Need to evacuate your colon (bowel
    movement)
Crabby / moody / irritable

***Support your morning by supporting your liver and digestive tract

Mid morning symptoms 9 a.m. - 1 p.m.

Tight chest
Heart double beating
Heart skipping a beat
Heart triple beating
Low back pain
Left shoulder pain

Left side of the neck pain
Joint pain
Ringing in the ears
High blood pressure
Slight fever (1 degree or less)

***Support your kidneys and heart via your kidneys.

Mid afternoon - Mid evening symptoms 1-11 p.m.

Bloating / gas
Blood pressure fluctuations
Low back pain
Bladder discomfort
Energy low or drifting / Lethargy

Moody / Irritable
Reproductive performance issues
Cold hands, feet or feeling cold
Feeling hot
Itching inner ear

***Support your digestive tract, kidneys and liver

Late night - Early morning symptoms 11 p.m. - 3 a.m.

Right side rib pain
Moody / Irritable
Eye irritation or blurring
Itchy skin
Insomnia
Restless sleep / Tossing and turning

Frequent urination
Right shoulder pain and stiffness
Left shoulder pain and stiffness
Leg cramps
Bloated or irritated abdomen
Pressure in the abdomen

19 Inner Anatomy Keys

As explained in the previous chapter, the body is executing exact processes at precise times of our 24-hour day. Early in the morning your body is going through a variety of processes that all involve starting the day. To rise with the sun we need oxygen, energy, less internal waste and finally vision to see the world. All of these systems are dependent on the liver for support. You may be one of the many people who wake up coughing or sneezing as if every day starts with an allergy. Your scalp or skin may itch as if you have fleas. You might be moody or tight lipped in the morning. You may struggle with mucus-filled eyes.

Your internal systems are just resetting themselves. A completely healthy system will not experience these issues. But once you and your energy are balanced, symptoms subside or never occur in the first place. Your symptoms directly correlate to your diet and lifestyle. The better you are the better you can be.

The 3 parts or your colon are: the ascending colon, starting just above your right hip and stretching up to the bottom of your rib cage on your right side; the transverse colon, starting just below the right side of your rib cage and crawling across your abdomen to the bottom of your left rib cage, and the descending colon starting just below the left side of your rib cage and drops down to the rectum, where evacuation takes place.

The colon needs to be lubricated for evacuation to take place. It must flush and process waste matter around the clock. Dedicated and routine morning intake of water / fresh juice is vital for proper colon / intestinal function. Again, the most important time to give your colon fluid is in the morning. Fluids need to be ingested little by little around the clock, but morning intake is critical.

Without question caffeine is one of the worst substances you can ever put in your body. Why? Because caffeine is a diuretic, a diuretic diverts water away from your colon causing your colon to paralyze. With caffeine present, your entire system crashes to rock solid standstill. Do not ever consume caffeine-bearing drinks. You cannot be at your healthiest with caffeine as health and caffeine are incongruous. The body must have plentiful amounts of water and fresh juices, period. The results of a body deprived of water are obvious as the body will be or experience: weakness, constipation, sluggishness, fatigue, weight gain, increased blood pressure, heart attacks, immune system dysfunction, kidney disorders including diabetes, aches /pains, bad moods, poor skin, poor sleep, insomnia, allergies and more.

By irrigating your system every morning with fluid (12 to 20 ounces or up to ? a liter of water or fresh juice), you give yourself the best chance to be healthy. Some people wait until their first elimination of the day before they eat anything solid. This does work, as it is a signal that your digestive tract has caught up on its work. Ideally you should never use something to cause the elimination, as you are only masking the problem, but not solving it. This does not mean that there is no application for a good colon formula or herb, but chronic use is never recommended. Recapping, the colon knows when it is ready to start the day and will signal you via elimination. A healthy colon runs itself.

The Stomach: In the morning, it is vital to give the stomach as little stress as possible. The wrong thing to do is eat a big meal in the morning. This does not negate the old standard that "Breakfast is the most important meal of the day." In reality, it is true, yet eating anything that needs any digestion in the morning is a mistake. Oatmeal, cereal, toast, eggs, all meat, pancakes, scrambled eggs, protein bars, protein drinks all need digestion, as does so much more.

The morning meal should consist of fresh fruit, juices and vegetables. You can also include freshly made smoothies from your favorite juice bar. For those who need more protein, include a raw egg or two in your smoothie. The reason for eating this way is to make the morning digestive process distress free. All of the above items digest themselves, and therefore require the body to do very little. Another great item in the morning is green salad (with no meat or cheese), which I eat every day. Salad is another item that due to its plentiful live enzymes allows the body to heal itself. Whenever you eat a meal that digests itself, the body uses its energy to correct its problems.

Recap: Eating easily digested fresh fruit, fresh juice, salads or water is necessary if you are to start your day successfully.

The Spleen: Sits behind the stomach and above the diaphragm. It is a somewhat misunderstood organ. It works hand in glove with the liver and kidneys to form the hub of our immune system. It produces antibodies whenever there is an infection. It is constantly monitoring the blood for such invaders. Without a healthy spleen even a common cold could be fatal. If you thought of the spleen as a pre-liver you would basically be right. Should your spleen be stressed with work during its repair cycle, you may feel weak, experience allergies or mild cold-like symptoms. The same successful treatments for the liver are also good for the spleen. Again, think of your spleen as a pre-liver, which is an accurate description.

The Heart: When it is healthy is about the size of your fist. It should beat 60 to 70 beats a minute for the average healthy person at rest. An athlete can have a resting pulse in the 40s. The only rest the heart gets is between beats. The fewer beats your heart executes per minute the less wear and tear it will experience. Amazingly, as the heart enters its repair cycle (as seen in the chart in the last chapter), 70% of all heart attacks occur (as per the Framingham study).

The Small Intestines: Your small intestines coils like a snake through 20 feet of your abdominal cavity. Its mass dominates your belly and is the culprit as soon as you are bloated. When you feel any discomfort in your abdomen, your small intestine is in some degree distressed. You may feel indigestion, bloating, pain, intense pressure or spasms. When the Ileoceco Valve (the connection between the small intestines and the ascending colon, just above the right hip) is blocked, you will feel pain or blockage in that region. Many people think this is a bladder issue or appendicitis. Some women who experience this believe it is a uterine issue when in actual fact it is just an Ileoceco valve blockage issue.

When the small intestine is running slow you may very well feel and look a bit fat. Either way, a proper diet is needed or the intestines will bloat and your midsection will become distended (you will look fat).

The Kidneys, Bladder, Pancreas: For thousands of years the Chinese have said that the kidneys are the master organs of the human body. Later, when you read all the function that they perform, you will wholeheartedly agree. Your kidneys filter all of the fluid of your body; regulate protein synthesis, spent protein removal, and collect lactic acid, uric acid and much more. Think of your kidneys as the water filter and pumping company for the body. If your joints or muscles need to be flushed, it is the kidneys that direct the clean up. As the body is 70% water, you can appreciate the importance of your kidneys. When the kidneys are going through their repair cycle, various symptoms may occur, such as: fatigue (needing a nap), sore muscles, left shoulder pain, ankle pain, intense craving for sweets, intense carving for meat, frequent urination, sore joints, reproductive failure or issues, ringing in the ears, vertigo (dizziness) and more. During these times, eat grapes, tomatoes and citrus, as these help to reset the kidneys and all that they regulate.

They regulate all mucus production and its pickup and disposal.

The Liver/Gallbladder/Endocrine System/Circulatory System: The liver sits just under and a little below the right side of the ribcage. It is a warehouse of chemicals and vitamins used to break down matter into usable food. It also works to dilute poisons and then excrete them from the body. It does not actually absorb or hold toxins; it is strictly a processing plant similar to a sewage facility. Along with the kidneys it regulates energy, clarity of thought, emotions, brightness of vision, right shoulder pain, skin, lungs, and the digestive tract. It also regulates the lungs, sinuses and sleep. The liver and kidneys modify the endocrine system. Yet the kidneys primarily regulate all glands including the Pituitary, Hypothalamus, Pineal, Thyroid and Parathyroid, Adrenals, Ovaries and Testes. All of these glands produce hormones that adjust temperature, blood flow, energy, muscle function and more. When these systems are off you may feel weaker, tired, exhausted, stressed, sleepless, task obsessed, restless, moody, hot or cold and off sexually. If you understand that all non-optimum functions of the body are caused by continual contact with toxins, then you are on your way to correcting your body and your life. These systems respond to citrus, i.e. oranges, grapefruit, tangerines, lemons, limes and fruit in general, including grapes and tomatoes.

20 Validating Herbal Safety

Every week I hear the same question from skeptics and goodhearted but uninformed individuals asking "are herbal formulas safe?" They then follow that musing with the following query, "how can we trust herbs if they are not regulated by the Food and Drug Administration (FDA)?"

Persistent rumors float around every day that creepy, dirty characters in filthy basement laboratories produce herbal products and sell them to the unsuspecting. These scandalous rumors are so twisted that they take on mythic proportion to the point of being "urban legend" material.

The basic questions that the public wants answered are:

- Are herbs and herbal formulas regulated?
- If they are regulated, who is doing it?
- How are herbal products produced?
- Is anyone policing how they are produced?

Those asking the above questions have an earnest concern that is rarely succinctly answered.

This chapter is offered to quell the chattering about herbal safety once and for all. Sit back and relax because in the next several paragraphs you are being presented with the esoteric truths that until now have been evading your awareness.

Traditional Medicine (TM) has been with man every step of recorded human history. 5000 years ago the only check and balance available was the test of life or death and sickness versus health. The wise man or wise woman of the tribe or group held the job because of his success handling the sick and treating wounds. If he or she failed, death by the hands of those offended was not far away.

The wise man / wise woman, medicine man / medicine woman or shamans were positions of untold respect and honor. They often presided over weddings, births, deaths and gave spiritual counsel. This position was earned based on results.

Imagine if we put to death all those who routinely failed us in healing. It would not be long before health care would be a very clean and very successful venture. Thousands of years ago health care was an oral tradition passed from one generation of "healers" to another. The same lessons that great grandma learned were passed on to her great granddaughter. If something worked it was used if it did not it was tossed in the scrap heap of good intentions gone a skew.

To many it comes as a great surprise when they find out, that the FDA oversees the herbal industry and has quietly done this job since about 1915. The idea that the FDA does not monitor herbs, herbal formulas and the labs that produce them is completely false.

The fact is that the FDA closely scrutinizes all herbals meant for ingestion. Prior to an herb being allowed to be put into an herbal formula or sold independently, it must be given Generally Accepted as Safe (GRAS) approval.

The GRAS list is a catalogue of botanicals / herbs that have been presented to the FDA along with extensive laboratory testing proving their safety.

This list is a collection of substances that have been extensively tested on animals to establish if they are toxic. The analysis is called the Lethal Dose 50 test (LD50) and has been rightly decried by animal rights groups such as PETA. The mode of testing involves giving an animal a large daily dose of the substance in question over a 60 day period. The test is concluded when at least 50% of the test animals have died. The 50 stands for the 50% death rate in the LD50 test. When this 50% death plateau has been reached the carcasses of the rats or animals are then watchfully dissected to establish the level of necropathy that ended their lives.

All testing does not result in death and this is of course an indicator of safety. Substances that kill rapidly and all substances that are found to have a lethal dose never make the GRAS list.

No company can legally make or sell a formula or herb unless it has been first approved by the FDA and is on the GRAS list.

Roger Bezanis

This is further policed in the United States by laboratories. Under the watchful eye of FDA regulators, labs will not make a formula or package an herb unless its components appear on the GRAS list. Further, the FDA makes surprise visits and examines the books of these laboratories. If an infraction is found arrests are made and the doors are closed.

These labs are also monitored by the state that they are located in. In California they are monitored by the California Department of Health.

Some people fear that anyone can make a formula in their bathtub or some such thing. This is an unfounded fear as it takes the purchase of pounds of raw material suitable for tableting and a tableting press. They would then have to acquire bottles, sealers, labels and all manner of packaging. Companies in the business of supplying large amounts of these items are also periodically reviewed.

These items are reported just as your bank must report large sums of cash being deposited into your checking, savings or business accounts.

With regard to the purchase of tableting machines, sales of these devices are closely scrutinized by the FDA and even more intensely at the state level. These checks and balances prevent unscrupulous products from ever reaching the public.

Should someone procure a tableting press; within two weeks of delivery they will be visited by authorities demanding an explanation of their purchase. Unless they have proper paperwork and can express a valid need for the machine; it is confiscated and a full investigation is launched.

The making of natural formulas is only handled by laboratories that pass all safety, ethics, cleanliness and quality standard inspections. Laboratories that make herbal formulas are each staffed by 100's of honest hard working men and women. Just like you and me they are sane and pursuing the greatest good for mankind. Chasing the quick buck offered by illegal product production is abhorrent. The mere thought of making an off GRAS list item is not only illegal it is unthinkable.

The only bone of contention in the use of the GRAS list is the inhumane treatment of animals that are subjected to the vehicle of validation for inclusion on the GRAS list.

Can testing be performed on humans sparing defenseless animals?

Yes, as PETA and other groups that fight for animal rights know all too well. Any number of tests are available yet the FDA only respects the LD50 test. "Smear tests" can be employed where a substance is smeared on the skin and then immune system response is monitored. Even though protests are loud the FDA continues to demand LD type testing.

There are many reasons to be unhappy with the FDA. The use of LD50 testing is just another one. Herbal formulators such as me and any good TM practitioner never administer or recommend any product that we have not extensively tested on ourselves.

I have taken doses so large that those around me wondered why I would do such a thing. The answer to this question is simple. If I cannot personally validate the safety of what I speak about I will not articulate it at all. The proviso being, that if anyone is going to die due to my work it will be me not someone I am helping.

To recap herbal safety

- The FDA approves all herbs via the GRAS list
- The GRAS list is validated via LD50 testing
- Herbs that fail LD50 testing do not make the GRAS list
- Laboratories only use ingredients that appear on the GRAS list
- The FDA monitors all laboratories
- Each state (California for example) monitors all laboratories

The rancor over herbal products and individual herbs is often very loud, but those who are making the noise have not been privy to the information in this chapter.

When you consider the simplicity of TM it is beyond reproach. For 5000 years it has consisted of the use of:

- Dietary change
- Herbs (food)
- Water
- Exercise

I am not in this chapter going to trash the forces which choose to oppose TM (i.e. allopathic medicine which is focused on drugs and surgery) as it is well known to be impudent, ineffective, dangerous and evil. Honestly I am not going to attack this group because it is not politically correct to harass any assembly staffed by brainwashed and insane people.

What is important to note is that TM is based on the history of man. Herbs are extensively used in Chinese, Indian, Middle Eastern, Japanese, Tibetan and all Asian medicine. More than 65% of the planet uses TM with rave results. The question you should be asking is why the West is so against this amazing approach to healing?

The answer is simple MONEY.

He who makes the rules makes the money.

Wrap your mind around the last sentence while you are thinking about the FDA, AMA and Big Pharma.

Now you know the truth and can concisely answer the next attacks that you receive on TM and your autonomous and honest approach to healing yourself, friends and family. Hippocrates said "Let the food be your medicine and your medicine be your food." Herbs are dried foods. Now you know what Hippocrates meant.

Be healthy.

Your Friend,
Roger Bezanis

21 Herbs by Their Action

I am forever being asked to explain the proper herb for the proper problem. Years of work, and hands on experience have revealed the following. A word of note, never use any herb or formula that forces the body to do something against its will. Example: using Uva Ursa Root to cleanse the kidneys is a bad idea as is an astringent and will cause the kidneys to spasm and release fluid.

To heal the body you must introduce substances to aid the body in naturally resetting itself, not forcing it off its schedule. I have attached some asterisks (*) to herbs that overpower the body. To be sure of their actions, look them up. There is no reason why you should not be an expert in healing yourself.

The only organs that can be safely flushed out are the colon, sinuses, lungs and skin. The liver regulates all of these organs.

LIVER

Dandelion	Dong Quai Root	Schizandra
Gentian	Peony Root	Chinese Skull Cap
Bupleurum	Hyssop Root	Reishi Mushroom
Beet Root	Chinese Mint Leaf	Hyssop
False Unicorn	Phyllanthus	Wasabi Japonica
Tribulus Terrestris	Artichoke	

KIDNEY

Gravel Root**	Bush clover	Plaintain
Uva Ursa Root**	California Poppy	Poke Root

False Unicorn	Canadian fleabane	Prickly Ash
Tribulus Terrestris	Cattail	St. John's Wort
Corn Silk**	Cedar	Saw palmetto
Cinnamon Bark	Celery seed**	Shepherd's purse
Borage	Chickweed	Silk Tassel
Cedar	Chlorophyll	Skullcap
Red Raspberry	Cleavers	Stoneroot**
Pygeum Bark	Cramp bark	Sweet sumac
Holy Basil	Horsetail-equisteum spp.	Wild hydrangea**
Beet Root	Irish moss	Irish yam**
Lycci Fructus	Juniper	Yarrow
Agrimony	Kava-kava**	Yellow Jessamine
Aspen	Mallow	Yellow pond lily
Astragalus	Marshmallow**	Yerba Santa
Black haw	Mullein root	Squawvine leaves
Buchu	Nettles	Damiana Leaves
Bugleweed	Oatstraw	Corydalis
Burdock	Parsley	

Many of these herbs for kidneys are diuretics that force the kidneys to expel fluid. This is not recommended. Your kidneys can and should run themselves. If they are not constantly poisoned with sugars, sodium and junk food, they will heal. Please use herbs and formulas for the kidneys that support their function rather than forcing them "off line" by either retaining fluid or expelling fluid. If allowed to be healthy, the kidneys keep you healthy.

INTESTINES AND COLON

Cascara Sagrada	Flax Seed	Psyllium Husk
Rhubarb Root	Burdock Root	Aloe
Buckthorn Bark	African Bird Peppers	Black Walnut Hulls
Habanero Pepper	Wormwood	Boldo Leaves
Senna	Buchu Leaves	Fedegosso
Slippery Elm Bark	Black Sesame Seeds	Fenugreek

Our immune system is supposed to recognize anything that is foreign and destroy it. But, depending on diet, it could be running at 30% of capacity, or worse. Cells in the circulatory and the lymphatic systems perform this recognition and destruction on an hourly basis. These cells are produced in the bone marrow and lymphatic tissue (thymus, lymph nodes, spleen and tonsils).

Whenever we take a part of the lymphatic system out, it is weakened. Prior to 1975, it was common to have the tonsils taken out. In recent years, the procedure is not nearly as common. These fearless cells are called "stem cells." Now that you know a little more about Stem Cells, forget what you know. Stem Cells without a body to work in are useless. A parachute is no good to a skydiver unless he is wearing it.

A healthy body produces all the stem cells it needs. The harvesting of Stem Cells for experimentation takes us down the road to Frankenstein's Castle. There is no point to goofing around with our chemistry if we understand the basics of life. Focus on the bigger picture of your WHOLE BODY. Remember, you can't see much of the elephant by studying its tail. When I speak of the immune system, I mean the whole body fighting a whole problem, not some fragmentation.

When we look at the body as a whole, and not as independent separate parts, as modern allopathic medicine does, we can solve issues in a sane manner. Holistic means whole, and the body is a whole organ with circuits and meridians that connect as a whole. If one part of the body is affected, every cell of the body is affected. In other words, what you do to your toe affects your hair as well. Our immune system is composed of the liver, kidneys, lungs, spleen, lymphatic system and more. When experts talk about organ detoxification or similar compartmentalization, they are making a fundamental error. The error is in breaking down bodily functions into segments rather than addressing the totality of the body.

GENERAL IMMUNE SYSTEM

Golden Seal Root	Hyssop	Echinacea Root
Una De gatp	Astragalus Root	Ashwagandha
Royal Jelly	Olive Leaf	White Peony Root
Lime Flower	Corydalis	Schizandra
Panax Ginseng	Lavender Flower	Figwort
Cats Claw	Poke Root	Suma
Juniper Berrier	Anise Seed	Red Clover

22 Why Diagnostic Face Reading™

When was the last time that your doctor told you what was wrong with you and you walked away wondering "what was he talking about?" Perhaps you have completely disagreed with his diagnosis whatever he told you the problem was with your body.

Getting upsetting news or a bum diagnosis from your doctor is no fun. For days you replay the words he used over and over in your head all the while wondering "huh?" You might have quietly gotten angry with his prognostication.

Diagnosing is a very tricky thing to do. It can cause all manner of upset even if it is done well. Right or wrong, a diagnosis is a very hard announcement to make and even harder to receive. That is why this book exists. Its sole purpose is to make you autonomous.

The only anyone seeks a professional for any reason is that they do not feel qualified to perform the job themselves. That is why we seek a professional.

If you are completely independent of your doctor by being able to diagnose yourself and then heal yourself you might ask "why do I need my doctor?" That is the right question to ask. I advise you to find a doctor who is familiar with my work and can work with you versus "work on you."

This book gives you the advanced tools to diagnose yourself from here to eternity. With all of the added tools such as fingernail analysis, tongue analysis, eyebrow analysis, hand analysis, scalp analysis, symptom analysis, iridology and face reading you are bullet proof from the horrors of being lied to or misled ever again.

Be Well

Your friend,
Roger Bezanis

23 Body / Health Indicators

Healing requires not book sense but human sense. One must use all of their faculties to understand the indicators or the body. Relying on idiot gauges (x-ray, MRI, microscopes, stethoscopes etc,) today's practitioners have gotten lazy and are not taught to observe. They are taught to study readouts but not their own patients. Today's doctors are educated in the theory of sickness and the administering of drugs but not how to restore health. To heal anyone, you must look, smell, touch and listen.

Step one: look at the color of the individual. What is his color? Is he pasty white? Grey? Is he ruddy? Is the skin almost transparent where veins are very clear and vivid? The more extreme the skin tone is from its ideal, the more unbalanced the individual is.

Step two: How long has this condition been present?

Step three: What has the person been eating? What we eat will affect us immediately. When bad eating habits are continually practiced, the body will break down faster. Often the current body complaints are directly tied to what we had in the last 24 hours or less.

Step four: Notice the smell of the body. Sickness does not smell healthy. It is pungent and stale. Does the body smell or is it just the breath? The less foul odor emanating from the body, the better indicator it is for a quick recovery.

Step five: Evaluate the posture. The more erect the stance, the stronger the will, and stronger the life energy of the body.

Step six: Eye color, are they grey or bright? The more grey and dull they are, the more the immune system is compromised.

Step seven: Back of hand skin elasticity. Hand should be flat / straight, not in a fist. Is the skin tension loose or taught? Does the skin immediately snap back to the hand or is it slow? The better the skin tension on the back of the hands the better. The right hand indicates the state of the liver and its corresponding organs and the left hand indicates the same data for the kidneys. The better the body is hydrated, the quicker the body will recover.

Step eight: Is the person hot (running a fever)? Fever is an obvious indicator of an infection being fought.

Step nine: Are there parts of the body that are cold? These areas are not receiving energy flow. If you understand what organ (liver or kidney) dominates this area of the body, you will further know what to correct.

Old time Osteopaths, Naturopaths and any good practitioner knew the value of these points and always used them. These simple observations are senior to x-rays, MRI's, Stethoscopes and other device dependent tests.

Doctors and healers from pre-history to 1940's often gave prescriptions that included rest, sun, water, fresh food, fresh juices and various herbs. They used nature to heal the body as the body was derived from nature and needed nature to heal.

Quant as this happens to sound; the above paragraph gives the key to understanding and healing the body. Allopathic doctors do not care about quaint or effective. They are focused on not being wrong based on insurance, laws suits and AMA membership and guidelines.

Armed with what you learn in this book, if you stay focused on face reading for diagnostic purposes and employ all the gifts that I give you, you cannot fail.

You will be amazed at what you can do and achieve.

When will you know that you are successful with these techniques and face reading? When what you observe leads to long-range, positive and accurate applications and gains. You can do this, and you can be expert in it.

Remember the last time you or a friend / loved one was sick? What did they look like? What was the color of their skin? What did their eyes look like? Did they look older? Did they look tired? We always look different when we are "off." Use these tools. Use these tools. Use these tools.

If you have noticed, the face always looks different depending on the following factors:

A.   How much sleep we have gotten.

B.   How much water we have consumed

C.   The use of caffeine

D.   Use of drugs

E.   Consumption of salt or sodium.

F.   What kind of diet we have had over a period of hours or years

G.   Heredity

H.   Environmental factors

I.   Habits and routines

J.   Use of tobacco

K.   Use of alcohol

When toxins physically tax us, we demonstrate the fact like a neon sign. Your internal organs are working overtime. From the early physicians such as Hippocrates, and the Shaman and Indian medicine men before him, healers used observation to diagnose.

These early practitioners were good because they practiced and honed their skills.

This book is dedicated to the precise time-proven, ancient technique of diagnostic analysis, via empirical observation. You can know what Hippocrates knew and of course what I know, as I am going to teach you through this book.

24 The History of Face Reading

Man has always tried to predict the future and control his environment. Lacking a deep perception of human motives and fear of the unknown, EARLY MAN was grasping at straws. How can anyone protect their family, personal interests and trust friends without a system of detection?

This was the plight of man. Create a system to identify who were friend or foe or risk danger and perhaps even death.

Some of the greatest minds in the ancient world took on these challenges. Since the face was how man was identified, it was logical to study the face and head for clues. Greek philosophers, Socrates (469-399 BC), Plato (427-347 BC), and Aristotle (384-322 BC) all speculated on the nature of man.

Aristotle appears to be the source of an early form of face reading called Physiognomy. It tried to predict actions and personality. For the first 1500 years or so man took many wayward attempts at prediction that led directly into fantasy.

The stirrings brought on by Socrates and passed down to Plato, who then instilled them in Aristotle, led him to speculate that a chart on face reading of a different sort was possible. His attempts compared man to beast and healthy to unhealthy.

Aristotle said that:

"Thick, bulbous noses belong to persons who are insensitive and swinish."

"Sharp-tipped noses belong to persons who are irritable and easily provoked, like dogs."

"Rounded noses belong to generous, lion-like individuals."

He was credited with the following formula:

Round foreheads add x 1% to honesty and x 2% to intellect

Large noses add x Y1% to will power.

Clearly, an esoteric formula, Aristotle's scribing proved basically nothing but did not tarnish his reputation. Nevertheless, even with the bizarre postulations in Aristotle's early work, his empirical study led to much advancement in the field of healing. The world of healing did not start with Aristotle and the Greeks, far from it. Man wanted to know about man long before this.

The concept of face reading is as old as man himself. Prior to man building monoliths and monuments, pyramids and palaces, there were caves and cave walls for painting. His own reflection in stream water was captivating, but his fellow man was fascinating. He had to understand. He also thirsted to know who he was and what made him tick. Early medicine was not enough. Even the casual observer could see that a sick man not only smelled different, he looked different. What was really at work? What did it all mean?

To appreciate DIAGNOSTIC FACE READING, you have to know what it is and what it is not.

BELOW IS WHAT DIAGNOSTIC FACE READING IS NOT.

PHYSIOGNOMY

From Webster's 1913 Dictionary:
Physiognomy, Phys`i*og"no*my\, n.; pl. {Physiognomies}. Etymology: OE.fisonomie, phisonomie, fisnamie, OF. phisonomie, F. physiognomie, physiognomonie, from Gr. ?; fy`sis nature + ? one who knows or examines, a judge, fr. ?, ?, to know.

1. The art and science of discovering the predominant temper, and other characteristic qualities of the mind, by the outward appearance, especially by the features—of the face.

PHRENOLOGY
From Webster's 1913 Dictionary:
Phrenology: \Phre*nol"o*gy\, n.
Etymology: Gr. ?, ?, the mind + -logy: cf. F. phr['e]nologie.

1. In popular usage, the physiological hypothesis of Gall that the mental faculties, and traits of character, are shown on the surface of the head or skull; craniology.

PERSONOLOGY
The Skeptics Dictionary
Personology is a recent "New Age" variant of the ancient pseudoscience of Physiognomy, which is closely related to the disproved study of Phrenology. It is a system of face reading that purports to show a correlation between a person's physical features and appearance, and the person's behavior, personality and character. Mainstream science considers Personology to be a wholly false pseudoscience.

The dirt on Personology: Edward Jones, who developed Personology in the 1930s, was a Los Angeles judge. According to Naomi Tickle, author of "It's all in the Face -The Key to Finding Your Life Purpose" (1997), "Jones became fascinated by those who appeared before him in court. He felt there was a relationship between facial features and behavior patterns" Jones believed there was a direct and undeniable correlation between what people looked like, and what they did in life. He was certain he knew who the criminals were on sight. His theories / musings became well known in the early 1930s.

When his practices were put to the test in a controlled trial, he failed miserably. Personology was dead by the end of 1935 and Jones, a laughing stock.

The true history of the above three attempts at "mankind prediction" are fascinating reading and important to understand as you again must know what DIAGNOSTIC FACE READING is to really understand what it is not.

The first book on record concerning face reading which devoted itself to the study and comparison of humans was Giovanni Battista Della Porta's De Humana Physiognomonia 1586. In this book, he made comparisons of humans to animals and attempted to predict aggressive behavior. This study of internal character from external appearances—most notably the face—

was a partly aesthetic and partly philosophical practice, which preceded phrenology. It's main advocate in the late eighteenth century was the Swiss clergyman J. G. Lavater (1741-1801) in his Physiognomical Fragments (1775-1778).

Thanks to his labors, he and his themes started to become popular. Much of the work in these early practices have been lost, some of the more recent advancements are still with us. Even though this book is not based or devoted to these earlier works, it is important to note them and understand something of them.

Battista Della Porta's vast work led to lectures and many later books by Charles Le Brun circa 1698 (the head of the French Academy). Physiognomy became popular thanks to the frenetic work of Le Brun and several other late 18th and 19th century French doctors who specialized and reveled in the subject.

It wasn't long until the new term Phrenology was coined. It is derived from the Greek roots: phren: "mind" and logos: "study/discourse." "[Before phrenology] all we knew about the brain was how to slice it..."
- R. Chenevix (phrenologist), 1828.

Phrenology was a forerunner to present day psychology and psychiatry. The term came into general use around 1819/1820 in Britain. The physician T.I.M. Forster coined phrenology, as a term. In fact if you take a look at the placement of this often sneered at pseudoscience, you will see its rise led directly to experiments on the brain including the lobotomy*, shock treatment and the frontal orbital leucotomy* (a procedure of shoving an ice pick up through the top of both eye sockets, then thrusting it into the frontal lobe of the brain using an arc motion, thus destroying vital nerve centers, leaving the patient dormant, intensely angry and often suicidal).

* I go into depth on both of these subjects in the chapter, YOUR LIVER AND MOODS.

Phrenology's brain studies eventually led to skull study. This because, as per phrenology, the indentations and bumps in the skull were studied in order to establish personality. These studies led to the disparaging term Bumpology. Ridicule was often levied at phrenology for two reasons,

1) It was a fairly ridiculous notion to read the ridges and low points of the skull to establish behavior.

2) Due to a relative lack of training needed to perform Phrenology, it attracted various rogue elements, which sought only to increase their reputation. With everybody from psychics to pub owners attempting to pick up the "skill", it lowered the perceived value of the entire movement. Misguided as they were, many of the 19th-century phrenologists called it "the only true science of mind." And now Phrenology had reached the Americas thanks to Viennese physician Franz.

Joseph Gall (1758-1828) From 1913 Encyclopedia Britannica, "Note: Gall marked out on his model of the head the places of twenty-six organs, as round enclosures with vacant interspaces. Spurzheim and Combe divided the whole scalp into oblong and conterminous patches."

Gall laid down the basic tenets of Phrenology, which were:

1. The brain is the organ of the mind.
2. The mind is composed of multiple distinct, innate faculties.
3. Because they are distinct, each faculty must have a separate seat or "organ" in the brain.
4. The size of an organ, other things being equal, is a measure of its power.
5. The shape of the brain is determined by the development of the various organs.
6. As the skull takes its shape from the brain, the surface of the skull can be read as an accurate index of psychological aptitudes and tendencies.

Number 1-5 above are clearly off in left field, ignoring the presence of a soul or life force that is free of the body, but most will agree that number 6 is not only off in left field, it is in left field in another state.

Remember "Bumpology"?

Physiognomy led to Phrenology, which led to the short-lived Personology.

But there were satellite studies that accidentally / intentionally linked previous work to anthropology which would later enhance Phrenology. Personology was coming next and, with a little imagination, you will be able to see the connection.

Simultaneously various European scientists studying anthropology such as Petrus Camper (1722-1789) started to blend with Physiognomy.

A Dutch naturalist, Camper, developed a similar physiognomical theory based on facial angle, which was a great influence on contemporary and nineteenth-century aesthetics and anthropology. Camper's facial angle was based on comparative anatomy and prescribed that the more vertical the angle of a straight line drawn from the chin to forehead, the closer to the ideal head, the classical head being assumed as the epitome of aesthetic and anatomical perfection.

Camper provided diagrams in his posthumous Über den natürlichen Unterschied der Gesichtszüge (1792) showing a scale of perfection from monkeys at the bottom of the scale, to an Apollo at the termination. Camper's facial angle would later be joined with phrenology in nineteenth-century racial anthropology.

Johann Friedrich Blumenbach (1752-1840), a German naturalist and anthropologist, introduced and developed the science of comparative anatomy in Germany. His De Generis Humani

Varietate Nativa (1775; tr. "On the Natural Varieties of Mankind", 1865, repr. 1969) marked the beginnings of physical anthropology and described the five divisions of mankind that have been the basis of all subsequent racial classifications. Via his foundation of his craniometrical research (analysis of human skulls, published as Collectio Craniorum Diversarum Gentium), he divided the human species into five races: the Caucasian or white race, the Mongolian or yellow, the Malayan or brown race, the Negro or black race, and the American or red race. Apart from physical characteristics, he assigned psychological characteristics.

In Blumenbach's day, physical characteristics like skin color, cranial profile, etc., went hand in hand with declarations of group character and aptitude. The "fairness" and relatively high brows of "Caucasians" were held to be apt physical expressions of a loftier mentality and a more generous spirit.

The epicanthic folds around the eyes of "Mongolians" and their slightly sallow outer epidermal layer bespoke their supposedly crafty, literal-minded nature. The dark skin and relatively sloping craniums of "Ethiopians" were taken as wholesale proof of a closer genetic proximity to the primates, despite the fact that the skin of chimpanzees and gorillas beneath the hair is whiter than the average "Caucasian" skin and that orangutans and some monkey species have foreheads fully as vertical as any human of any race.

The work was mysterious and fostered much curiosity. This calls to mind what the great Greek philosopher Plato said, "Everything that deceives may be said to enchant." Due to this mystery, it became the temporary rage of Europe and the Americas. The aforementioned researchers arduously labored to establish "Body types" for predicting personality, character traits, honesty, capacity to rear children and more.

In the early 1900s, the work of Orson Squire Fowler (1809-1887) was used as the new Personology / Phrenology springboard. Criminologists often attempted to use facial analysis for spotting criminals, with faulty results.

This brings us full circle back to our laughable 1930s judge, Edward Jones. People's criminal motives while at times being sensed, do not show up on the face. With his public failures and embarrassment, it is a wonder that face reading, even on a diagnostic health front, didn't die altogether.

Some of the old terminology found in Phrenology is still in use today. At present, there are still Phrenology terms found in our language such as, "High / Low Brow", "Bull Headed" etc. Now these phrases have a completely different meaning and have no application here. For the purposes of this book, we are going to ignore most, if not all, of those earlier quaint and flawed works.

When you discuss Diagnostic Face Reading with others, if they try to bring up Physiognomy / Phrenology / Personology, you are now armed. If someone should challenge you in any way, you know the history of what really happened.

25 What Your Face Really Says

You have now learned the bombastic and even dangerous beginnings of this thing called face reading. The earlier works on the subject, while not being complete hoaxes, were fraught with folly. Time has an interesting way of sifting to the bottom of truth.

The face and the eyes, through thousands of years of literature, poetry and music, are clearly the center of our emotional universe. Look at Shakespeare, or consider the volumes of love songs, the popularity of plastic surgery and the amount of beauty creams sold every day. The face really is the center of our universe. Thousands of years of woman have been sold the notion that facial youth and beauty is what it takes to be alluring and sexy. That statement is very interesting when you consider when I was first exposed to face reading.

I ran across my first face reading chart at health care conference in 1991. I was at the San Jose Skin Care convention where Estheticians (skin care experts) came to learn new techniques and examine new products. While there I noticed a Homeopathic Medicine doctor was exhibiting. Looking at his promotional pieces, I spotted a very colorful yet very confusing face reading chart. I was drawn to it.

Immediately understanding what he was doing, I knew it could be done better. He was trying to convey that the face reflected the state of the internal organs. And that through internal work the face will change (which is true).

His presentation though was very confusing. Yet I was intrigued. I went home and started researching the subject. Every original (not melting pot) culture on the planet had its own chart for the purpose of predicting health. Every Asian country had a chart and sometimes two or three. I collected all of these charts and realized that they often argued on the exact same points. One would say this area is the liver while another chart said it was the kidneys and so on.

I had to develop a way to be sure what part of the face represented what organ. The question was how to do it! I realized that I had to do as scientific a study as possible. Choosing one organ (the kidneys), I collected two hundred people with known kidney issues and studied their faces. This revealed absolutely nothing. I could not honestly detect anything from just this observation. Examining two hundred people without kidney issues revealed zero as well.

The only way to establish where the kidneys were was to treat them and look for changes. It was not until I gave the whole group herbs and herbal combinations for the kidneys (one at a time over days) that I saw anything of significance.

Eventually it was clear that the exact same points on the face were being affected. I had uncovered the location of the kidneys! This empirical study was paying accurate dividends. I then worked through every major organ of the body using this exact technique to establish the organ map of the face.

Anyone could have conducted this empirical study; I was just the one who did it. These results have been verified thousands of times over the last eight years. They are routinely validated on a daily basis.

To be very clear, this is my personal face reading technique. It is not drawn from any of the known works. This book is a laser precise unveiling of the truth regarding all aspects of your health. This has been a work in progress since I was a teenager. No group owns this work or me. My allegiance is to you the reader and to what works to make you healthy.

I take my hat off to all the thinkers and sages that have came before me. I applaud them. My work may have never taken place unless someone developed them first thousands of years ago. I have no illusions as regards discovering these amazing techniques or analysis. I am sure that I have rediscovered data lost long ago. If we dig deep enough maybe one day we will find the authors of my work. In the mean time I present it to you here.

The face reveals three very distinct pieces of data:

- The predisposition to organ weakness.
- A current weakened organ or system that is inflamed or troublesome right now.
- An area of weakness that has strengthened yet is still a weak link and may be a problem in the future.

Summation: Your face tells you moment to moment just how healthy you are and how healthy you are going to be. It is that simple.

26 Laws of Face Reading

LAW 1 - Aging and looking older are not synonymous. One has nothing to do with the other. You have seen people who are in their '70s, '80s and '90s with snow white hair and yet smooth wrinkle free skin. How is that possible if "WE MUST LOOK OLDER AS WE AGE"? It is not possible as it is a lie.

We look older for a variety of factors but age is not one of them.

LAW 2 - When you look at someone you are seeing the whole of their ancestry and habits represented from ear to ear and chin to scalp. The face does not lie.

LAW 3 - All wrinkles, blemishes, pimples, moles, bumps, red spots, brown spots, age spots, flaking, dry areas, peeling areas, scars, pockmarks, growths and discoloration are realized in areas of the face that are connected to irritated organs or organs that have an inherent weakness.

LAW 4 – All moles lay over areas connected to a weakened or a potentially weak organ or organ system. Should a mole or growth lay over the kidneys or bladder area, the mole / growth often represents a growth on the organ in the same location in the body.

LAW 5 – All redness, flaking and irritation, including dry skin, indicate that the organ is irritated and not getting proper circulation and water.

LAW 6 – All scars on the face should heal. When they do not, it is an indicator that the corresponding organ to that part of the face is weak. To validate this point, why have some of your pockmarks healed and others did not? Scars are a road map to organ weakness.

LAW 7 – Acne always represents temporary irritations of corresponding organs to the part of the face affected.

LAW 8 – The human face is not set; it constantly changes from moment to moment and hour to hour. Remember the last time you woke and looked terrible? It was just a few minutes after your shower that you looked rested and felt rejuvenated. Your body balances and reflects changes rapidly.

LAW 9 - The only reason the skin of our face is not smooth, supple and perfect, is due to drugs, chemicals, excess hormones, a poor diet or heredity. Sun also damages the skin of the face and the body. Anything in excess can cause damage to the human body.

LAW 10 - Piercings on the face, including the ears, create weakness in the organs where the piercing took place.

LAW 11 – All swelling or puffy regions of the face represent a swollen, irritated or enlarged region of the body associated with the face.

LAW 12 – Discolorations of the skin represent damage or potential damage in the associated organ for that region of the face.

LAW 13 – All damage to the body (unless surgery or accident has removed an organ, etc) can be repaired. The only caveat being the length of time it will take to do it. The same is true for the face.

LAW 14 – Face reading gives you notice of problems months and years in advance of the events manifesting themselves. If you apply what is in this book you can spot and handle these tribulations before they slow you down.

Heredity: We have all been handed our genetic makeup from our parents and their parents. There is nothing you can do to change that. Therefore, how you look has been influenced by their habits. What happens after that is entirely your choice. If you learn to listen to your body, you will look and feel AS FIRST-RATE AS POSSIBLE. Should your organs start giving you problems, it is incumbent upon you to get to the bottom of the difficulty and correct it.

Rule 1 - If the face has wrinkles, blemishes, pimples, moles, bumps, red spots, brown spots, age spots, flaking, dry areas, peeling areas, scars, pockmarks, growths or discoloration, it is solely due to drugs, chemicals, excess hormones, sun, poor diet or heredity.

Rule 2- If the face does not improve when you treat it, you are not treating the correct organ, what you are using is faulty or you are trying to treat a hereditary state that has not manifested itself yet.

Rule 3 – In treating any condition always consult the symptoms of the body. Symptoms indicate the presence and severity of the issue being addressed

Rule 4 – Anyone who is treated will feel better and look improved when the correct food or herbal is applied to the organ in question.

27 Parts of the Face

NOTE: *Many of the internal organs have the same shape as the areas of the face that represent them.*

NOTE: *Face reading extends from the jawbone to the ears and includes the scalp. It does not include anything below the jaw line (such as the neck).*

NOTE: You will be looking for wrinkles, blemishes, pimples, moles, bumps, red spots, brown spots, age spots, flaking, dry areas, peeling areas, scars, pockmarks, growths or discoloration.

NOTE: The ileocecal valve is located just above the right hip and is a valve that connects the small intestines to the ascending colon.

Two major organs govern not only the body but also the look of the face. These two organs, the liver and kidneys (as you read in the History of the Kidneys and Liver) regulate every function of the human body. If the parent organ is running well, the system will function at its optimum level.

VITAL NOTE OF COMPLIANCE: *The descriptions of the face that you are about to read are*

somewhat esoteric (understood by few). READ THIS SECTION WHILE REFERRING to a mirror. If you hope to fully grasp each part of the face, do not just read these explanations. Study them again and again. Do not go on to the next description until you fully understand the last one. You are building your future success in face reading. Take your time.

Starting at the top and working our way down the face, we find:

THE SCALP
The scalp is a representation of the **BLADDER & REPRODUCTIVE SYSTEM. The Kidneys regulate the entire area**.

MIDDLE OF THE FOREHEAD
The middle of the forehead represents the SMALL INTESTINES. Have you ever noticed the creases of the forehead that snake across its surface? Your intestinal tract looks similar in its construction. **The LIVER regulates the entire area.**

RIGHT & LEFT CORNERS OF YOUR FOREHEAD
The right and left corners of your forehead represent the right and left side of your **BLADDER**. Imagine a line stretching from the innermost point of your eyebrow (nearest your nose) that backtracks across your eyebrow to your hairline. Now imagine another line stretching from the same inside point of your eyebrow (nearest your nose) and stretching diagonally back over the brow to the corner of your hairline (where the hair on the side of your head meets the hair on the top). These two triangle-shaped areas are the right and left side of the bladder. The kidneys, via the bladder, supervise these two areas. **The Kidneys regulate the entire area.**

THE ENTIRE OUTER RIM OF THE RIGHT AND LEFT EARS
The entire outer rim of the right and left ears represents the **KIDNEYS**.

THE ENTIRE EARLOBE OF THE RIGHT AND LEFT EAR
The entire earlobe of the right and left ears represents your HEART. **The Kidneys regulate the entire area.**

THE ENTIRE RIGHT AND LEFT EYE (EYE BALL ONLY)
The entire right and left eyeball represents the state of the **LIVER**.

BRIDGE OF THE NOSE BETWEEN THE EYEBROWS
The center space at the bridge of the nose between the eyebrows represents the **LIVER**.

THE CROW'S-FEET AREA TO THE LEFT AND RIGHT OF EACH EYE
The crow's-feet area to the left and right of each eye represent the **LIVER**.

THE HALF MOON UNDER THE RIGHT AND LEFT EYE
The half moon under the right eye and left eye represents the **RIGHT AND LEFT KIDNEY**. The outer most area (near the crows feet portion of the face) is the **ADRENAL GLAND** on the right

and left kidney. When irritated, this area can appear swollen like a black-eyed pea.

The Kidneys regulate the entire area.

THE ENTIRE NOSE AND UPPER LIP FROM SMILE LINE TO SMILE LINE
The entire nose and upper lip area from smile line to smile line is a representation of the
HEART. The Kidneys regulate the entire area.

THE RIGHT AND LEFT CHEEKBONES
The right and left cheekbones are a representation of the **STOMACH. The LIVER regulates the
entire area.**

RIGHT AND LEFT SMILE LINES
The right and left smile lines represent the **ASSENDING COLON/ILEOCECAL VALVE** (nearest the
nose), the **TRANSVERSE COLON**, in the middle of the smile line and the **DECENDING COLON**
closest to the top of the upper lip. **The LIVER regulates the entire area.**

RIGHT AND LEFT HOLLOW OF THE CHEEK
The right and left hollow of the cheek represents the **RIGHT AND LEFT LUNG. The LIVER
regulates this entire area.**

THE ENDOCRINE STRIP
The Endocrine Strip starts at the innermost bottom corner of the right and left eye and stretches
down next to the half moons under each eye, along the nose, outer smile lines, next the stomach
(cheekbones), and lungs (hallows of the cheeks) down to the jaw line. This area is a representation
of the **ENDOCRINE SYSTEM. The KIDNEYS** and **LIVER** regulate the endocrine system.

THE CHIN AND LOWER LIP
The entire chin and lower lip, stretching across the chin, from Endocrine Strip to Endocrine
Strip, Represents the **MALE AND FEMALE REPRODUCTIVE SYSTEM. The Kidneys regulate the
entire area.**

28 How to Read the Face

You are assessing the person's wrinkles, blemishes, pimples, moles, bumps, red spots, brown
spots, age spots, flaking, dry areas, peeling areas, scars, pockmarks, growths or discolorations,
against perfection. Perfection equals none of the above and is practically impossible to find.

The reason you are learning face reading is either for your own personal needs, your family or in
your business (practitioner of some sort). Understanding that, it is very important to recognize
the power that you are wielding. What you say will be very personal to the individual you are

working with. You are predicting the person's future and reading secrets that they did not know they were revealing. Face reading is very powerful. Do not misuse it.

Guideline 1: Be gentle; do not crush someone with your investigation or observations. Some people are very sensitive. All you are trying to do is bring about an understanding that how a person feels directly corresponds to how they look.

Guideline 2: Unless you are doing a full assessment from ear to ear and chin to scalp, stop when you have interested the person in changing something about them. When you have accomplished this, the person will want to get better. After you have discovered the core issue for the person, direct them to a solution.

Step 1 – Have the person stand in good lighting.

Step 2 - He or she should remain still as you observe them.

Step 3 – Be sure the individual being observed is not smiling or frowning. Nothing can be seen unless the face is calm and relaxed.

Step 4 – Briefly enlighten the person being observed about what you are about to do.

Step 5 – Hand the individual being observed a hand mirror so that he or she can follow what you are pointing out.

Step 6 – Quickly look over the face and observe what jumps out at you. The worst area is always the lynch pin of their problems.

Step 7 – A-Start at the hairline and cover the entire face one area at a time. Picking one area at a time fully investigates it. Your job is to be a good detective.

Step 7 - B-Zero in on the top 4 (or 4 worst) areas of the face and indicate them to the individual in ascending order (smallest problem to the largest). Remember, you are looking for wrinkles, blemishes, pimples, red spots, brown spots, age spots, flaking, dry areas, peeling, moles, scars, growths, swelling and discolorations. You will almost always see puffiness, bagging and or dark circles under the eyes.

Step 8 – With this book as a reference, let them use the hand mirror and compare their face to the face-reading gallery in the book and see if their assessment agrees with yours.

Based on your findings, use the questions that follow later to find out just what are the person's problems based on what you are observing. Do not make the person wrong; gently probe to get to the bottom of what you are looking at. It is always good to make note of what you have spotted and the answers they have given you. Probe gently; the answers are always there.

Offer them a solution based on diet or supplements or both.

29 Accessing What You Are Looking At

When you find wrinkles, blemishes, pimples, moles, bumps, red spots, brown spots, age spots, flaking, dry areas, peeling areas, scars, pockmarks, growths or discolorations on the face, compare these areas to each other to determine the severity of the condition or potential condition.

Areas of comparison will tell you how severe the problem or potential problem is.

BLADDER ISSUES / REPRODUCTIVE ISSUES
Scalp
Bladder areas above each eye
Chin and lower lip area

DIGESTIVE DISTURBANCE
Intestines (center forehead)
Stomach (cheekbones)
Colon (smile lines left and right)

STOMACH ISSUES
Cheekbones

COLON ISSUES
Entire smile line, both sides (these lines break down into three parts, see below)

ASSENDING COLON / ILEOCECAL VALVE
Portion of the smile line connecting at the nostrils of the nose

TRANSVERSE COLON
The middle of the smile line

DESCENDING COLON
The lowest part of the smile line nearest the mouth

LUNG ISSUES
Hollow of each left and right cheek

LIVER ISSUES
Area between the eyebrows at the bridge of the nose
Eyes themselves
Crow's feet area to the outer left and right eye

HEART ISSUES
The entire nose
The left and right earlobe
The entire upper lip area, from smile line to smile line is the heart

** % Percentage rate for each affected area toward a heart condition:

20%   Affected nose

20%   Affected upper lip region

30%   Right earlobe

30%   Left earlobe

Therefore if a person has an affected nose and right earlobe, their chances of having a heart condition are 50% (nose = 20% + earlobe = 30% = 50%)

ENDOCRINE SYSTEM
Endocrine Strip (see last chapter)

REPRODUCTIVE ISSUES
Entire chin (reproductive system)
Scalp (reproductive system and bladder)
Half Moons under the eyes (kidneys)

KIDNEY ISSUES
Kidney issues are represented in the half moon area under the left and right eyes as well as the upper rim of the left and right ear.

30 Notes on Face Reading

Face reading cures nothing and is solely a diagnostic tool for detecting areas of inner body stress. The liver and kidneys dominate the body and therefore the face.

When examining any one part of the face or organ system, always look to compare organ systems on the face that are in the same bracket. Regularly, multiple areas in the bracket are affected at the same time.

LIVER BRACKETS

*Liver issues also look at:

Small Intestines	Colon
Eyes	Lungs
Stomach	

*Small intestine issues also look at:

Liver	Colon
Eyes	Lungs
Stomach	

*Eye issues also look at:

Small intestines	Colon
Liver	Lungs
Stomach	

*Stomach issues also look at:

Small intestines	Colon
Liver	Lungs
Eyes	

*Colon issues also look at:

Small intestines	Stomach
Liver	Lungs
Eyes	

*Lung issues also look at:

Small intestines	Stomach
Liver	Colon
Eyes	

KIDNEY BRACKET

*Bladder issues also check:

All areas related to the bladder
Kidneys
Adrenal glands
Endocrine system
Heart (all areas related to the heart)
Reproductive system (all areas related to the Reproductive system)

*Kidney issues also check:
Bladder (all areas related to the bladder)
Adrenal glands
Endocrine system
Heart (all areas related to the heart)
Reproductive system (all areas related to the Reproductive system)

*Adrenal Gland issues also check:
Bladder (all areas related to the bladder)
Kidneys
Endocrine system
Heart (all areas related to the heart)
Reproductive system (all areas related to the Reproductive system)

*Endocrine System issues also check:
Bladder (all areas related to the bladder)
Kidneys
Adrenal glands
Heart (all areas related to the heart)
Reproductive system (all areas related to the Reproductive system)

*Heart issues also check:
Bladder (all areas related to the bladder)
Kidneys
Adrenal glands
Endocrine system
All areas related to the heart
Reproductive system (all areas related to the Reproductive system)

*Reproductive System also check:
Bladder (all areas related to the bladder)
Kidneys
Adrenal glands
Endocrine system
All areas related to the heart
All areas related to the Reproductive system

When looking at the face "think" in groups. When one area is affected, it is normal to find one or more of the "other" areas affected under the same control (i.e. kidney / liver).

The next step is to compare what you see on the face to the symptoms on the energy-balancing chart. These symptoms will tell you whether you are looking at a weakness or full-blown irritation. Remember, no matter what technique you use to get to the source of a problem, the symptom analysis from the Energy Balancing Technique will always guide you correctly. Never neglect the fact that symptoms are always immediate and 100% accurate. The body never imagines pain. Never discount the power of the body's symptoms, as they are how the body speaks to you. To ignore a symptom is tantamount to turning your back on helping someone in need.

31 Face Reading Interview Questions

This section is devoted to teaching you what questions to ask to reveal the severity of any condition you are assessing. These questions probe deeply but are of little use if they are not employed. Before you start questioning your patient, be very sure your patient is willing to speak to you honestly. If your patient is trying to convince you that everything is fantastic, you will not get very far. This is normally not an issue but can surprise you when you least expect it. Speaking to a patient who is interested in your help is rejuvenating. The opposite is worse than pulling teeth.

The symptoms / questions on this list have been developed over the last 10 years. Every one of these questions is valid in uncovering an actual problem in the affected organ.

Conducting Your Interview for Anything Kidney Related

Trust these questions; they UNCOVER THE SYMPTOMS RELATED TO THE EXACT QUESTION UNDER THE HEADING OFFERED. Once a person is interested in their personal condition they will allow you to help them. This is the complete purpose of face reading.

Regulated by the kidneys are: the bladder, blood pressure, ovaries, ovum production, estrogen, period cramps, testicles, testosterone, sperm production, uterus, prostate, sex drive, pancreas, spleen, lymphatic system, heart, left elbow, all ligaments*, all tendons*, all joints*, ears, scalp, left side of your neck, right and left low back, mid back, left upper back, left shoulder, left deltoid, left trapezoid, left pectoral muscle, left scapula, left latissimus dorsi muscle (lat for short), both forearms, both biceps, both wrists, both hands, both thumbs, both sets of fingers, both hips, both thighs, both hamstrings, both knees, both calves, both ankles, both feet, both sets of toes and soles of both feet. The right shoulder, which includes the right trapezoid, right side of your neck, right deltoid muscle, right pectoral muscle, right scapula and the right lat are all regulated by the liver and will be discussed later.

* Except the right elbow, the stomach regulates this point only.

The upcoming section can be used verbatim. It is written the same way that I have done this testing for the past 10 years. Once you have one or several yes answers, you can move on to the ENERGY BALANCING TECHNIQUE (coming up in a later chapter).

NOTE TO DOCTORS: *If you are taking a patient history, note all of your patients symptoms and file them along with a picture taken of them today (digital or Polaroid) with whatever therapy you are going to give them (adjustment, herbal supplements, vitamins, exercise, diet, etc.). Thirty days later bring your patient back in to be looked at again. Take a new history and take a new picture and compare the two. The results can be staggering.* At this point you have already performed a full-face reading.

*Have your patient rate each area of irritation on a 1-10 scale, 10 being worst and 0 being the best or most desirable. If kidney issues show up on the face that you are looking at, do the following:

Questions to ask to establish KIDNEY weakness

WHAT YOU MIGHT SEE WITH A PERSON LIKE THIS - *Darkness or puffiness under or around the eyes. You may also see growths, wrinkles or discolorations in the right or left eye bag region under each eye.*

Do you feel pain or stiffness or soreness in the left side of your neck?

Have you been told you have Tempro-Mandibular Joint (TMJ) issues?

Do you feel pain or stiffness or soreness in the left trapezoid muscle?

Do you feel pain or stiffness or soreness in the left pectoral?

Do you feel pain or stiffness or soreness in the left scapula?

Do you feel pain or stiffness or soreness in the left bicep?

Do you feel pain or stiffness or soreness in the left triceps?

Do you feel pain or stiffness or soreness in the left elbow?

Do you feel pain or stiffness or soreness in the left upper forearm?

Do you feel pain or stiffness or soreness in the RIGHT lower forearm?

Do you feel pain or stiffness or soreness in the left lower forearm?

Do you feel pain or stiffness or soreness in the left wrist?

Do you feel pain or stiffness or soreness in the RIGHT wrist?

Have you been told that you have carpel tunnel syndrome in either wrist?

Do you feel pain or stiffness or soreness in the left hand?

Do you feel pain or stiffness or soreness in the RIGHT hand?

Do you feel pain or stiffness or soreness in the left fingers or thumb?

Do you feel pain or stiffness or soreness in the RIGHT fingers or thumb?

Do you feel pain or stiffness or soreness in the upper left back area?

Do you feel pain or stiffness or soreness in the center mid back area?

Do you feel pain or stiffness or soreness in the left center back area?

Do you feel pain or stiffness or soreness in the RIGHT lower back area?

Do you feel pain or stiffness or soreness in the left lower back area?

Do you feel pain or stiffness or soreness in the RIGHT hip area?

Do you feel pain or stiffness or soreness in the left hip area?

Do you feel pain or stiffness or soreness in the left hamstring area?

Do you feel pain or stiffness or soreness in the RIGHT hamstring area?

Do you feel pain or stiffness or soreness in the left front thigh area?
Do you feel pain or stiffness or soreness in the RIGHT thigh area?
Do you feel pain or stiffness or soreness in the left knee area?
Do you feel pain or stiffness or soreness in the RIGHT knee area?
Do you feel pain or stiffness or soreness in the left calf area?
Do you feel pain or stiffness or soreness in the RIGHT calf area?
Do you feel pain or stiffness or soreness in the left ankle area?
Do you feel pain or stiffness or soreness in the RIGHT ankle area?
Do you feel pain or stiffness or soreness in the left foot area?
Do you feel pain or stiffness or soreness in the Right foot area?
Do you feel pain or stiffness or soreness in the left foot toes?
Do you feel pain or stiffness or soreness in the Right foot toes?
Do you have dizziness / vertigo in the left ear?
Do you have dizziness / vertigo in the right ear?
Do you have ringing / tinnitus in the left ear?
Do you have ringing / tinnitus in the right ear?
Have you ever had kidney stones?
Are you prone to kidney stones?
Do you frequently urinate during the night (more than once)?
Do you experience arthritis- like symptoms in your joints?
Have you had any swollen joints (with or without pain)?
Do you have floaters (clear shapes) cross your field of vision?
Do you have or have you had weak nails that chip or break?
Do you have high blood pressure?
Have you had gout?
Have you been told you have diabetes?
Are you aware of having any "diabetic" symptoms?
Are any of your muscles ever numb or tingly?
Do you eat a diet high in meat protein?
Do you eat a diet high in peanuts, walnuts, almonds, cashews, pistachios or other nuts?
Are you exhausted a short time after eating?
Are you exhausted from 3 pm till 11 pm daily?
Do you find that your energy is often depleted throughout the day?
Do you need a nap before bedtime?
Do you need a nap before dinner?
Have you been told that you have weak adrenal glands?
Do you consume caffeine?
Do you consume sodium?
Do you consume salt?
Are you retaining water?
Is there a history of kidney problems in your family?
**Have you taken or used Ephedra (Ma Wang)?

**Have you taken or used cocaine?
**Have you taken stimulants?
**Do you take stimulants?
**Have you taken Cialis, Levitra, Viagra or like substances?
**Have you taken any other cocaine like substances?

** These substances are damaging to the kidneys, as they are heavy stimulants.
NOTE: *Kidney issues often present themselves as pain, weakness or stiffness of the left side of the body first.*

The above are the questions you would ask to establish kidney weakness.

Questions to ask to establish a BLADDER (run by the kidneys) problem:

WHAT YOU MIGHT SEE WITH A PERSON LIKE THIS - *Corners of the forehead broken out or creased, puffy or discolored. You may also notice a receding hairline or little or no hair on the head.*

Do you have pain or discomfort in the bladder?
Do you have trouble urinating?
Do you feel intense pressure when urinating?
Do you frequently have to urinate?
Have you ever had a bladder infection?
Do you have a history of bladder infections?
Has urination caused pain, burning or itching?
Does your bladder swell?
Is your bladder swollen?
Do you have trouble with the leaking of urine (incontinence)?
Is your scalp frequently itchy?
Is your scalp frequently broken out?
Is your scalp dry?
Have you suddenly started to lose your hair?
Do you consume caffeine?
Do you consume sodium?
Do you consume salt?
Are you retaining water?
Is there a history of bladder problems in your family?
**Have you taken or used Ephedra (Ma Wang)?
**Have you taken or used cocaine?
**Have you taken stimulants?
**Do you take stimulants?
**Have you taken Cialis, Levitra, Viagra or like substances?
**Have you taken any other cocaine like substances?

** These substances are damaging to the bladder, as they are heavy stimulants.

The above are the questions you would ask to establish a bladder weakness.

Questions to ask to establish a HEART weakness (run by the kidneys):

WHAT YOU MIGHT SEE WITH A PERSON LIKE THIS - *Deep furrows or creases on the earlobes, a red or irritated nose, scars, blemishes or moles on the nose, redness, blemishes or wrinkling on the upper lip.*

Does your heart double beat?
Does your heart skip a beat?
Does your heart flutter?
Have you had any discomfort in the chest?
Do you feel faint from time to time?
Do you feel severe pounding in your chest during some light activities?
Have you had heart surgery?
Do you have congestive heart failure?
Are you taking heart medications?
Have you had a heart attack?
Have you had a stroke?
Does your heart pound late at night for no apparent reason?
Is there a history of heart problems in your family?
Do you consume caffeine?
Do you consume sodium?
Do you consume salt?
Are you retaining water?
**Have you taken or used Ephedra (Ma Wang)?
**Have you taken or used cocaine?
**Have you taken stimulants?
**Do you take stimulants?
**Have you taken Cialis, Levitra, Viagra or like substances?
**Have you taken any other cocaine like substances?

** These substances are damaging to the heart, as they are heavy stimulants.

The above are the questions you would ask to establish a heart weakness.

Questions to ask to establish a REPRODUCTIVE SYSTEM weakness (run by the kidneys)

WHAT YOU MIGHT SEE WITH A PERSON LIKE THIS - *The chin may be heavily creased, red, irritated with acne, scars, swelling or moles.*

Have you experienced sexual performance issues?
Do you have a difficult time staying aroused?
Do you suffer with a lack of interest in sex?
Do you suffer with a lack of lubrication during sex?
Do you suffer from a lack of orgasm during sex?
Do you experience unexpected pain during sex?
Do you have a low sperm count?
Do you have trouble getting pregnant?
Have you had an abortion?
Have you taken fertility drugs?
Do you have heavy bleeding during your period?
Do you have ovarian cysts?
Do you have uterine cysts?
Do you experience unusual vaginal discharge?
Have you had issues related to the uterus?
Do you experience heavy cramps during your period?
Is your scrotum overly sensitive to the touch?
Do you experience a lack of sensation in the penis?
Do you often have low back pain?
Do you have dull or sharp pain in the groin area?
**Have you taken or used Ephedra (Ma Wang)?
**Have you taken or used cocaine?
**Have you taken stimulants?
**Do you take stimulants?
**Have you taken Cialis, Levitra, Viagra or like substances?
**Have you taken any other cocaine like substances?
The above covers the questions you would ask to establish a reproductive system weakness.

Questions to ask to establish a LIVER WEAKNESS

WHAT YOU MIGHT SEE WITH A PERSON LIKE THIS - *Deep furrow or blemishes between the eyebrows, deep crow's feet, blemishes on the left or right outside of either eye, red, burning, watery or irritated eyes.*

Do you feel pain stiffness or soreness in the RIGHT side of your neck?
Do you feel pain stiffness or soreness in the RIGHT base of your skull?
Do you feel pain stiffness or soreness in the RIGHT trapezoid muscle?
Do you feel pain stiffness or soreness in the RIGHT rotator cuff region of your shoulder?
Do you feel pain stiffness or soreness in the RIGHT deltoid region of your shoulder?

Do you feel pain stiffness or soreness in the RIGHT scapula area?
Do you feel pain stiffness or soreness in the RIGHT pectoral muscle?
Do you feel pain stiffness or soreness in the RIGHT Latissimus Dorsi muscle?
Do you feel pain stiffness or soreness in the RIGHT area just under the RIGHT rib cage?
Do you feel pain stiffness or soreness in the RIGHT rib cage area?
Do you feel pain stiffness or soreness in the RIGHT bicep?
Do you feel pain stiffness or soreness in the RIGHT Triceps?
Do you have a hard time sleeping between 11pm and 5 am?
Do you get unexpectedly depressed or does your depression linger?
Do you get angry at times?
Are you moody?
Do you get irritable?
Does your energy fluctuate off and on all daylong?
Do you need a nap during the day?
Do you get fearful or paranoid?
Are you obsessive or compulsive about situations in life?
Do you find it hard to stay in a good mood?
Do you have brief outbursts?
Do you have long outbursts?
Do you stay angry longer than you should?
Does it take a superhuman effort to control your anger?
When you get upset do your ears get hot?
Do you warm all over when you are upset?
Do you have a hard time concentrating?
Do you have a poor memory?
Do you feel drugged at times?
Do you feel dull at times?
Do you have fuzzy vision at times?
Do your eyes itch or burn during the day?
Do your eyes water?
Does the room seem dimly lit at times?
Do you wake up sneezing?
Does your nose frequently run?
Does your nose get stuffy?
Do your sinuses get full or stuffy?
Do you get sinus headaches?
Do your lungs get congested?
Do you wake up coughing?
Do your eyes burn or itch on waking?
Do you always want to rub your eyes?
Do you have sneezing fits without warning?
Do you have random headaches that quickly disappear?

Does your skin burn anywhere?
Are you prone to rashes?
Is your skin sensitive?
Does cologne make you sneeze?
Does perfume make you sneeze?
Does cigarette smoke make you sneeze?
Are there other substances that make you sneeze?
Do certain scents make you groggy?
Does your tongue burn?
Does the inside of your mouth burn?
Does your throat burn?
Do you have skin that is numb anywhere?
Do you have skin that tingles anywhere?
Do you have skin that itches or is routinely itchy in a certain place?
Have you been told that you have high cholesterol?
Have you been told that you have high liver enzymes?
Have you been told that you have gallstones?
Do you have liver spots?
Do you have age spots?
Do you have skin tags?
Do you have strawberry marks?
Do you have acne?
Do you have boils?
Do you have allergies?

The above covers the questions you would ask to establish a liver weakness.

Questions to ask to establish a LUNG WEAKNESS

WHAT YOU MIGHT SEE WITH A PERSON LIKE THIS - *Deep furrow, blemishes, creasing, age spots, sun spots, liver spots, growths, acne, boils, redness flaking or irritation in on the hollow of either cheek.*

Do you experience pain in the right side of your chest?
Do you experience pain in the left side of your chest?
Do you get short of breath?
Does it hurt to take a deep breath?
Is something restricting your breathing?
Do you cough in the morning?
Do you cough during the day?
Do you wake up coughing at night?
Do you cough up discharge from your lungs?

Have you been diagnosed with emphysema?
Have you had pneumonia?
Have you been told that you have tuberculosis?
Have you been told that you have lung cancer?
Do you have bronchitis?
Have you been told that you have pulmonary fibrosis?
Have you been told that you have Sarcoidosis?
Have you been diagnosed with respiratory failure?
Do you have asthma?
Are you out of breath easily?
Do you smoke?
Are you around air borne toxins?
Do you use an inhaler?

The above covers the questions you would ask to establish a lung weakness.

Questions to ask to establish a STOMACH WEAKNESS

Do you have a stiff right elbow?
Do you have right forearm pain?
Do you have right forearm soreness?
Do you have ulcers?
Do you have gas?
Do you experience heartburn?
Do you experience acid reflux?
Do you experience GERD (Gastroesophgeal Reflux Disease)?
Do you experience indigestion?
Do you use antacids?
Do certain foods set you off?
Do you often have an upset stomach?
Do you get bloated?
Do get abdominal distention?
Do you belch more than a little after you eat?
Do you feel tired after you eat?
Do you have a Hiatal hernia?

The above covers the questions you would ask to establish a stomach weakness.

Questions to ask to establish an INTESTINAL WEAKNESS (small intestines)

Do you have a stiff right elbow?
Do you experience pain / cramping just above the right hip?
Do you experience abdominal pain or soreness?
Do you experience abdominal spasms?
Is your abdomen sensitive to direct pressure?
Do you have gas?
Is your abdomen distended (bloated)?
Do you carry your weight in your abdominal area?
Are you overweight?
Are you constipated less-than-one-elimination-per-mea-eaten?
Do you experience indigestion?
Do certain foods set you off?

The above covers the questions you would ask to establish an intestinal weakness.

Questions to ask to establish a COLON WEAKNESS

Do you have a stiff right elbow?
Do you experience pain / cramping just above the right hip (ileocecal valve)?
Do you experience abdominal pain or soreness?
Do you experience abdominal spasms?
Have you been told that you have leaky gut syndrome?
Have you been told that you have polyps?
Have you been told that you have ulcerative colitis?
Have you been told that you have diverticulitis?
Have you been told that you have diverticulosis?
Have you been told that you have IBS (irritable bowel syndrome)?
Have you been told that you have Crohn's disease?
Have you been told that you have chronic fatigue syndrome?
Have you been told that you have Epstein-Barr?
Have you been told that you have Sprue?
Have you been told that you have H. pylori (Heliobacter pylori)?
Do you suffer with hemorrhoids?
Do you have candida?
Do you have bloody stools?
Do you have painful stools?
Do you have foul smelling stools?
Do you have foul gas?
Do you have to use laxatives to eliminate?
Is your abdomen sensitive to direct pressure?
Is your abdomen distended (bloated)?
Do you carry your weight in your abdominal area?

Are you constipated less-than-one-elimination-per-meal-eaten?

The above covers the questions you would ask to establish a colon weakness.

Questions to ask to establish an ENDOCRINE SYSTEM challenge

Do you often feel extremely hot?
Do you often feel extremely cold?
Do you often feel dizzy?
Do you often lose your balance?
Do you often feel faint at times?
Do you sometimes faint?
If you do not eat right away do you feel faint?
Do you sometimes feel light headed?
Do you often feel overwhelmingly exhausted?
Do you often feel overwhelmingly hyper energized?
Do you often feel wired or jumpy?
Do you have low blood pressure?
Does your heart suddenly race for no reason?
Do you suddenly start sweating for no reason?
Can you not put on weight?
Do you never feel hungry?
When hungry, is your vision dark or cloudy?
Is your thinking often cloudy?
Do you suddenly have poor concentration?
Do you become forgetful?
Are you always forgetful?
Can you suddenly get very moody?
Are your armpits often sore or swollen?
Is either side of your groin area often sore or swollen?
Do you often see clear shapes (floaters) in your vision?
Do your breasts produce milk long after pregnancy?
Do you have a persistent infection?
Do you have a persistent allergy?
Do you have a persistent cold symptom?

SPECIAL NOTE: *It is not unusual to find the Endocrine Strip red and irritated when a person has a history of drinking alcohol or has a diet high in oils or protein derived from nuts. These oils coat not only the liver (see chapter Oil a Life Obsession) but block all major glands of the body.*

The above covers the questions you would ask to establish an endocrine system weakness.

32 Face Reading Gallery

The following photos are examples of what can be seen and diagnosed with the use of Face Reading. Utilize this section of my book to interest your patients in face reading. Hand them this book opened to the gallery section and tell them to look at the pictures and descriptions. Direct them to a mirror so that they can compare their face to the photos. With these photos you have the tools and the power to understand and change your own personal conditions. These photos are a gift that you can use or ignore. But once you read this book, to turn your back on what you have learned is tantamount to committing treason against yourself.

Since you are your own best friend, I hope that is not the case.

ORIGIN
The origin of face reading is unknown.

DEFINITIONS

FACE: Etymology: Middle English, from Old French, from (assumed) Vulgar Latin facia, from Latin facies make, form, face, from facere to make, do—more at DO.
1 a: the front part of the human head including the chin, mouth, nose, cheeks, eyes, and usually the forehead.
b: the face as a means of identification: COUNTENANCE <would know that face anywhere>

READING
Etymology: Middle English redden; to advise interpret, read, from Old English raedan; akin to Old High German; Atan to advise form Sanskrit Adhnoti he achieves, prepares.
1 a (1): to receive or take in the sense of (as letters or symbols) especially by sight or touch (2): to study the movements of (as lips) with mental formulation of the communication expressed:

UNDERSTAND, COMPREHEND
2 a: to interpret the meaning or significance of <read palms> b: FORETELL, PREDICT <able to read his fortune>

FACE READING
The study or observation of the face used to detect the state of a current health or a predisposition of future health of the organs of the body.

FACE READING™ MAP

1

3

2

2

4

4

4

6

5

5

6

8

8

7

7

11

11

7

10

10

9

12

7

12

9

13

"The face is not set; it constantly changes based on the health of our organs".

DIAGNOSTIC FACE READING™ MAP KEY

1. BLADDER/REPRODUCTIVE SYSTEM/KIDNEYS:
The BLADDER is represented by the entire scalp from hairline to neck (with or without hair).

2. RIGHT AND LEFT SIDE OF THE BLADDER:
The RIGHT and LEFT SIDE of the BLADDER is represented by the Triangular shaped areas above the RIGHT and LEFT eyebrows. The area stretches diagonally from the connection point at the bridge of the nose and the eyebrow, to the upper corner of the hairline and down to the temple.

3. THE SMALL INTESTINE:
This is represented by the middle section of the forehead extending up to the hairline.

4. THE LIVER:
Is found in 5 separate areas of the face at the bridge of the nose between the eyebrows, the crows feet area at the corners of the eyes and the eyes themselves.

5. THE KIDNEYS:
The RIGHT and LEFT kidneys are represented as the half moon area above the eye lids and the half moon area that is often puffy (kidney eye bag) below the eyes.

6. THE ADRENAL GLANDS:
The RIGHT and LEFT adrenal glands are found at the lower outside corner of the RIGHT and LEFT kidney eye bags. They are seen as a raised area the shape of a black-eyed pea.

7. THE HEART:
The HEART is found in THREE places. THE NOSE, THE AREA BELOW THE NOSE including the UPPER LIP, stretching from smile line to smile line and the EARLOBES.

8. THE STOMACH:
Is represented by the right and left cheekbones.

9. THE LUNGS:
The RIGHT and LEFT LUNGS are represented as the RIGHT and LEFT hollow of each cheek.

10. THE COLON:
The colon is found at the smile lines stretching from the nose to the mouth.

11. THE ILEOCECAL VALVE:
The deep crease or shadow behind the flare of the nose where it connects the skin of the face.

12. THE ENDOCRINE SYSTEM:
The ENDOCRINE SYSTEM is represented by a strip that stretches from the inside corner of the eye and nose junction, down to the jaw line. It is boarded by the kidneys, heart (nose), stomach, colon, lungs and reproductive system.

13. THE REPRODUCTIVE SYSTEM:
This is represented by the bottom lip and entire chin area between the right and left ENDOCRINE SYSTEM STRIPS.

NOTES:
- The face should not look older as it ages. Looking older is a function of organ breakdown.
- All wrinkles, acne, moles, redness, irritations and dry areas indicate organ weakness.
- The face should not have acne, accident or sickness scars (like Chicken Pox).
- If some part of the face is red, this indicates that the associated organ is heated due to stress.
- The human face is not set, it constantly changes based on the health of our internal organs.
- All white graying hair is a function of weak kidneys. Hair color often changes back.
- Always study the person you are reading with a relaxed (not smiling) face
- When reading the face, start at the scalp and work your way down area by area.

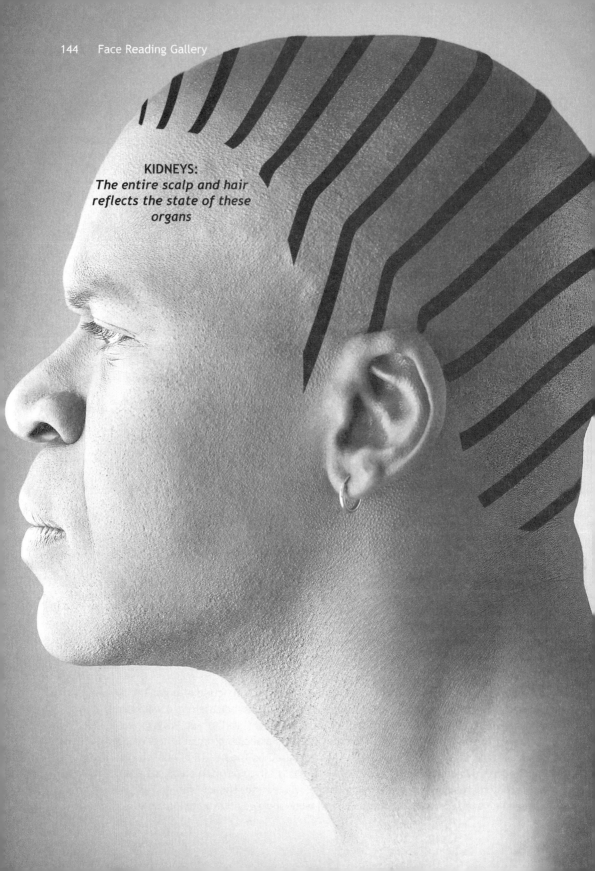

KIDNEYS:
The entire scalp and hair reflects the state of these organs

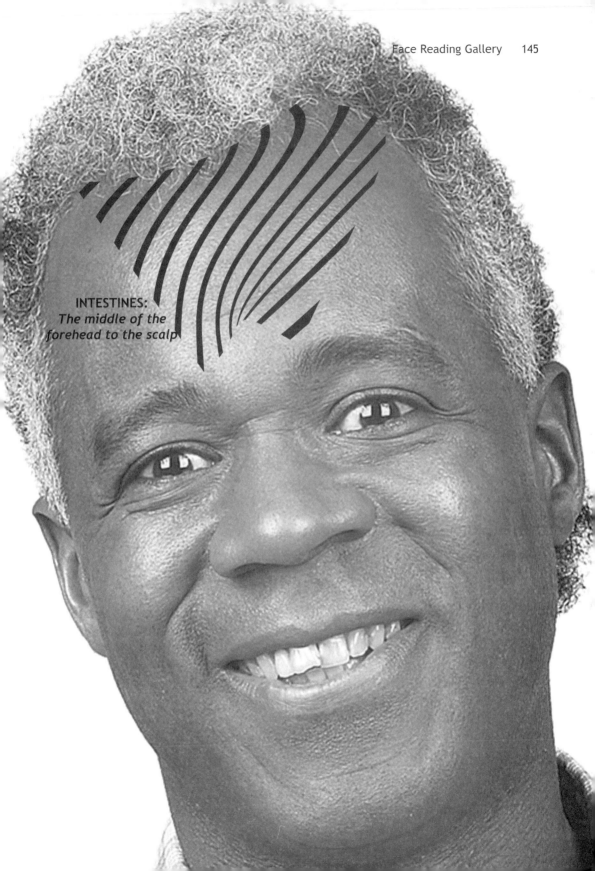

INTESTINES:
*The middle of the
forehead to the scalp*

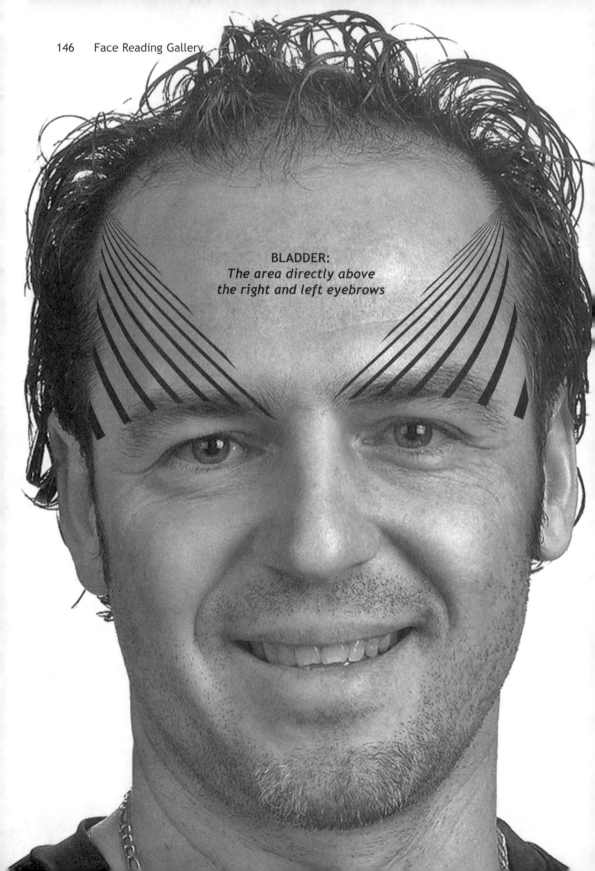

BLADDER:
*The area directly above
the right and left eyebrows*

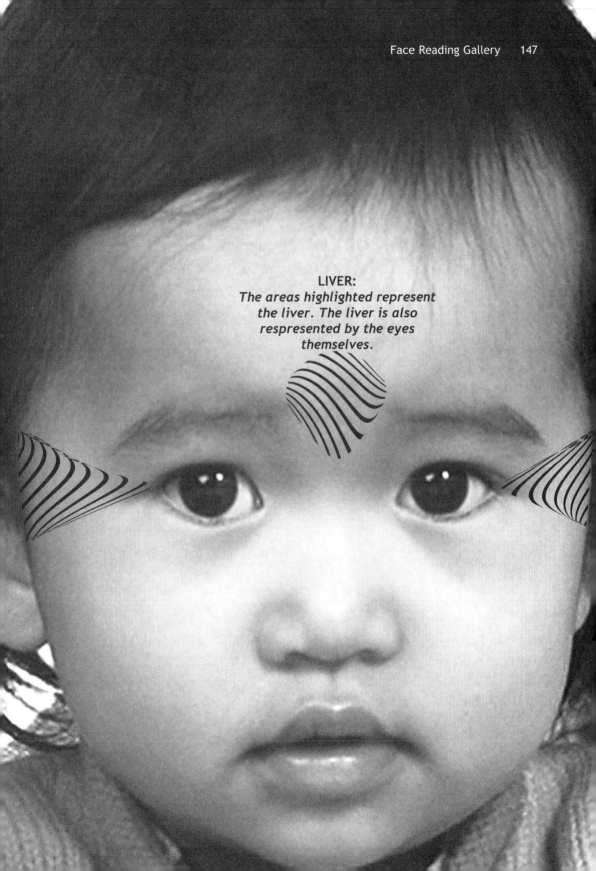

LIVER:
The areas highlighted represent the liver. The liver is also respresented by the eyes themselves.

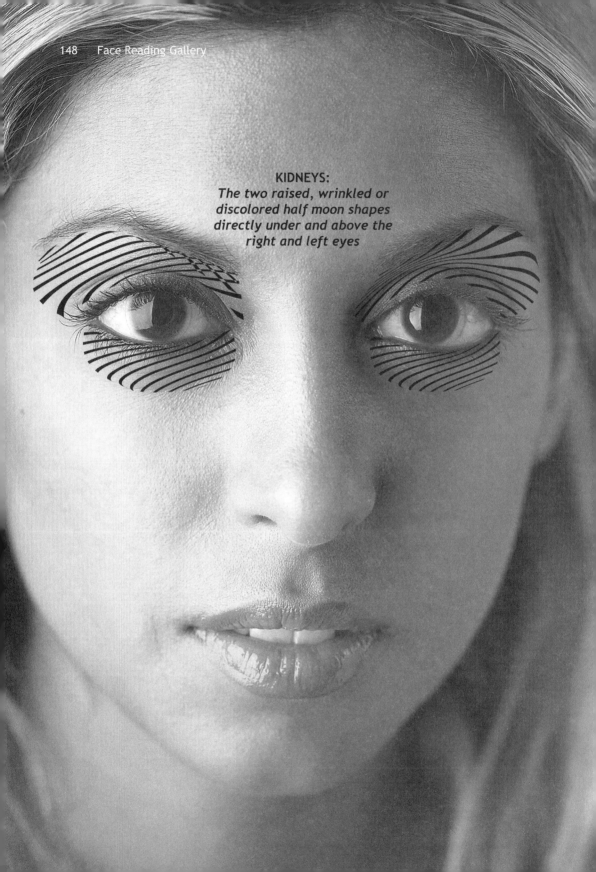

KIDNEYS:
The two raised, wrinkled or discolored half moon shapes directly under and above the right and left eyes

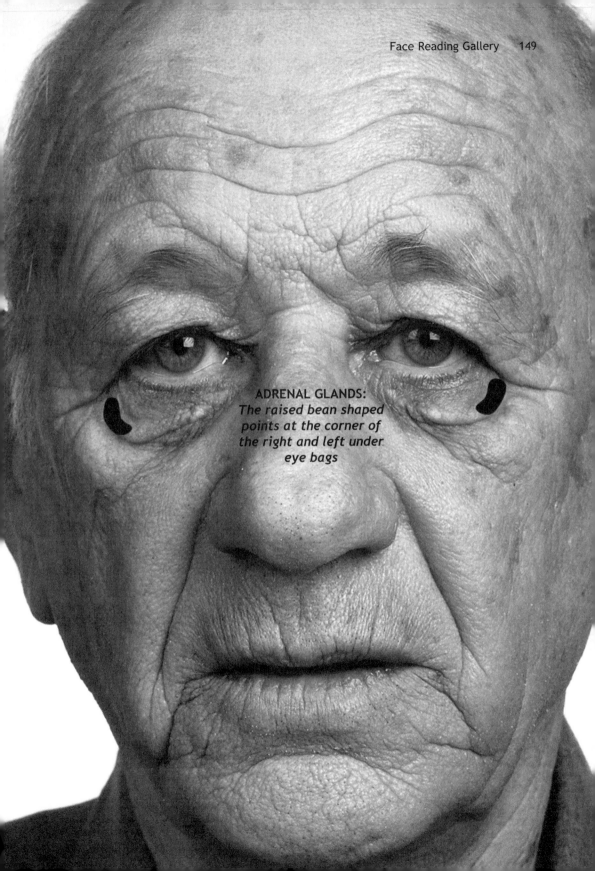

ADRENAL GLANDS:
The raised bean shaped points at the corner of the right and left under eye bags

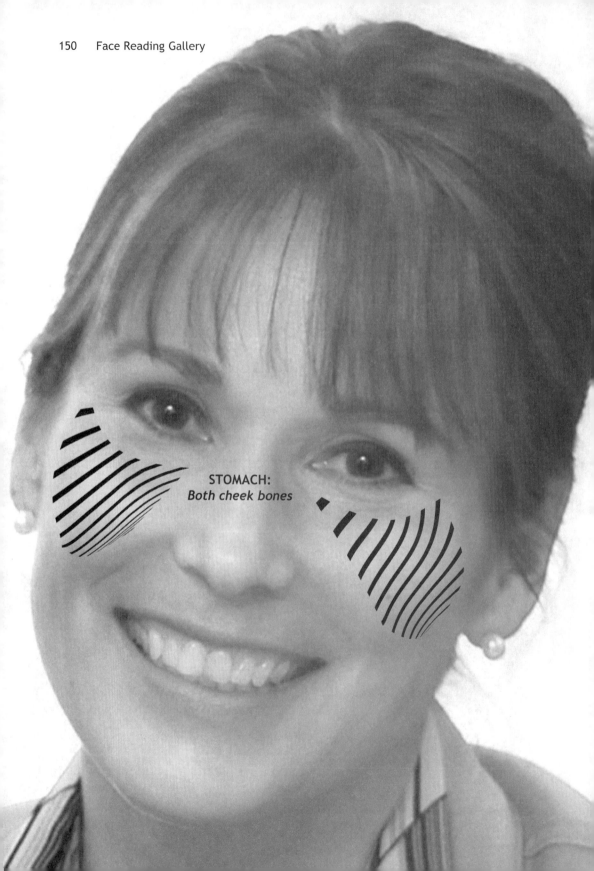

STOMACH:
Both cheek bones

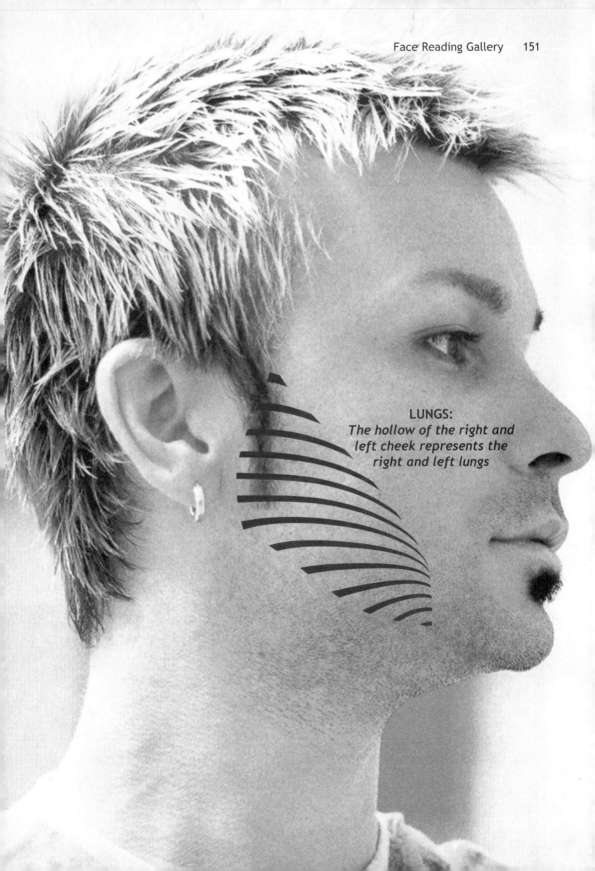

LUNGS:
The hollow of the right and left cheek represents the right and left lungs

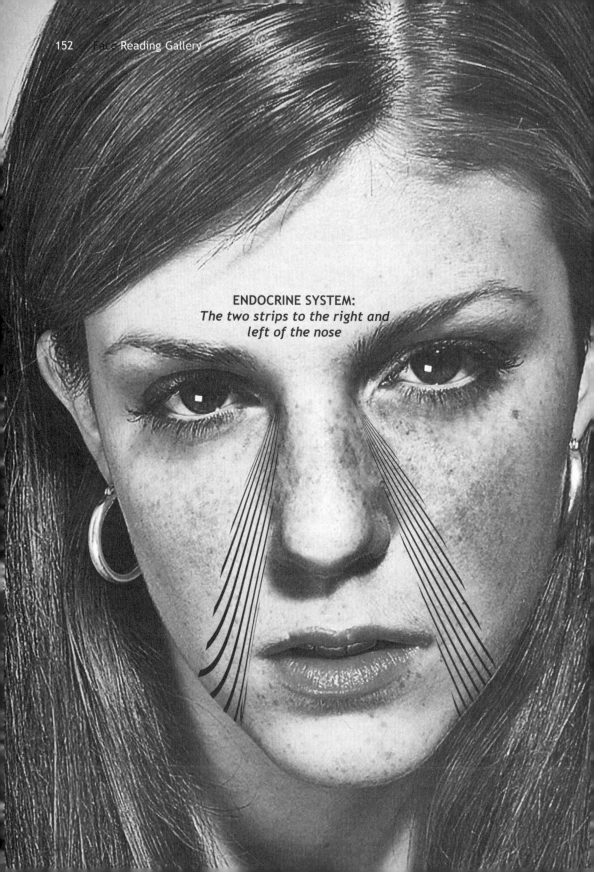

ENDOCRINE SYSTEM:
*The two strips to the right and
left of the nose*

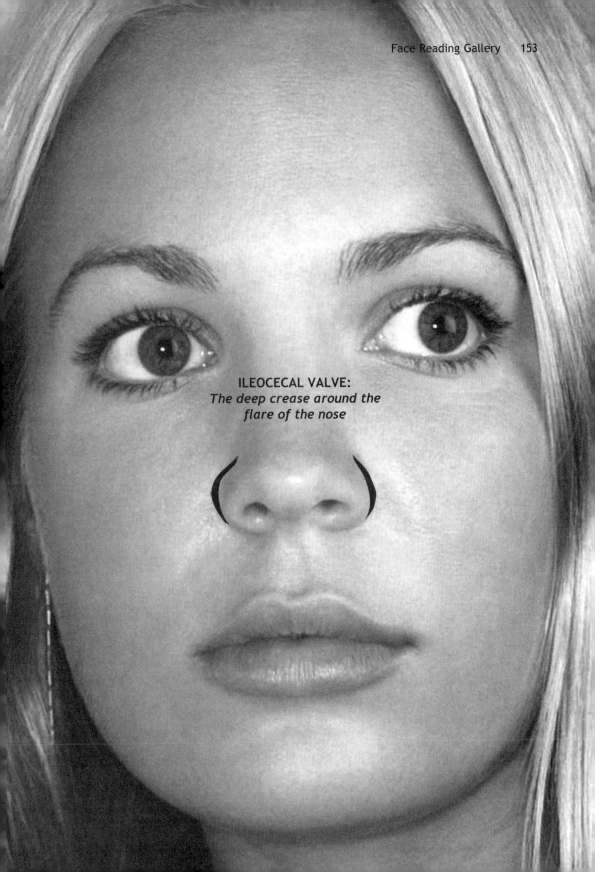

ILEOCECAL VALVE:
*The deep crease around the
flare of the nose*

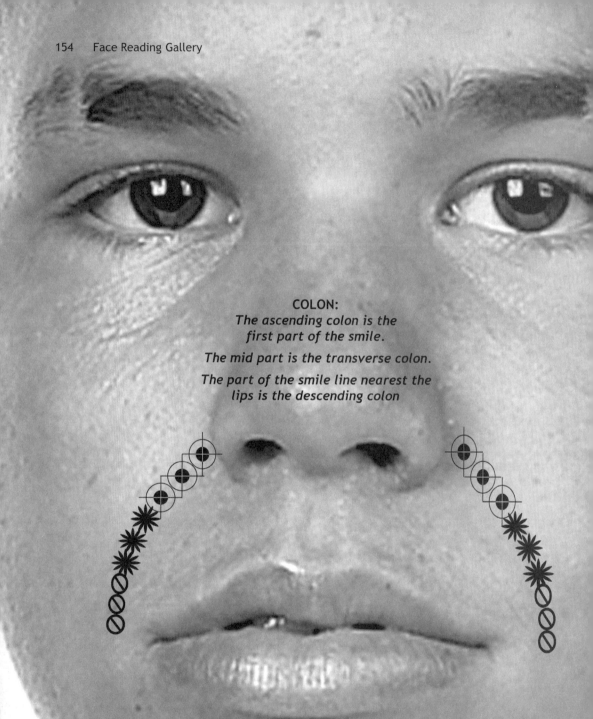

COLON:
*The ascending colon is the
first part of the smile.*

The mid part is the transverse colon.

*The part of the smile line nearest the
lips is the descending colon*

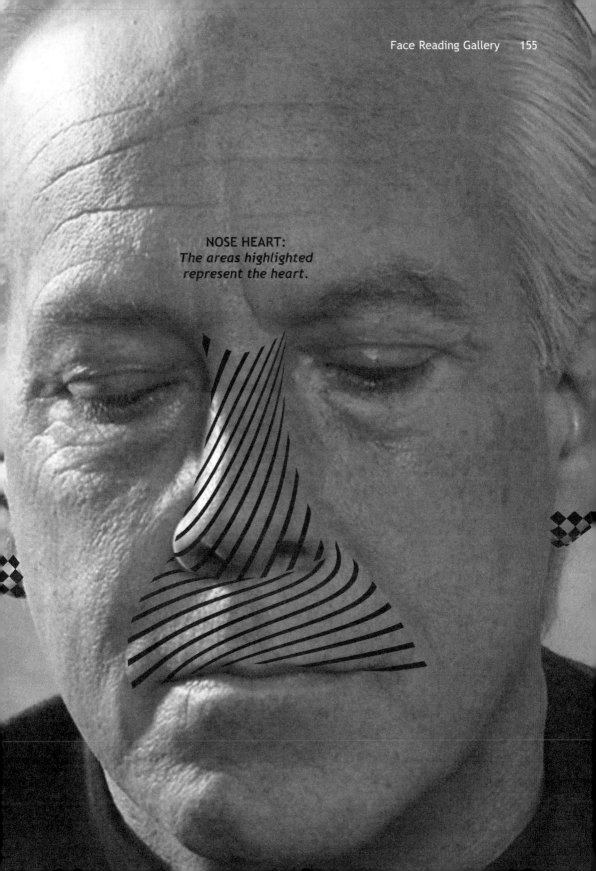

NOSE HEART:
*The areas highlighted
represent the heart.*

REPRODUCTIVE SYSTEM:
*The bottom lip and the area
below the bottom lip extending
down to the jaw line.*

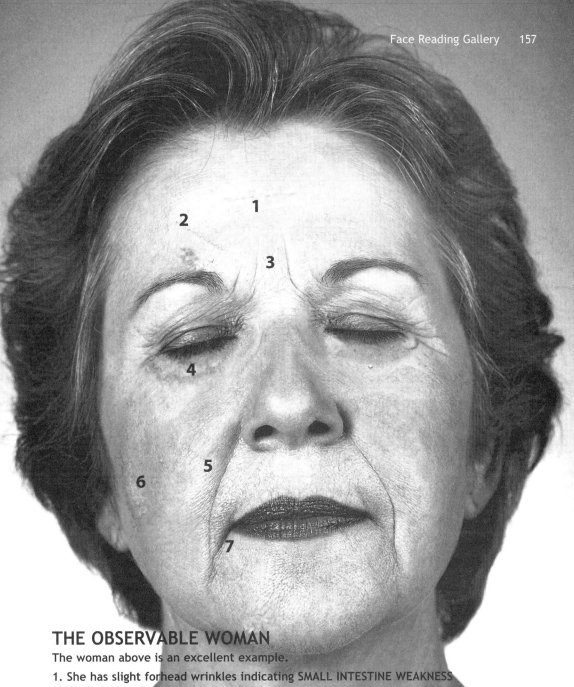

THE OBSERVABLE WOMAN

The woman above is an excellent example.

1. She has slight forhead wrinkles indicating SMALL INTESTINE WEAKNESS
2. The blemish above her RIGHT EYEBROW indicates BLADDER WEAKNESS
3. She has deep creases at the bridge of her nose indicating LIVER WEAKNESS
4. She has half moon discolorations under her right and left eye that indicate KIDNEY WEAKNESS
5. She has deep smile lines indicating COLON WEAKNESS
6. She has swelling in the hollow of right check indicating LUNG WEAKNESS
7. Her smile lines dip below the corners of her mouth indicating hemorrhoids

When I look at a face I always start at the top and work my way down. I always consult with the person about anything that I find so that I can establish if the condition is current or not.

Anyone can learn face reading, it just takes a bit of practice.

Face: Scar at hairline or upper forehead (intestines), left under eye swelling (kidney), right endocrine strip (immune system / virus issues), and slight indentations at the lower smile line (descending colon).

Problem: Built in weakness in the intestines not yet realized. There is also left kidney and adrenal gland weakness. Hemorrhoids are present and causing routine irritation.

Solution: Protect intestines via a diet rich in whole foods. Whole foods such as grapes, tomatoes, leafy green vegetables and citrus heal the kidneys and will correct her hemorrhoids.

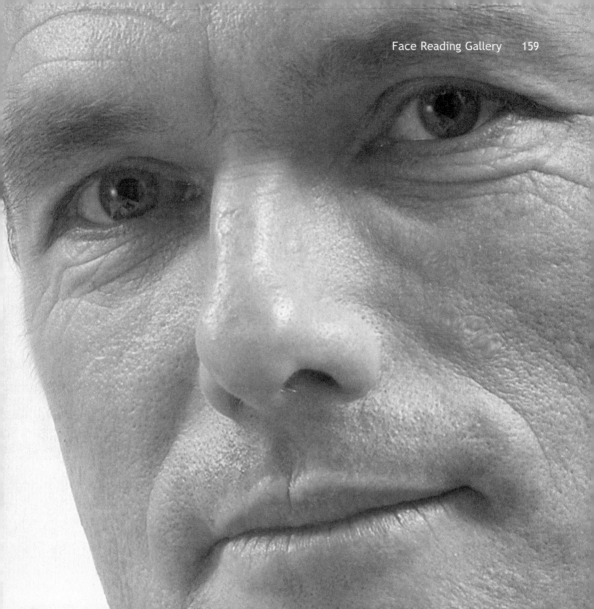

Face: Crease above right eye (bladder). Furrow at the bridge of the nose (liver). See the puffiness under both eyes (right and left kidneys). Notice the swelling in the endocrine strip near the nose (Immune system / virus issues). Defined smile lines (colon). Crease on the chin (reproductive).

Problem: The colon is blocked and irritating the entire system. Uses of prostate "healing" drugs and male virility tonics have made his condition worse.

Solution: Eliminate all breads, candy, energy drinks, alcohol, tobacco and cut down on processed meats. Do an entire body detox (a deep systemic cleanse). Eat fresh fruit, especially melons, apples, pears, plums and pineapple.

THIRTEEN AND ALREADY IN TROUBLE!

Face: Upper middle forehead blemishes (intestines). Slight wrinkling above left eye (bladder). Eyebrow ring in left brow (bladder / kidneys). There are blemishes and discoloring at bridge of the nose. She is dark under each eye (adrenal glands / kidneys). She has blemishes in the right endocrine strip (immune system). There are blemishes and discolorations on her nose (heart). She has deep smile lines (all three parts of the colon). There is a deep furrow and blemish on her chin (reproductive system / uterine / ovary irritation).

Problem: Popular caffeine loaded drinks have greatly affected her kidney function. Since she is hyper from the caffeine, her parents put her on RITALIN (which is destroying her liver, kidneys, emotions and digestive tract). Processed foods have further blocked her colon and affected her reproductive system (she is now prone to ovarian cysts). Her sleep problems are due to the caffeine; Ritalin and sugar in her diet, thus causing adrenal gland burnout.

Solution: Immediately cease Ritalin use. Cut out all caffeine and processed sugar intake including breads and pasta. Eliminate breads, pasta, rice cakes and crackers (all convert to sugar). Add fresh fruit, vegetables and juices (not juice drinks). Use liver, kidney and circulation herbs frequently 4-5 times a day as needed.

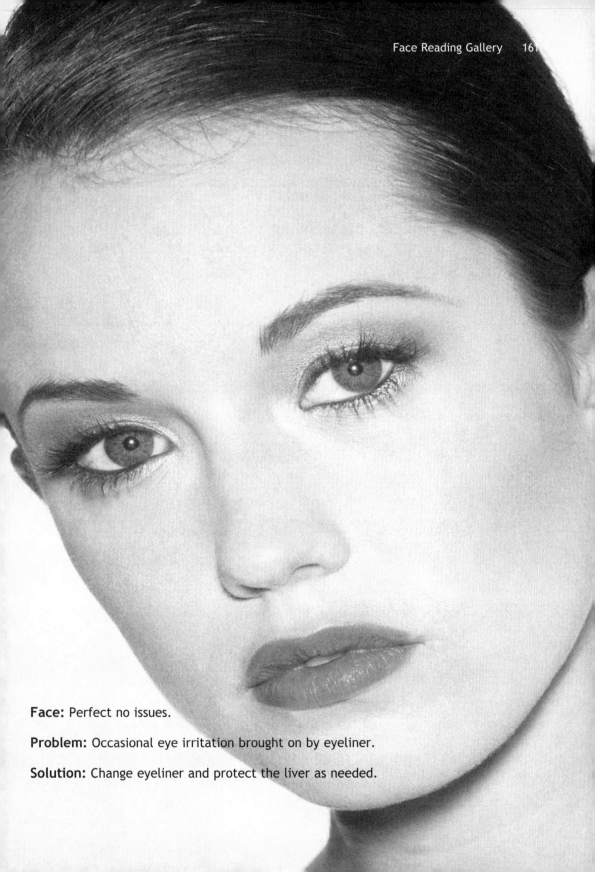

Face: Perfect no issues.

Problem: Occasional eye irritation brought on by eyeliner.

Solution: Change eyeliner and protect the liver as needed.

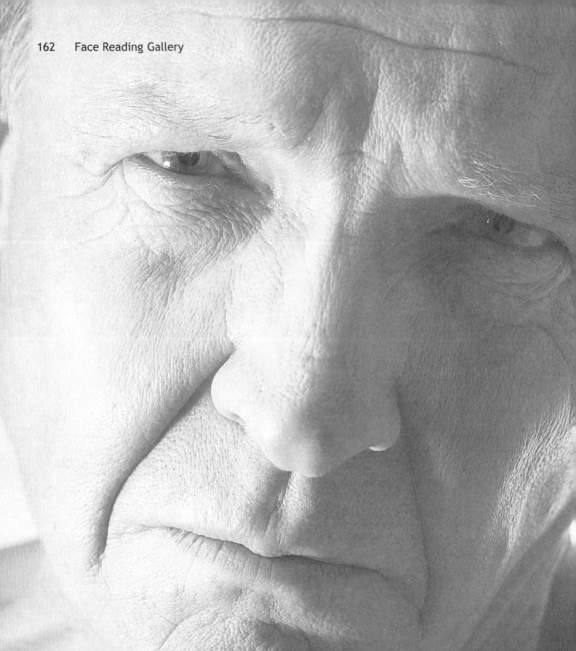

Face: Furrow on forehead (intestines), puffy under each eye (kidney), furrow at bridge of nose (liver), crow's feet (liver), deep smile lines (all three parts of the colon, deep philtrum (heart), swelling on chin (reproductive system).

Problem: Bloating, indigestion, kidney stones (right kidney) and weak prostate.

Solution: Total body cleanse, give up caffeine, smoking, dairy products and cocktails (alcohol) before bedtime.

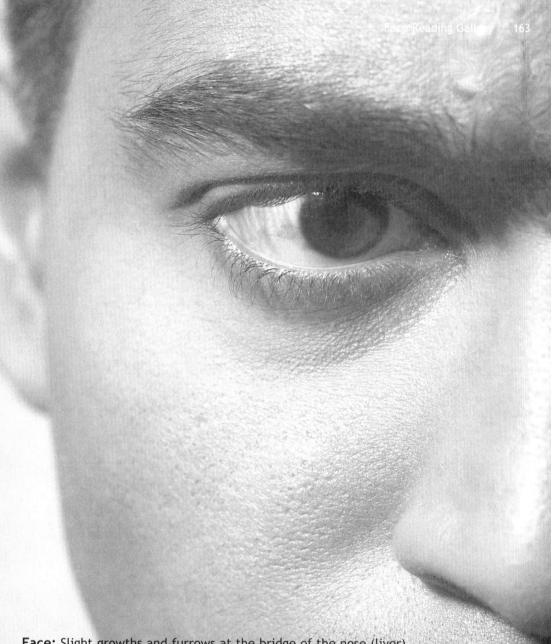

Face: Slight growths and furrows at the bridge of the nose (liver).

Problem: Poor moods brought on by use of Tylenol and other liver irritants. There is also soreness under the right ribcage.

Solution: Use of bupleurum, gentian and other beneficial liver strengthening herbs, citrus, increased water consumption, skin brushing, hot showers and elimination of all processed oils.

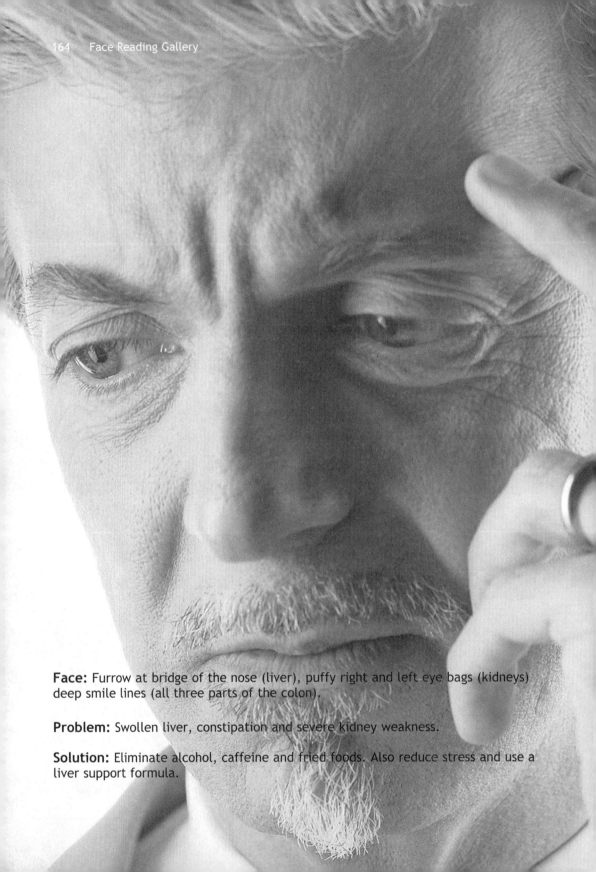

Face: Furrow at bridge of the nose (liver), puffy right and left eye bags (kidneys) deep smile lines (all three parts of the colon).

Problem: Swollen liver, constipation and severe kidney weakness.

Solution: Eliminate alcohol, caffeine and fried foods. Also reduce stress and use a liver support formula.

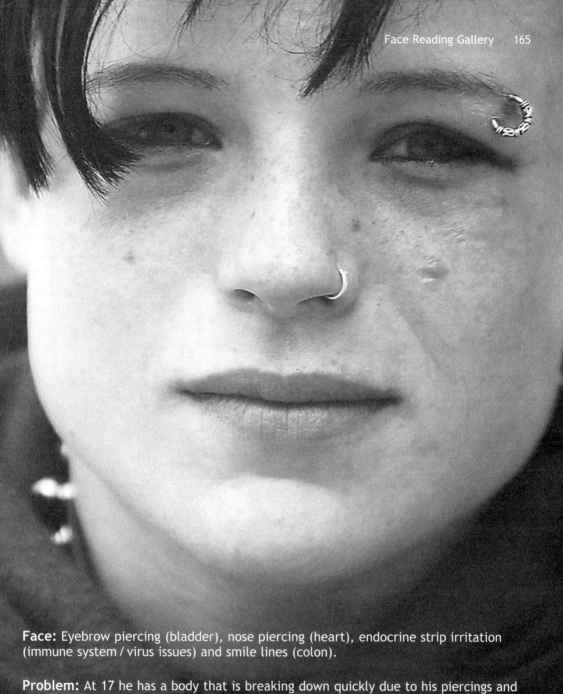

Face: Eyebrow piercing (bladder), nose piercing (heart), endocrine strip irritation (immune system / virus issues) and smile lines (colon).

Problem: At 17 he has a body that is breaking down quickly due to his piercings and tattoos. His diet is terrible and full of sugar and caffeine.

Solution: Take out all piercings, do a full liver support program, use herbs to support his immune system and completely upgrade his diet. He needs to flush and rebuild with fresh fruit and veggies.

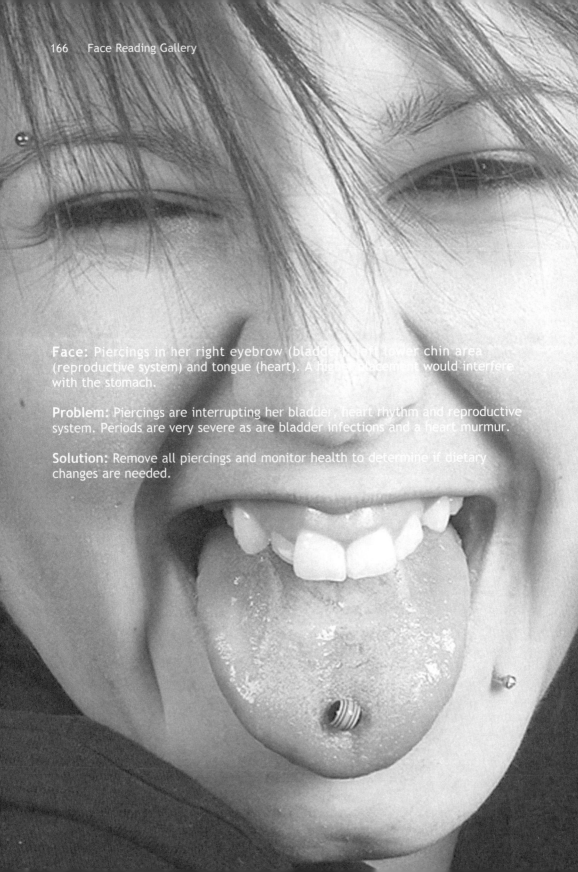

Face: Piercings in her right eyebrow (bladder), left lower chin area (reproductive system) and tongue (heart). A higher placement would interfere with the stomach.

Problem: Piercings are interrupting her bladder, heart rhythm and reproductive system. Periods are very severe as are bladder infections and a heart murmur.

Solution: Remove all piercings and monitor health to determine if dietary changes are needed.

Face: Horizontal and diagonal creases on the left and right corner of the forehead (bladder right and left side). Deep furrows across the middle of the forehead (intestines). Deep furrows at the bridge of the nose (liver). Notice the crow's feet at the outside of each eye (liver). Very puffy eye bags (right and left kidney). Dimple in the chin (reproductive system).

Problem: His bladder and kidneys are very weak and he is susceptible to kidney stones. The kidneys are very swollen which gives him "arthritis-like" symptoms all over his body. His prostate is swollen as his kidneys regulate it.

Solution: Lose forty pounds via diet and exercise (after a physical). Eliminate caffeine, salt, white sugar and all artificial sweeteners. No more alcoholic "nightcaps" before bedtime. No eating six hours before bedtime unless it is fresh fruit or juice.

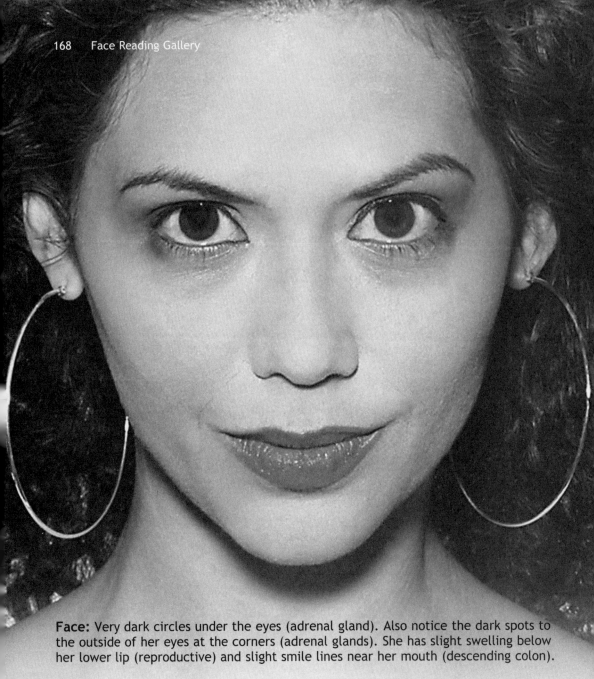

Face: Very dark circles under the eyes (adrenal gland). Also notice the dark spots to the outside of her eyes at the corners (adrenal glands). She has slight swelling below her lower lip (reproductive) and slight smile lines near her mouth (descending colon).

Problem: Caffeine and a lack of sleep are burning out her adrenal glands causing low back pain and left shoulder pain. Her diet is full of rice and grains and they are congesting her colon and irritating her reproductive system.

Solution: Get off coffee and all sweetened drinks. Consume grapes, tomatoes, citrus and fruit juices. Use herbs to support her kidneys.

Face: Scar on the tip of the nose (heart), middle and low smile lines (transverse and descending colon).

Problem: Slight weakness in the heart (double beating and skipping a beat), slight constipation.

Solution: Cayenne, Hawthorne Berry, Wasabi Japonica and various heart and circulation aiding herbs. Constipation aided by increased water consumption and fewer processed foods (bread, cookies, rice, pasta and cereals).

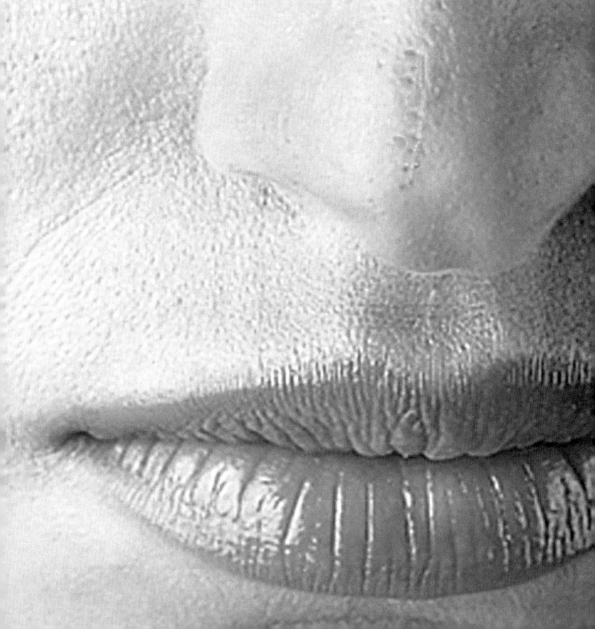

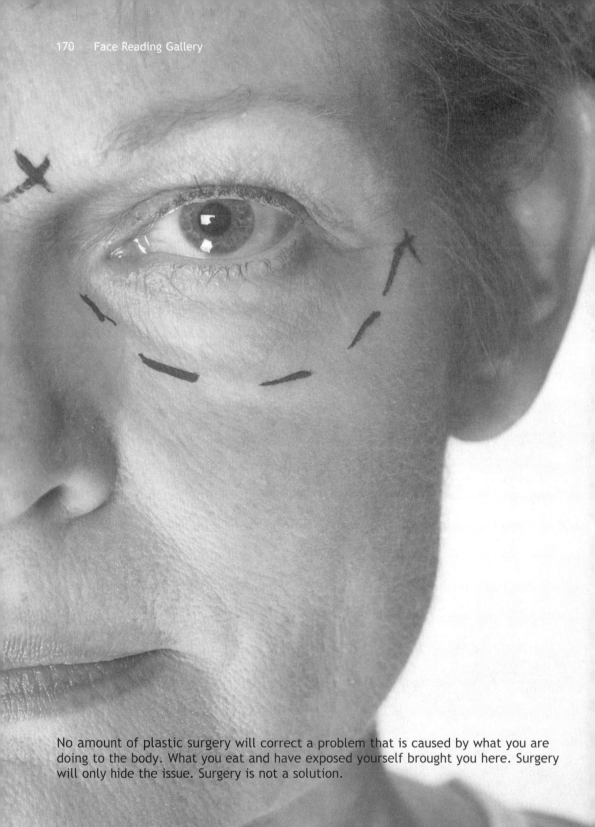

No amount of plastic surgery will correct a problem that is caused by what you are doing to the body. What you eat and have exposed yourself brought you here. Surgery will only hide the issue. Surgery is not a solution.

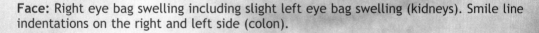

Face: Right eye bag swelling including slight left eye bag swelling (kidneys). Smile line indentations on the right and left side (colon).

Problem: Medium right kidney swelling and slight left kidney swelling. Colon congestion is present and frequent constipation including hemorrhoids.

Solution: Cut out use of ephedra for weight control and eliminate green tea (full of caffeine). Start using grape juice to help purge the colon. Also reduce salt intake.

Face: Slight creasing above the left eyebrow (left side of the bladder). Notice the small growth at the left nostril of her nose (heart = 20% chance of trouble). She has a deep or defined philtrum (indentation on the upper lip below her nose – heart = 20% chance of trouble) Near the mouth, notice the deep crease (descending colon and hemorrhoids). Notice the irritation on her chin (reproductive system).

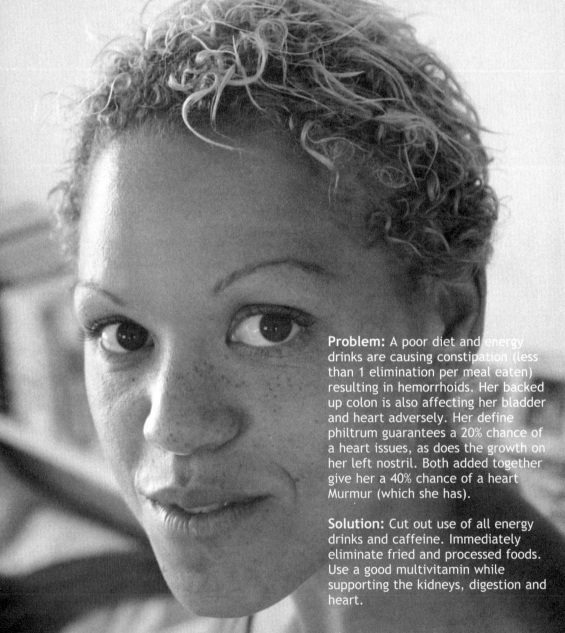

Problem: A poor diet and energy drinks are causing constipation (less than 1 elimination per meal eaten) resulting in hemorrhoids. Her backed up colon is also affecting her bladder and heart adversely. Her define philtrum guarantees a 20% chance of a heart issues, as does the growth on her left nostril. Both added together give her a 40% chance of a heart Murmur (which she has).

Solution: Cut out use of all energy drinks and caffeine. Immediately eliminate fried and processed foods. Use a good multivitamin while supporting the kidneys, digestion and heart.

Heart Murmur = Double beating and or skipping a beat to varying degrees.

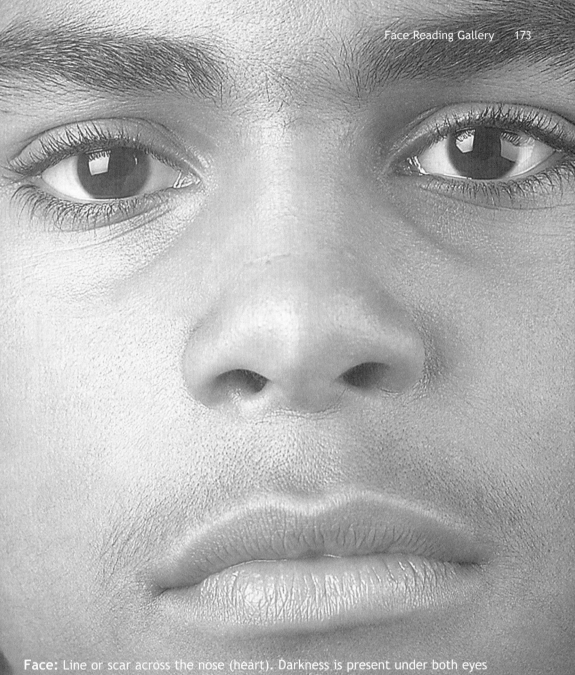

Face: Line or scar across the nose (heart). Darkness is present under both eyes (kidneys). Notice the slight puffiness on the chin (reproductive system).

Problem: He has a slight weakness in his heart that was inherited. His kidneys are also a bit weak as is his reproductive system.

Solution: Cut out all caffeinated beverages, fried foods, fast foods and white sugar.

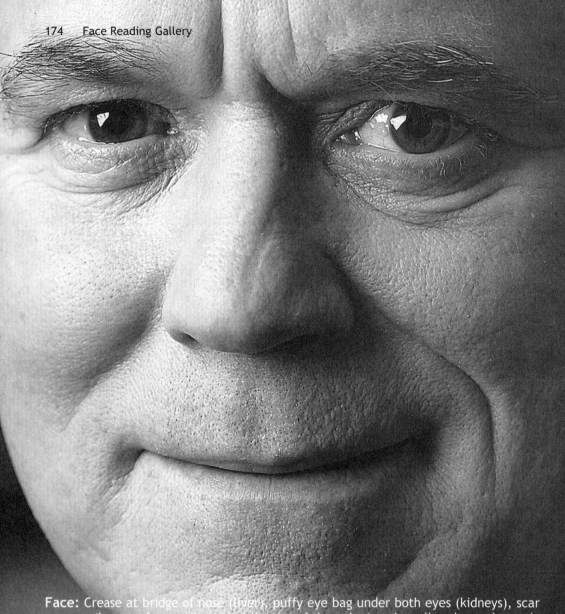

Face: Crease at bridge of nose (liver), puffy eye bag under both eyes (kidneys), scar on nose (heart), deep smile lines (all parts of the colon) and small moles and creasing on his chin (reproductive system).

Problem: Drinking has caused severe liver and kidney issues; his poor diet full of meat protein has clogged his colon and his reproductive system is in near shut down for the same reasons. His heart is moderately weak as well.

Solution: Cut out all alcohol; switch over to a raw food diet and use a colon formula to open up his congested colon. His heart will respond to cinnamon and grapes, as will his kidneys.

Face: Blemish at bridge of nose (liver), growths and darkness under left eye (kidney), small growths in the endocrine strip (immune issues / virus issues).

Problem: Poor moods, insomnia, irritated eyes, left shoulder pain. Left low back pain, routine lumbar and low thoracic subluxations. There are also immune system and glandular issues (i.e. hypoglycemia) present.

Solution: Stop drinking beer and smoking marijuana; drink more water, employ citrus, cut out white sugar, added salt and get more sleep. Use herbs to repair circulation, oxygen and energy movement in the body. Use them further to repair kidney function.

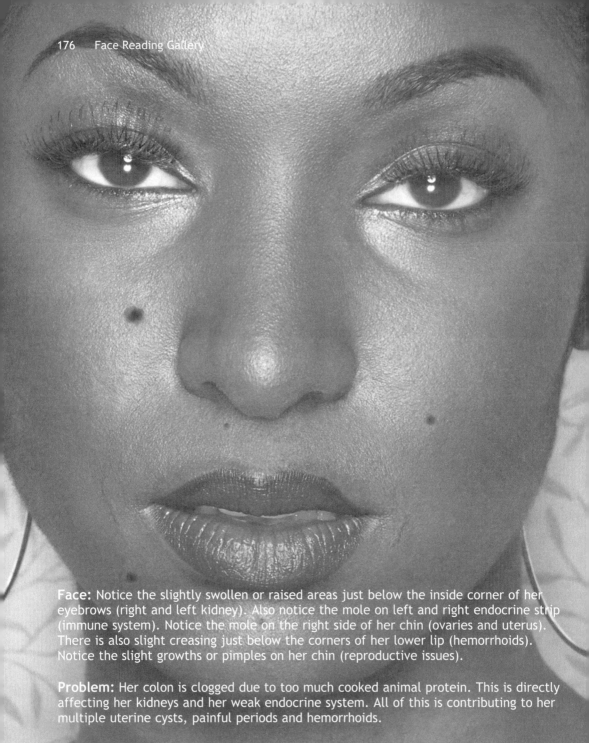

Face: Notice the slightly swollen or raised areas just below the inside corner of her eyebrows (right and left kidney). Also notice the mole on left and right endocrine strip (immune system). Notice the mole on the right side of her chin (ovaries and uterus). There is also slight creasing just below the corners of her lower lip (hemorrhoids). Notice the slight growths or pimples on her chin (reproductive issues).

Problem: Her colon is clogged due to too much cooked animal protein. This is directly affecting her kidneys and her weak endocrine system. All of this is contributing to her multiple uterine cysts, painful periods and hemorrhoids.

Solution: Eliminate cooked animal protein and watch the cysts to detect if there are other factors (birth control pills, caffeine, etc.) irritating these conditions. Use various herbs for the kidneys as they regulate the reproductive system of both sexes. Eliminate caffeine; drink juices and plentiful amounts of water (dependant on activity level and climate).

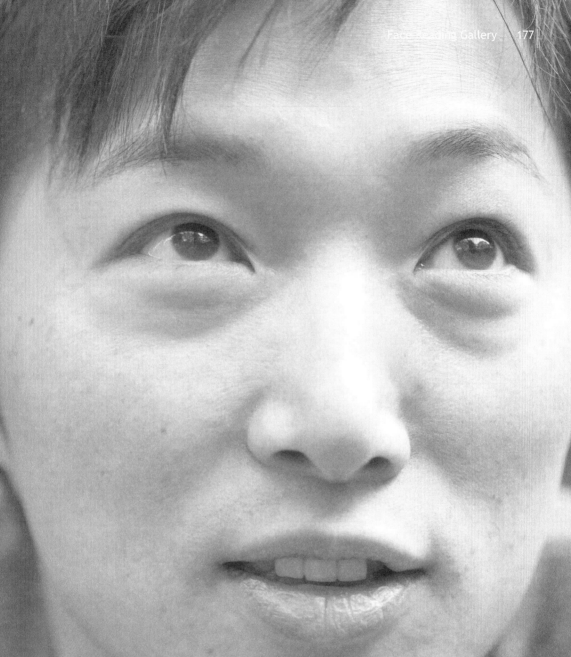

Face: Puffy right and left eye bags (kidneys), upper smile line puffy (ileocecal valve)

Problem: Right and left kidney swollen, blocked ileocecal valve (causing spasms above right hip).

Solution: Eliminate sugar, caffeine and excess salt. Eat citrus 4-5 times a day and after meals. Use a colon cleanser as needed.

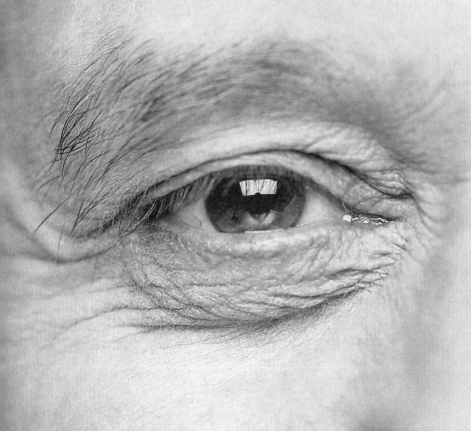

Face: Crows feet (liver), puffy under eye (kidney), deep smile line (colon).

Problem: Severe colon overloads leading to liver and kidney congestion.

Solution: Eliminate sugar, coffee, breads and dairy products. Increase water consumption and do a good colon cleansing.

Face: Deep furrow between eyes at bridge of nose (liver), smile lines (colon).

Problem: Liver overwhelm, ascending colon and descending colon blockages.

Solution: Liver support, fresh fruit especially citrus, melons and a good cellular detox. She must also stop taking over the counter sleep aids and diet aids.

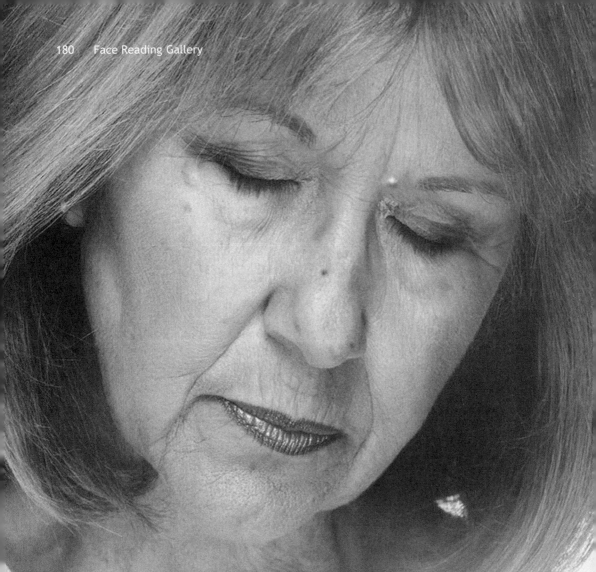

Face: Deep furrows and growth at the bridge nose (liver). Bags und both eyes (kidneys). The right corner of the right eye bag area is raised (adrenal gland). Notice the spots on the nose (heart). Notice the creases on the upper lip (heart from a mild stroke). Deep smile lines (colon). The chin area is puff and creased (reproductive issues). Hollow of the right cheek (right lung).

Problem: A mild stroke has affected her whole system and was brought on by smoking, alcohol, caffeine and a poor diet of processed foods. Constipation is also severe.

Solution: Eliminate caffeine, smoking, processed foods including dairy and replace with fresh fruit and vegetables with some egg and avocado protein. Use something to open up and repair circulation. Also use a liver, kidney and heart formula along with a good colon formula.

Face: Deep indentations at the flare of the nose (ileocecal valve), deep indentations at the lower end of the smile line nearest to mouth (descending colon). There is a slight irritation on the right endocrine strip (Immune system / virus issues). Including a small growth on the left side of the cheek (upper stomach).

Problem: Clogged ileocecal valve causing cramping above the right hip. Descending colon is weakened. Upper stomach and esophagus is irritated, including acid reflux.

Solution: Breads and cooked proteins must be eliminated. Water intake increased to 80 - 90 ounces a day (depending on activity level). Use of breads and caffeine eliminated.

Face: Swollen endocrine strip (Immune system / virus issues). The hollow of the cheeks (lungs).

Problem: Viral / endocrine weakness due to parasites (Giardia). Chemical exposure and smoking has caused lung weakness.

Solution: Eliminate parasites and support lung function with turmeric, pleurisy root, etc.

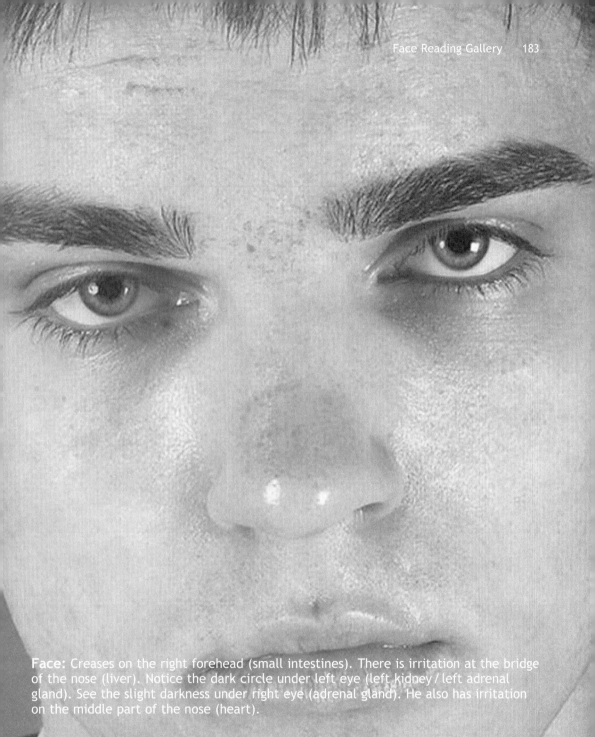

Face: Creases on the right forehead (small intestines). There is irritation at the bridge of the nose (liver). Notice the dark circle under left eye (left kidney / left adrenal gland). See the slight darkness under right eye (adrenal gland). He also has irritation on the middle part of the nose (heart).

Problem: Alcohol, marijuana use and illegal stimulants are raping his system.

Solution: Eliminate the items listed above and address the diet as needed.

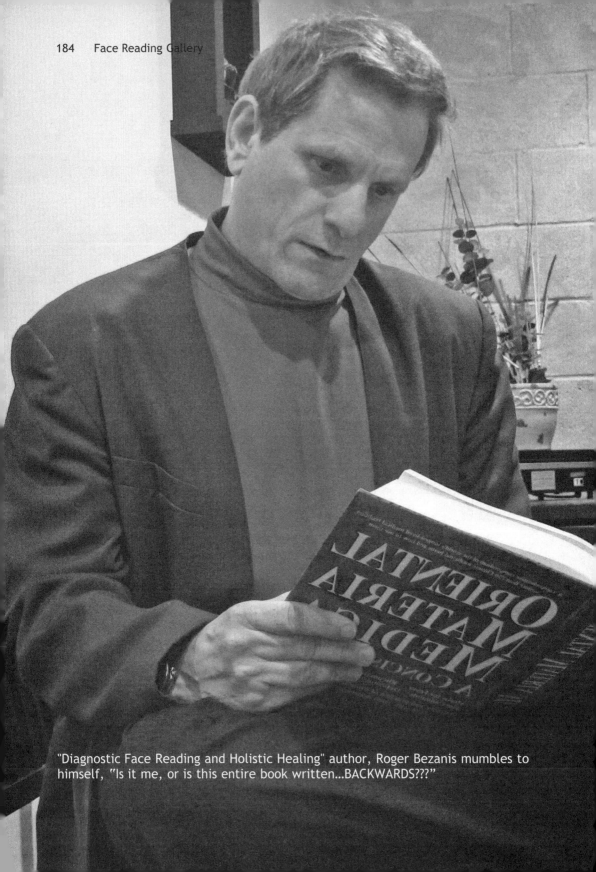

"Diagnostic Face Reading and Holistic Healing" author, Roger Bezanis mumbles to himself, "Is it me, or is this entire book written...BACKWARDS???"

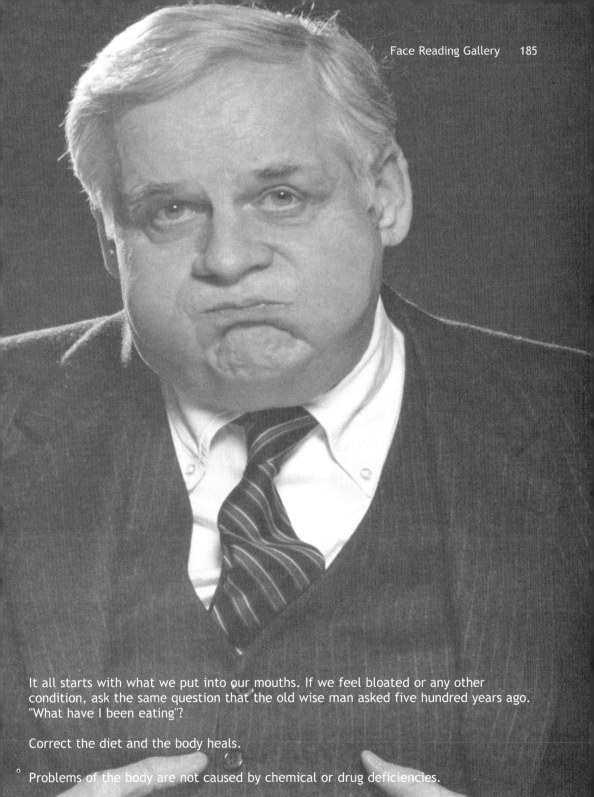

It all starts with what we put into our mouths. If we feel bloated or any other condition, ask the same question that the old wise man asked five hundred years ago. "What have I been eating"?

Correct the diet and the body heals.

Problems of the body are not caused by chemical or drug deficiencies.

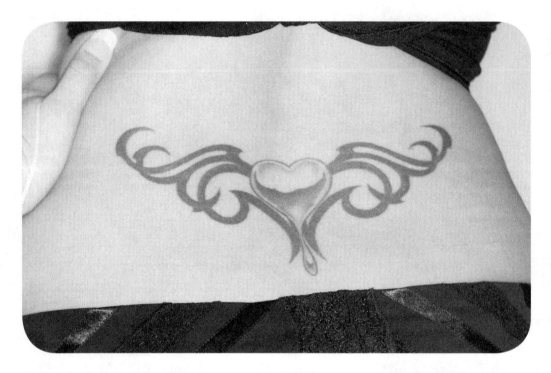

Tattoos attack the liver as it regulates the skin. Over time tattoo ink is absorbed via the skin and attacks the liver. Because the liver is slowly digesting tattoo ink, they eventually fade and disappear. Tattoo ink is so powerful that it alone can cause hepatitis.

Every human on the planet is lactose intolerant. We are the only species on the planet that consumes dairy from another species. Only humans and to lesser degree primates, eat solely for pleasure. We can kid ourselves but the state of our health is our responsibility alone.

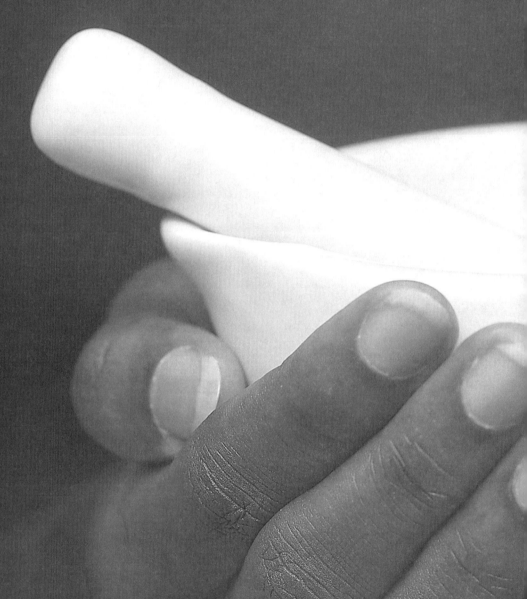

This is what poor circulation looks like on the fingernail moons. Notice there are none. Each finger (except the pinky on both hands) should have a moon. The largest is the thumb moon to the smallest at the ring finger. This problem is solved via a general detox of the system. It is best to include cayenne, wasabi japonica, cinnamon bark and turmeric along with B-vitamins, liver and kidney support.

This is what healthy circulation looks like as represented by the nail-moons. Notice that all the nails have moons except the pinky. This is what your nails should look like. To keep your nails and circulation strong it is advisable to take: cayenne, turmeric, wasabi japonica, cinnamon bark with liver and kidney support and B-vitamins.

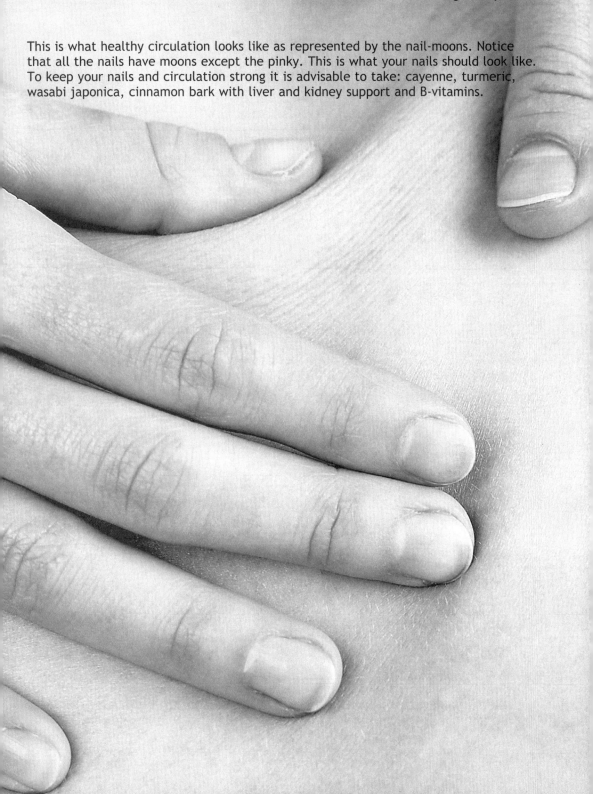

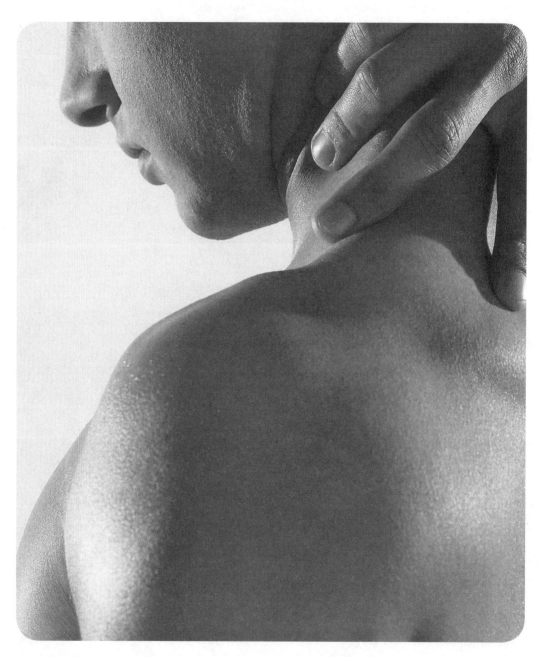

Upper left shoulder pain is always a current kidney issue. Kidney issues are demonstrated by upper left shoulder, low back, joint and various muscle pains.

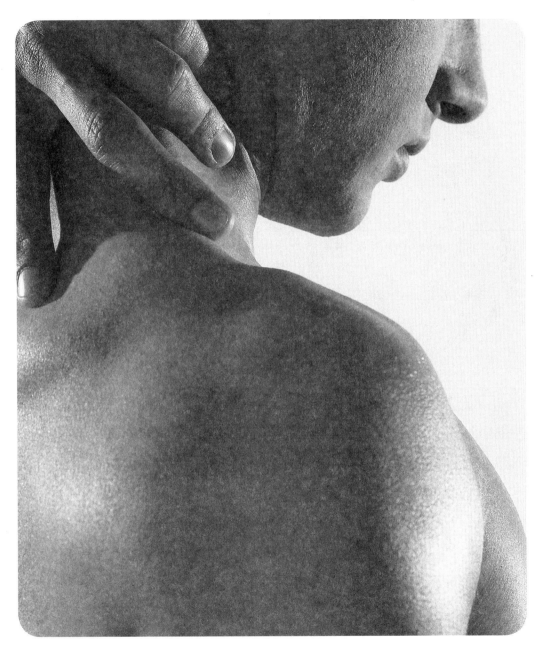

Upper right shoulder pain is always a signal of a current liver issue. Soreness can also be present in the right side of the neck, right pectoral, right bicep and triceps muscle.

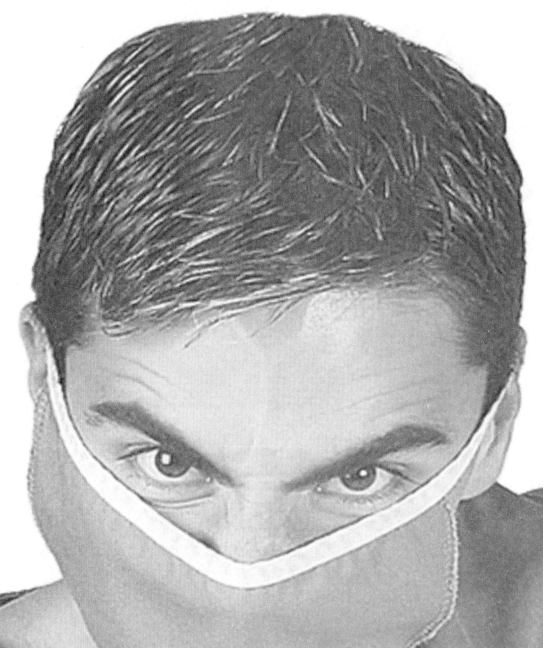

Who is the surgeon behind the mask? What motivates him? Is he a free thinker? Is he beholding to an organization that dictates what he does? Does he have your best interest in mind or a new Mercedes? Maybe you should see a chiropractor first.

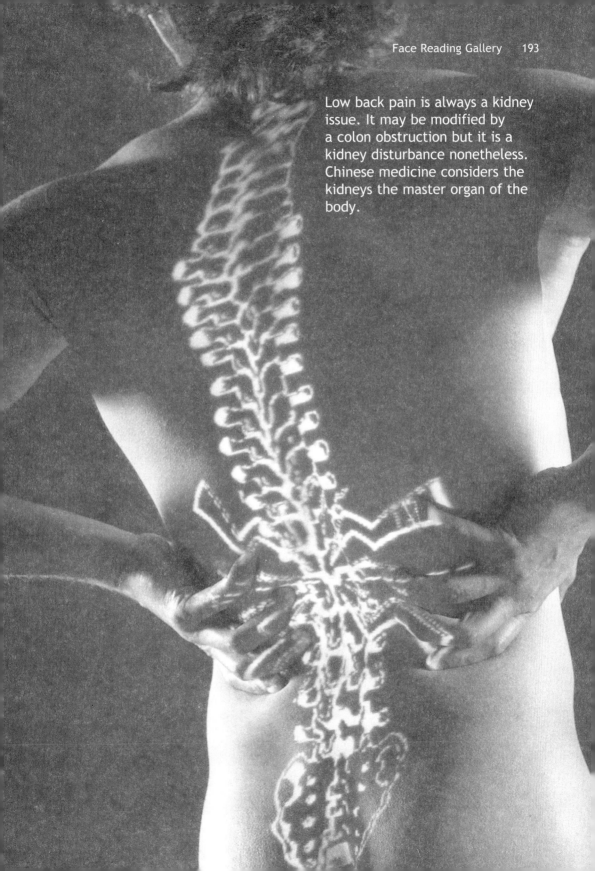

Low back pain is always a kidney issue. It may be modified by a colon obstruction but it is a kidney disturbance nonetheless. Chinese medicine considers the kidneys the master organ of the body.

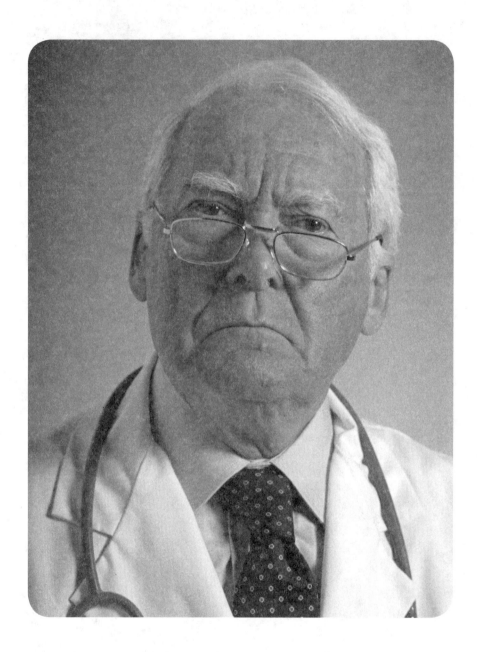

A doctor who does not listen to you and is not interested in letting you participate in your own healing is not a good doctor. You deserve respect.

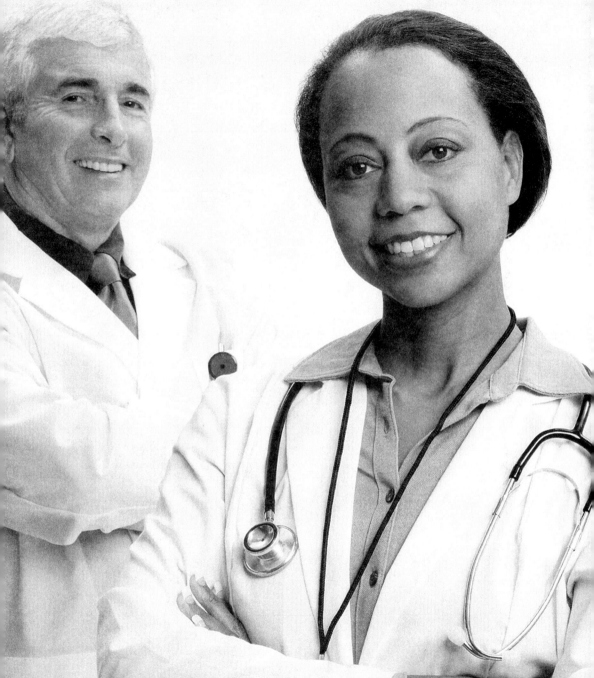

A good doctor listens to you and cares about what you think. He is not anxious to send you in for surgery. Your doctor should be interested in alternative treatments and you should be willing to learn. Your doctor should never look down on you or belittle you.

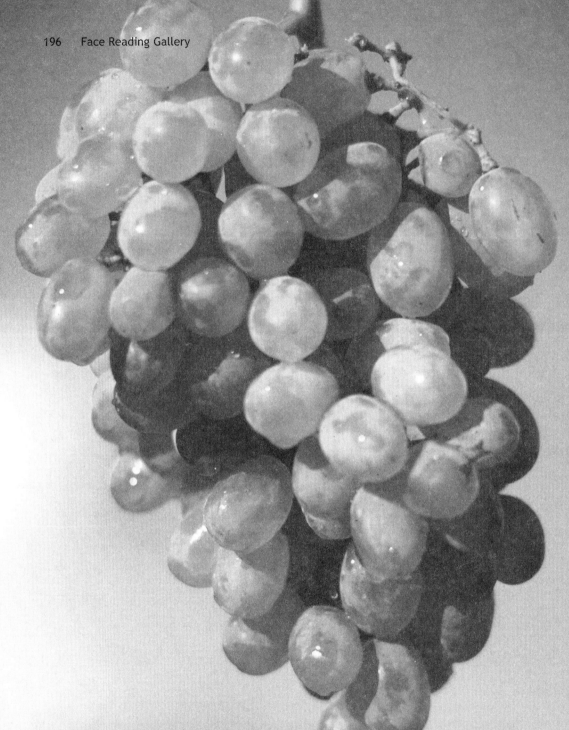

The most important food on the planet to eat for kidney health is grapes. They protect and feed the kidneys. They help the body correct the most dramatic problems imaginable including vertigo. The type of grapes consumed does not seem to matter.

The best food for digestion is Clementine Tangerines. Indigestion is improved or made a non-factor within minutes upon eating them. They are also very good for liver health.

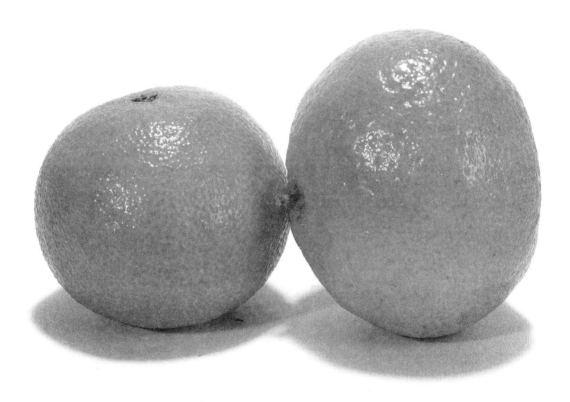

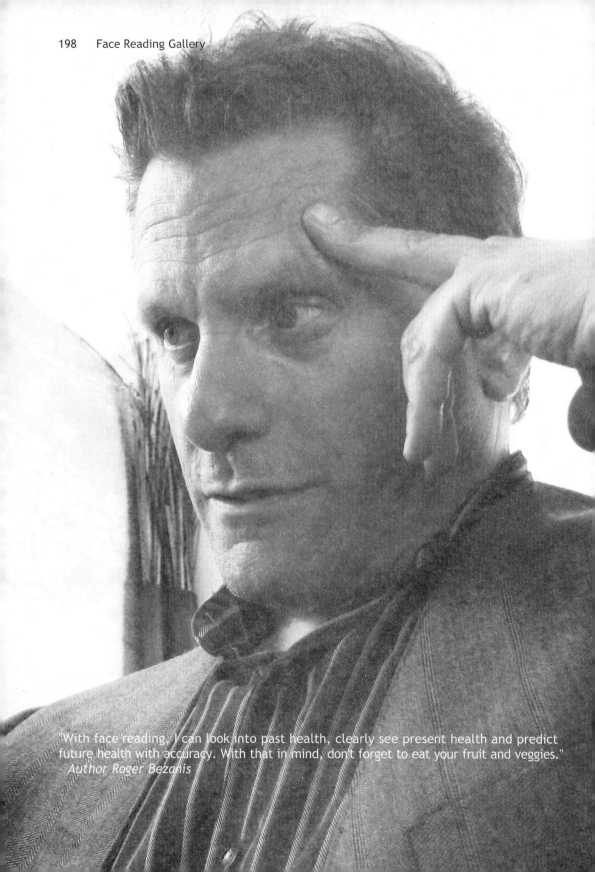

"With face reading, I can look into past health, clearly see present health and predict future health with accuracy. With that in mind, don't forget to eat your fruit and veggies."
- *Author Roger Bezanis*

Fresh vegetables are God's medicine and if consumed in plentiful amounts, they make the body almost impervious to sickness.

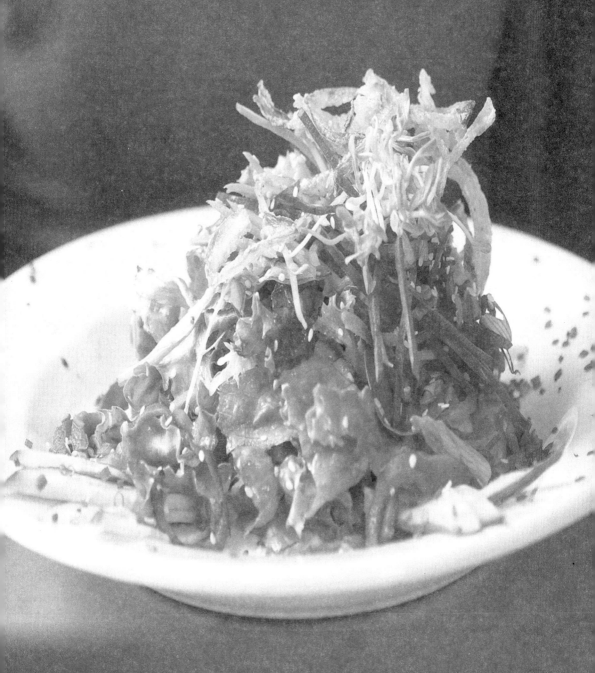

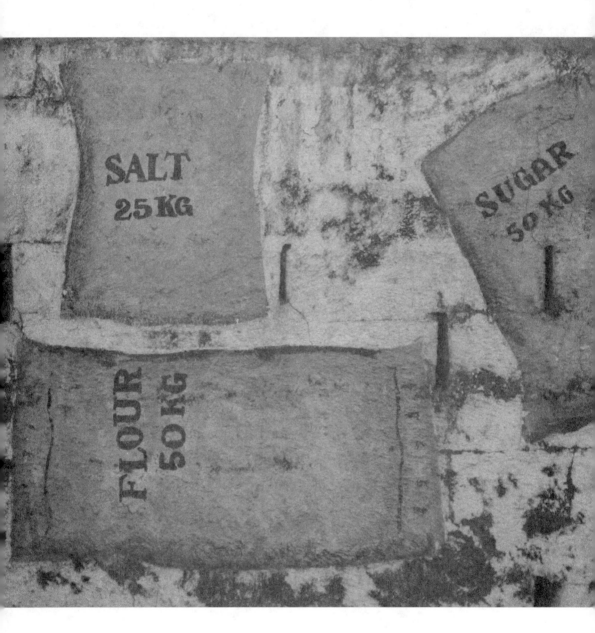

Meet the "3-Amigos" of poor health; sugar, flour and salt. Sugar is deadly in all processed forms as is flour which converts to sugar. Salt is a mineral that is only useful when it is ingested in a natural or whole food form. Table salt is not a natural form of salt as it was processed. Salt naturally occurring in a tomato, etc., is fine.

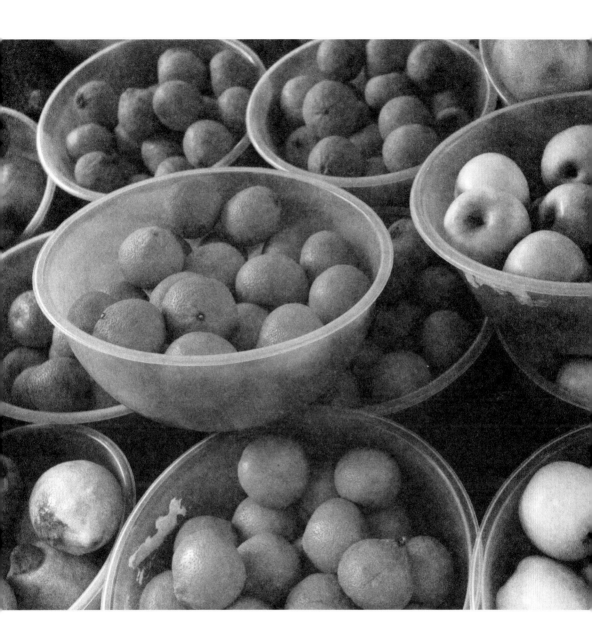

The best friend your body can have is "nature's candy": fruit. Do not be afraid to indulge. If you can, get it organically grown. Nevertheless, eat fruit.

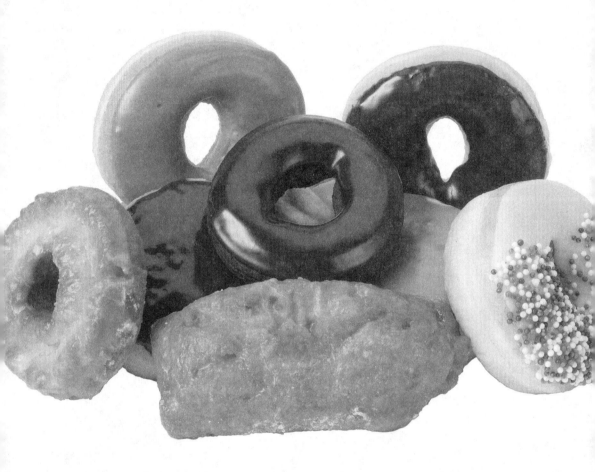

This so-called food is addicting and deadly to the system. We are burning-out our kidneys at an alarming rate thanks to poisons like these. More people are addicted to sugar than heroin and cocaine combined.

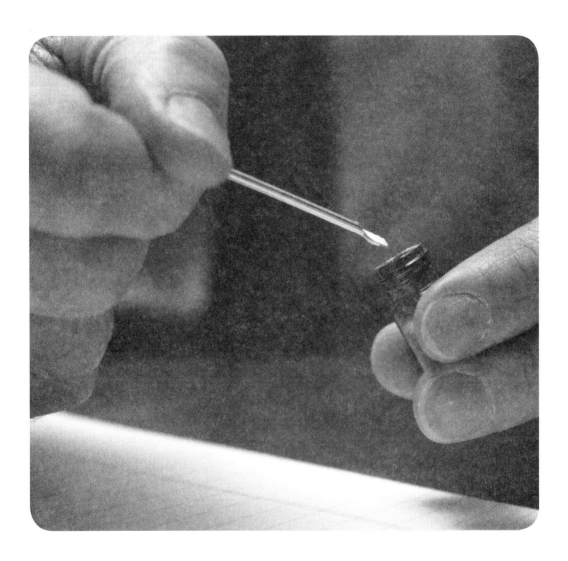

Cocaine is not the most addictive substance on the planet. But sugar, salt and flour are. Everyone you meet is addicted to the 3-Amigos of poor health.

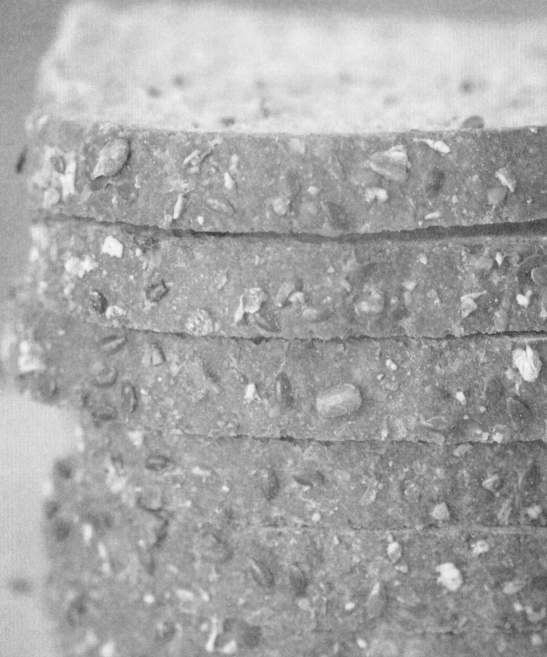

Whole wheat bread is worthless to the body. Once grains are made into flour, they are toxic to the body. The cracked wheat you see adorning the crust of this bread is also worthless. Once the wheat kernel is cracked, the germ inside is dead. Bakers create bread by cooking flour until everything healthy in it is destroyed.

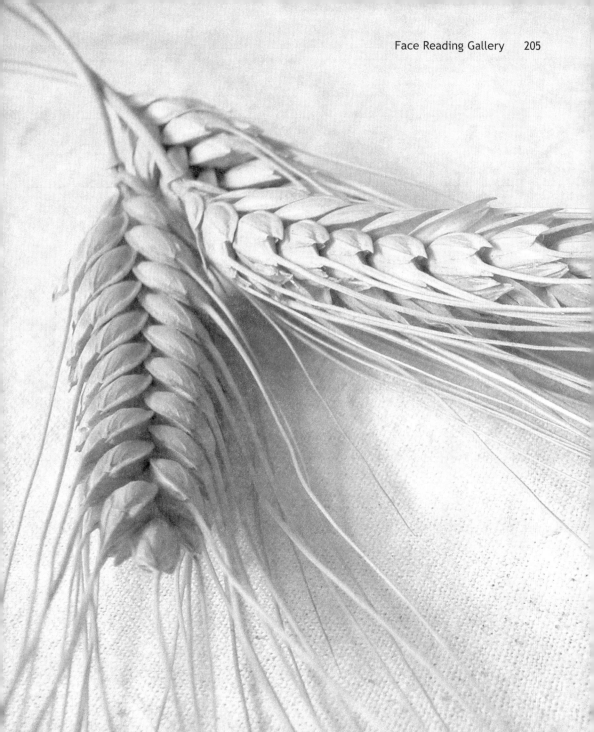

This is what whole wheat looks like. If you were really eating "whole wheat" you would be gnawing on a stalk of wheat like this. If you planted a stalk of wheat, you could grow wheat. Planting bread may grow mold.

Caffeine is the most dangerous daily use substance on the planet. It is a poison and must not be consumed. Because of this my book will never be sold at Starbucks, Seattle's Best, Peet's or _____(fill in the blank).

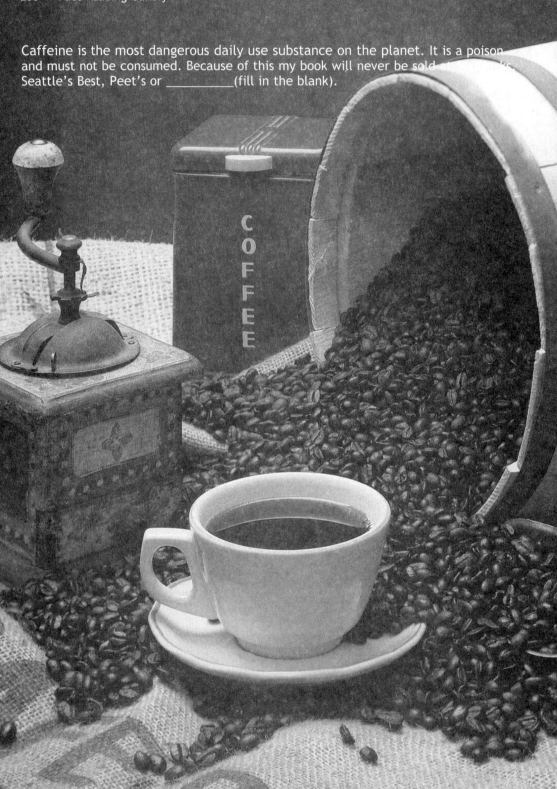

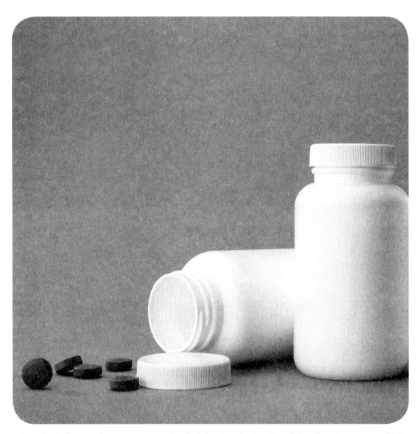

Herbal formulas are wonderful but whole food is the true medicine.
Herbals are only temporary substitutes until you correct the source of
your dietary issues. We eat ourselves into ill health. Caffeine is deadly
and it is best removed from the body by a full 3-month detox.

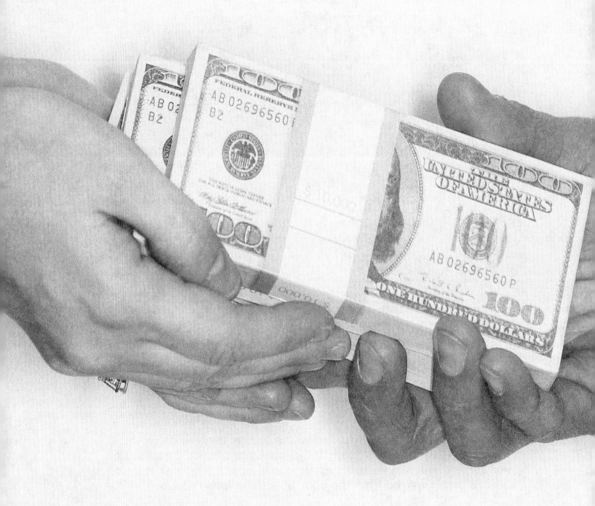

The FDA (a government agency) takes 800 million dollars to approve a drug for sale. They issue a seven-year patent and then turn a blind eye to complaints until the patent runs out. To be truly useful to the government, you must be on drugs and in need of surgery.

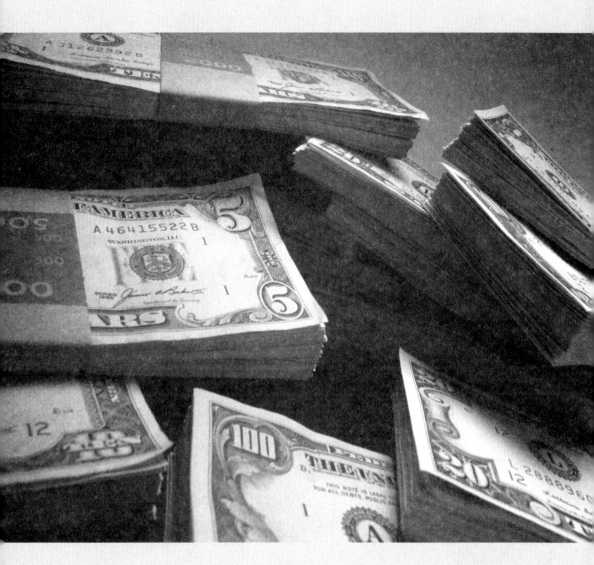

Insurance companies, the FDA, AMA and American Psychiatric Association see you like a commodity to be spent. Your health is worthless, your sickness is a priceless goldmine, your insurance is a treasure chest to be plundered, your free will must be controlled and your ability to think must be suppressed.

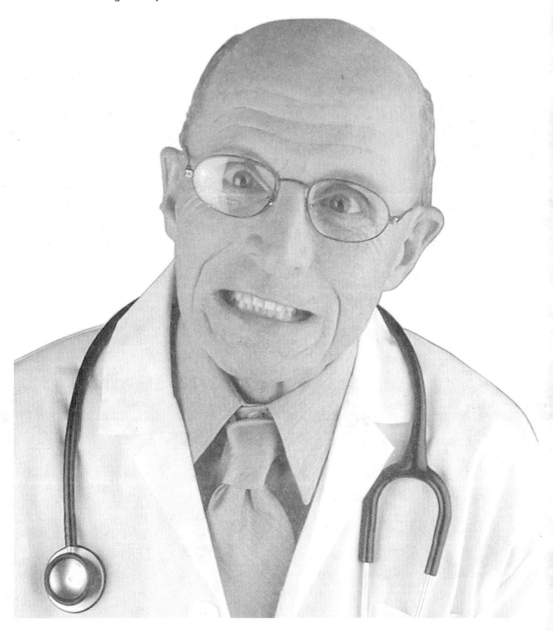

Psychiatry is an inhuman practice performed by insane doctors who want nothing more than to drug and control you. If you are taking drugs for a condition that is slowly made worse by their use, you will never recover. Remember Virginia Tech? Do you remember Columbine? Psychiatric drugs created all of the aforementioned.

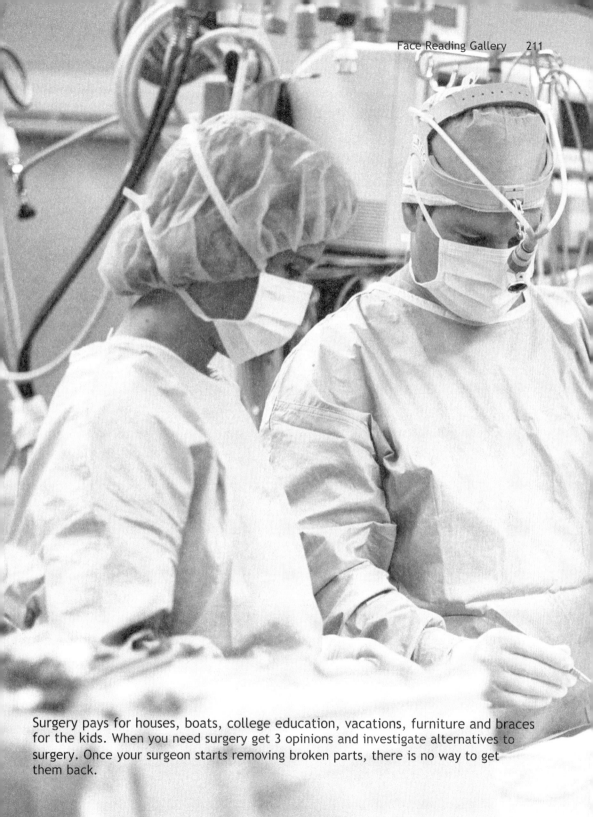

Surgery pays for houses, boats, college education, vacations, furniture and braces for the kids. When you need surgery get 3 opinions and investigate alternatives to surgery. Once your surgeon starts removing broken parts, there is no way to get them back.

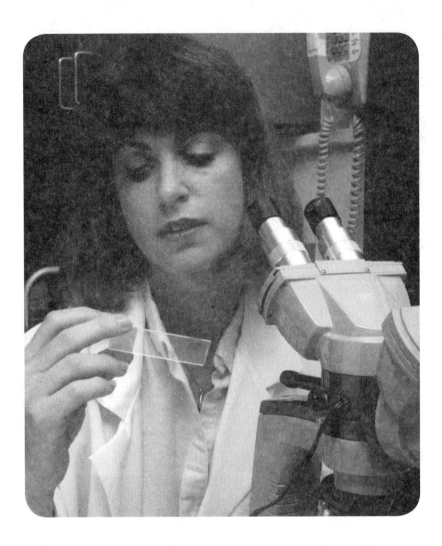

AIDS, cancer, flu and diabetes cannot be isolated under a microscope and are just a huge scary sales pitch. When you hear that x-million dollars is being dropped into research on some nebulous problem, the problem is smoke and mirrors.

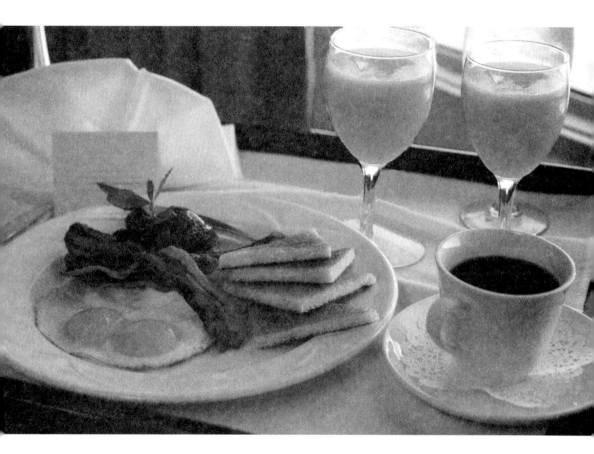

This is not a healthy breakfast unless you only drank the juice.

Healthy Sources of Protein

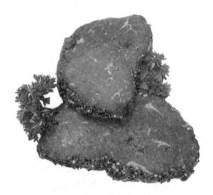

Beef
Rare or raw steak (steak tartare)
is fully bio-available to the body.

Avocados
Raw avocados are very
friendly to the body.
They also contain oils
that when consumed raw
are very healthy.

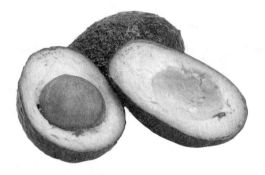

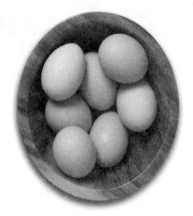

Eggs
Eggs can be readily consumed
raw in fruit drinks or smoothies.
Cooking destroys protein that
then becomes an irritant
to the kidneys, liver
and endocrine system.

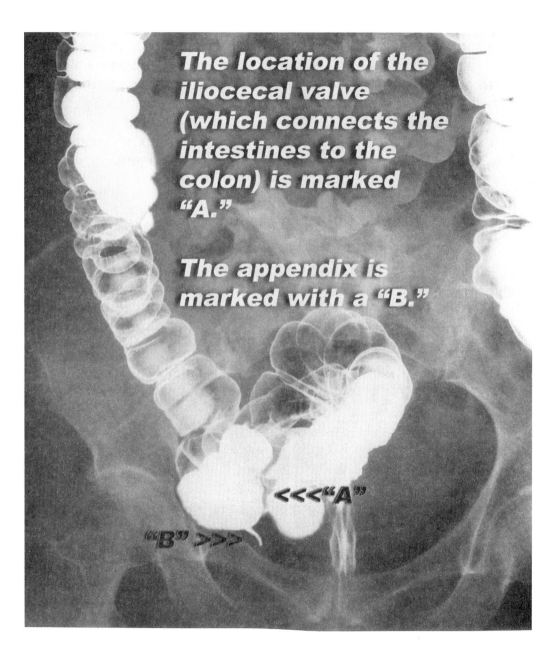

LIVER/KIDNEY BODY SYMPTOM CHART

Kidney-Muscle-Joint symptoms appear in throughout the rest of the body in all of the black areas. They include aches, pains, soreness and stiffness.

Liver-Muscle-Joint symptoms appear in limited locations on the right side in the shaded areas only. They include aches, pains, soreness and stiffness.

If the right elbow is sore, stiff or aches, this indicates a digestive disturbance.

If the right ankle is sore, this indicates that the heart and kidneys are irritated.

MAJOR ORGAN LAYOUT

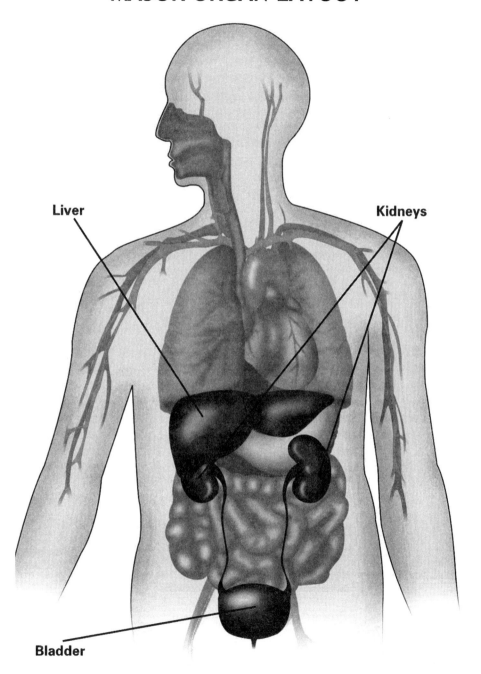

33 Additional Notes on Face Reading

Red face or parts of the face that are red:

This always means that the organ associated with that part of the face is running hot. In other words that organ is stressed due to some problem that the body is experiencing.

The actual temperature of that organ is elevated.

The Nose represents the right and left side of the heart

The right side of the nose represents the right side of the heart and the left side is the left side of the heart.

Ear Lobes and the heart

The right ear lobe represents the right side of the heart and the left ear lobe represents the left side of the heart.

Scoring system for possible heart issues

Left ear lobe crease = 30% chance of a current or future heart issue.
Right ear lobe crease = 30% chance of a current or future heart issue.
Either side of the nose = 20% chance of a current or future heart issue.
The upper lip area below the nose = 20% chance of a current or future heart issue.

Repairing problems found on the face during face readings

There are no death sentences with face reading. All face reading does is give us a place to look. It does not diagnose a problem. It alerts us to something to be aware of. All of these problems no matter how bad, are reversible by way of diet, detox and exercise.

Face reading is a fantastic tool that alerts us of possible weakness so that we may use other techniques to fully evaluate the issue.

I have symptoms but my face does not show problems in that area

This sort of comment comes up every now and again. This condition is very easy to handle. It indicates that the diet and or lifestyle are not supporting this person's body. All that needs to be done is a correct diet handling and the removal of any other bad habits. The good news is that, based on his or her face, they are genetically very healthy.

Smile lines show us our colon at birth and the current state of our colon

The smile line on the right side of the face represents the state of our colon when we were born. The left side represents it today. A deep smile line crease on the left and a faint one on the right indicate that this person has eaten themselves into a problem.

Ileocecal Valve as it appears on the face

The nostril flairs of the nose are not all the same from person to person. If you look through the face reading gallery you will see this very clearly. Some nostril flairs are large and produce a shadow around the edge of the nostril. It may appear that the smile line crawls up and all the way around the nose.

The more pronounced the nostril flair is, the more the Ileocecal valve is irritated.

When the ileocecal valve is irritated or spasming, the more the area above the right hip will hurt. This is the location of the ileocecal valve. It connects the small intestines to the ascending colon.

Gray Hair Update

Gray hair can reverse. It happens all the time. It is well known that people have gone gray prior to their natural color hair falling out. In other words, the hair can be gray or full color from day to day.

The factor is what we eat. The hair is a representation of the bladder and reproductive system as regulated by the kidneys. When hair is turning gray, it is due to the kidneys getting weak.

Adrenal Glands

The adrenal glands show up as a black-eyed-pea shaped raised spot to the outside of the kidney eye bag area. The raised area is right next to the crows' feet area and is close to the lower eye lashes of the eye in question.

Roger Bezanis

If this is raised then adrenal fatigue is present. This may very well have been brought on by the ingesting of sugar or caffeine.

Smile lines that dip below the mouth

This is almost always an indicator of hemorrhoids.

Endocrine strip

The endocrine stretches from the junction of the nose and inside corner of the eye nearest the nose, down along the nose and then smile line down to the jaw. It is bordered on the other side by the kidney eye bag, stomach and lungs.

If it is swollen, red, discolored or has pimples on it, then the immune system is fighting some sort of battle.

If the pimples or redness is localized and near the nose and eyes then this indicates that the lymph nodes at the armpits or above are being impacted.

If the irritation is across from the center of the nose then it is the kidneys, spleen or pancreas that is at issue.

If the irritation is across from the bottom of the nose and upper lip then it is the lymph nodes of the groin on either side. The groin is the junction where the abdomen and thigh join.

Upper eye region above the eye lid and below the eyebrow

This area is a valid place to look for kidney issues. The eye lid should never droop down and cover the actual eye lid.

If one eye lid is covered by sagging skin and one is not, the one that is covered is the weaker of the two kidneys.

34 Validating Face Reading Effectiveness

Again, use these Diagnostic Face Reading photos in your office by simply directing your patients to really look at them. The effect of these photos and this book is really quite amazing. You will of course need to keep extra copies of this book at your office. When patients see these photos, they always want their own copy.

To really help your patients, use my Diagnostic Face Reading Charts (24 x 36) side by side on your wall with a good sized mirror between the two charts.

- Point out the charts on your wall to your patients. Tell them to:
- "Look in the mirror and compare your face to the charts on the wall and tell me what you think is wrong."

They will turn to you and say

- "Doctor, is my _____ a problem?"
- It is then up to you and your patient to determine the best course of action.
- Get a full history of what symptoms your patient has present today (using the questions in the Energy Balancing Technique section or get an Energy Balancing Technique cheat card to help).
- Pick a therapy that will help your patient i.e. herb, diet etc.
- Take a picture (Polaroid or digital) of the patients face as it appears today.
- Put this picture and their current list of symptoms in their file.
- Send them home with what you two have decided is the best course of action.
- 30-45 days later have the patient return.
- Take a new picture and compare their new picture to the old one.
- Take a new patient full history of symptoms.
- Compare the new picture to the old one. Show the patient how they have changed.
- Do a new patient full history of symptoms; compare the new list to the old list. It will have reduced from 20 items to perhaps 9.

This simple approach validates that what you are doing is really working. In this day and age it is important to prove that what you are doing is safe and effective. Face reading and symptom reduction are the keys to your success.

Roger Bezanis

35 Quantum Physics and the Body

About now you might be asking yourself "What does quantum physics have to do with face reading and the human body"? Your answer is EVERYTHING.

The body is an energetic organism made of material or mass. Read on.

Some of the greatest minds on the planet have toiled in the subject of Quantum Physics. The history of the study essentially started with quantum mechanics. This groundwork was the forerunner of quantum physics and took place in 1838 with Michael Faraday. Max Planck furthered it with the 1900 paper on blackbody radiation.

In a nutshell, Quantum Physics is the study of mass and its relationship to energy. In any structure (such as the human body), when there are equal amounts of mass and energy present, a state of optimum health is the result or balance is achieved. When there is an overabundance of mass or energy, the body gets sick and can die. If an imbalanced condition persists long enough, without fail the body will die.

Simple quantum physics formula: **Equal Mass + Equal Energy = Balance**

Quantum physics is so basic in its balancing aspect of life. It permeates all parts of life, even our language and government, stretching ad infinitum (infinity). For example, black and white, hot and cold, dry and wet, forward and backward, soft and hard, acid and alkaline, etc., are all statements of balance.

On the road to further illustrate how mass and energy coexists, look at your dinner table or bed. Why do they not get up and walk away? The answer is: they do not possess energy available in sufficient quantity to accomplish the task of movement. All inanimate objects possess potential energy that can be ignited from an outside source. In the human body, a complete absence of energy would be called death.

A complete overwhelming amount of energy in the body can also cause death. This is commonly associated with a drug or chemical overdose. This is furthermore where we get the terms hyper-hypo and attack.

Organ overwhelm, caused by too much mass or energy, is different from failure as failing organs are experiencing very little or no energy.

The absolute expression of pure energy would be nuclear fission. A near absolute expression of energy would be a common fire. This is clearly only a near absolute expression of energy as this type of fire leaves ashes and cinders. The more complete the energy expression is, the more ability it has to destroy all mass.

This formula of mass versus energy explains why drugs are so harmful to the body. Drugs are, due to their processing, mass deficient and energy rich. Later I will dig deeper into this subject, with the focus on cocaine. You can now think with this concept; you are now starting to see mass / energy errors all about you.

Any organ or organ system that cannot process mass or energy / waste at its optimum capacity is failing and eventually will shut down. This fact is irrefutable and inevitable.

Consequently, is CANCER nothing but a mass that is not interfacing with and not being monitored by energy? That is exactly what it is. Hence, any health remedy for a so-called cancer must at its heart reestablish the flow of energy and mass at the affected site.

The body must be in communication with itself at every level 100 percent of the time to survive at an optimum echelon. All life is dependent upon these factors.

All life is trying to balance its mass and energy. The next chapter (Energy Balancing Technique) will explain this complex relationship.

36 Energy Balancing Technique (EBT)

Following on the heels of quantum physics is my energy balancing technique. EBT is the realization of real time quantum physics on the human body.

When I introduced the Energy Balancing Technique (EBT) almost 8 years ago, it was met with understandable skepticism. The technique was the outcrop of observations that I could not otherwise explain. Since I am in the business of explaining everything, I had to get to work.

First and foremost, I am an observer of life, and second, a formulator of herbal supplements. Testing my formulas almost a decade ago revealed that people claimed they felt better just holding the formulas before they even took them. I had not asked or probed for these observations. My test groups just kept offering them up.

Knowing that such "instant response" was impossible, I ignored the comments for weeks. Yet after 60-100 such comments I became very curious. Were these people all hallucinating?

Still not letting on that I was the least bit interested in these comments, I started testing the group with placebos. Suddenly the pleasant amazed comments detailing relief from aches, emotional improvement, enhanced vision, improved breathing, diminished pains and such, fell by 85%.

With instant response, I had achieved the impossible!

Still not sure what I had achieved, I began working on another formula. This mixture would be for the kidneys. I was certain nothing like this could ever happen again. Yet, I was not opposed to the idea.

A few months later I was back at it, with a new formula for kidneys. I was merrily testing away when I started hearing the comments again. Nevertheless, these comments were different. I checked my oriental medical references and in the descriptions were clues to what I was seeing.

Empirical data was proving that what was put in the LEFT HAND had a distinctly different affect than what was put in the RIGHT HAND.

Herbs put in the right hand affected all areas of the body directed by the liver. What was put in the left hand was directing all things regulated by the kidneys. When I switched formulas from one had to the other the affect would disappear. In other words, the hands were sensing for different systems of the body. This was the beginning of The Energy Balancing Technique.

Certainly what I have discovered is not something new. This must be very old. My guess is that it is more than 3000 years old as there is no mention of it. Regardless of its origins or how deeply it was buried in the sands of time, I present it to you now.

PRECEPT: The body has a constant flow of energy running through it.

PRECEPT: Whenever the flow of energy is interrupted in the body there will be a reaction of pain, discomfort, tightness, etc.

EBT AXIOM 1 - Your body is a sentient being (it is alive and conscious)

EBT AXIOM 2 - Your body is dependent on you for its survival.

EBT AXIOM 3 - Your body communicates to you 24 hours a day via sensation (pain, hot, cold, hunger etc)

EBT AXIOM 4 - Your body reacts in real time to all stimuli good or bad.

EBT AXIOM 5 - All aches, pains, swellings and other sensations are communications from your body to you.

EBT AXIOM 6 - Aches and Pains are requests for help from the body.

EBT AXIOM 7 - Man and his body communicate to the world via touch.

EBT AXIOM 8 - Touch is the most important sense humans have. Without it, man would perish.

With a few exceptions like hunger, and need for sleep, man & his body are not in communication.

At the moment of touch we will feel better, worse / hotter, colder, etc, instantly. If used, this technique evaluates any food or supplement in real time.

FACT: The body has two major test plates (or areas) that directly connect to our major organs for quick assessment.

TEST PLATE - RIGHT HAND (all organs and functions directed by the LIVER)

TEST PLATE - LEFT HAND (all organs and functions directed by the KIDNEYS)

SHORT LIST — RIGHT HAND LIVER — LEFT HAND KIDNEYS

RIGHT HAND **LIVER:**
    Liver
    Gallbladder
    Right shoulder / neck
    Stomach
    Small Intestines
    Colon
    Eyes
    Lungs
    Head / Brain
    *Lymphatic System
    **Parasites

LEFT HAND **KIDNEYS:**
    Kidneys
    Heart
    Left Shoulder / neck
    Most joints
    Low Back
    Adrenal glands
    Leg Muscles
    Prostate / Ovaries
    Bladder
    **Lymphatic System
    **Parasites

LIVER / LIVER / LIVER
FULL LIST FULL LIST FULL LIST

RIGHT HAND
(RIGHT SIDE OF YOUR BODY ONLY)

Roger Bezanis

Shoulder pain soreness or stiffness
Deltoid pain soreness or stiffness
Rotator cuff pain soreness or stiffness
Trapezoid pain soreness or stiffness
Neck (right side only) pain soreness or stiffness
Bicep pain soreness or stiffness
Triceps pain soreness or stiffness
Scapula pain soreness or stiffness
Latissimus Dorsi muscle soreness or stiffness
Right pectoral muscle pain soreness or stiffness
Fuzzy vision
Foggy vision
Irritated eyes
Stinging eyes
Watery eyes
Red eyes
Stinging tongue
Stinging or sore mouth (inside)
Congestion or pain in your nose
Congestion or pain in your sinuses
Congestion or pain in your chest
Bad moods
Mood swings
Irritable
Nervousness
PMS
Depression
Post partum depression
Obsessive behavior
Hot flashes
Insomnia

Trouble falling asleep
Trouble staying asleep
Headaches
Tiredness (is both a liver and kidney problem)
Itchy skin
Skin irritations
Skin tags
Strawberry spots
Acne
Boils
Numb skin
Tingling skin
Age spots
Liver spots
Lung irritation
Asthma
Pneumonia
Pain in the right side of your chest
Pain in the left side of your chest
Short of breath
Restricting breathing
Coughing
Emphysema
Tuberculosis
Lung cancer
Bronchitis
Pulmonary fibrosis
Sarcoidosis
Respiratory failure
Out of breath, easily
Gallstones
H. pylori (Heliobacter pylori)
Chronic fatigue syndrome
Epstein-Barr

STOMACH / COLON / INTESTINES
FULL LIST FULL LIST FULL LIST

RIGHT HAND

Right elbow pain
Right elbow stiffness
Right elbow soreness
Right forearm pain
Right forearm soreness
Gas
Bloating
Acid Reflux
GERD (Gastroesophgeal Reflux Disease)
Acid indigestion
Heartburn
Indigestion
Abdominal discomfort
Abdominal spasms
Ulcers
Gas
Upset stomach
Abdominal distention
Hiatal hernia
Pain just above the right hip

Soreness just above the right hip
Cramping just above the right hip
Leaky gut syndrome
Polyps
Ulcerative colitis
Diverticulitis
Diverticulosis
IBS (irritable bowel Syndrome)
Crohn's disease
Sprue
H. pylori (Heliobacter pylori)
Hemorrhoids
Candida
Bloody stool
Painful stools
Foul smelling stools
Abdomen sensitive to direct pressure
Constipated less-than-one-elimination-per-meal-eaten

KIDNEYS / KIDNEYS / KIDNEYS
FULL LIST FULL LIST FULL LIST

LEFT HAND

Right kidney
Left kidney
Pain, stiffness or soreness in the left side of your neck
Pain, stiffness or soreness in the left trapezoid muscle
Pain, stiffness or soreness in the left pectoral
Pain, stiffness or soreness in the left scapula
Pain, stiffness or soreness in the left bicep
Pain, stiffness or soreness in the left triceps
Pain, stiffness or soreness in the left elbow
Pain, stiffness or soreness in the left upper forearm
Pain, stiffness or soreness in the RIGHT lower forearm
Pain, stiffness or soreness in the left lower forearm
Pain, stiffness or soreness in the left wrist
Pain, stiffness or soreness in the RIGHT wrist
Carpel tunnel syndrome in RIGHT wrist

Carpel tunnel syndrome in LEFT wrist
Pain, stiffness or soreness in the left hand
Pain, stiffness or soreness in the RIGHT hand
Pain, stiffness or soreness in the left fingers or thumb
Pain, stiffness or soreness in the RIGHT fingers or thumb
Pain, stiffness or soreness in the upper left back area
Pain, stiffness or soreness in the center mid back area
Pain, stiffness or soreness in the left center back area
Pain, stiffness or soreness in the RIGHT lower back area
Pain, stiffness or soreness in the left lower back area
Pain, stiffness or soreness in the RIGHT hip area
Pain, stiffness or soreness in the left hip area
Pain, stiffness or soreness in the left hamstring area
Pain, stiffness or soreness in the RIGHT hamstring area
Pain, stiffness or soreness in the left front thigh area
Pain stiffness or soreness in the RIGHT thigh area
Pain stiffness or soreness in the left knee area
Pain stiffness or soreness in the RIGHT knee area
Pain stiffness or soreness in the left calf area
Pain stiffness or soreness in the RIGHT calf area
Pain stiffness or soreness in the left ankle area
Pain stiffness or soreness in the RIGHT ankle area
Pain stiffness or soreness in the left foot area
Pain stiffness or soreness in the Right foot area
Pain stiffness or soreness in the left foot toes
Pain stiffness or soreness in the Right foot toes
Dizziness / vertigo in the left ear
Dizziness / vvertigo in the right ear
Ringing / tinnitus in the left ear
Ringing / tinnitus in the right ear
Kidney stones
Frequent urination during the night (more than once)
Frequent urination
Arthritis
Swollen joints (with or without pain)
Floaters (clear shapes) cross your field of vision
Weak nails that chip or break
High blood pressure
Gout
Diabetes

Numb or tingling muscles
Foamy morning urine (men only)
Exhausted a short time after eating
Exhausted from any time during the day (liver and kidney symptom)
Weak adrenal glands
Sexual performance issues
Difficult time staying aroused during sex
Lack of interest in sex
Lack of lubrication during sex
Lack of orgasm during sex
Unexpected pain during sex
Low sperm count
Trouble getting pregnant
Problems with fertility
Heavy bleeding during your period
Ovarian cysts
Uterine cysts
Uterine fibroid tumors
Unusual vaginal discharge
Heavy period cramps
Scrotum overly sensitive to the touch
Lack of sensation in the penis
Dull or sharp pain in the groin area
Heart double beat
Heart skips a beat
Heart flutter
Discomfort in the chest
Feel faint from time to time
Feel severe pounding in your chest during some light activities
Congestive heart failure
Heart attack
Stroke
Heart pound late at night for no apparent reason

When in contact with any substance, the body changes

Quantum physics clearly states this fact. We choose to ignore that a live organism (us) exists in a chemically hostile environment.

Man has neglected and denied this fact. Why?

Ergo, man believes he is intelligent and that his body is stupid. He misunderstands the language the body speaks and finds these "communications" annoying. So much so that he suppresses these communications with painkillers and sedatives.

Imagine walking into your boss' office and telling him that the building is on fire. Ignoring you, he jabs a hypodermic needle full of morphine in your arm and depresses the plunger. You are now blissfully unconscious. Like your boss, you too are now clueless to the danger that the building is on fire.

Sounds silly, doesn't it? Yet the above describes our relationship with our body. We constantly ignore and sedate it.

Man's instant response to stimuli is unavoidable, undeniable, unrelenting and irrefutable. You are going to test this and validate it for yourself.

Man reacts to:

All Foods	Water
All herbals	Oxygen
All chemicals	

Earlier in this book, I made mention of how the body changes when it is in contact with any substance. It will feel:

Better	Retain waste
Worse	Release water
Neutral - No change.	Retain water
Get hotter	Relax
Get colder	Become tense
Contract / tighten	Oxygenate
Expand / loosen	Deoxygenate
Feel more pain	Awaken / more energy
Feel less pain	Sedate / less energy
Accelerate or speed up	Lighter
Decelerate or slow down	Heavier
Release waste	

To test these phenomena, look at the KIDNEY LIST from this chapter.

SHORT KIDNEY TEST

- Turn your head from the left to the right
  Notice how stiff and sore the LEFT SIDE of your NECK was just now
  Rate the irritation on a 1-10 scale, 10 being the worst_____

- Move your LEFT ARM over your head and behind you
  Notice how stiff and sore the LEFT SIDE of your SHOULDER was just now
  Rate the irritation on a 1-10 scale, 10 being the worst_____

- Bend your LEFT ELBOW all round, twist it and torque it
  Notice how stiff and sore the LEFT ELBOW was just now
  Rate the irritation on a 1-10 scale, 10 being the worst_____

- Turn and flex your RIGHT and LEFT WRISTS
  Notice how stiff and sore the RIGHT WRIST was just now
  Rate the irritation on a 1-10 scale, 10 being the worst (R)_____
  Notice how stiff the LEFT WRIST WAS
  Rate the irritation on a 1-10 scale, 10 being the worst (L)_____

- Flex your RIGHT and LEFT FINGERS
  Notice how stiff and sore the RIGHT FINGERS were just now
  Rate the irritation on a 1-10 scale, 10 being the worst (R)_____
  Notice how stiff and sore the LEFT FINGERS were just now
  Rate the irritation on a 1-10 scale, 10 being the worst (L)_____

- BEND AT THE WAIST left, right, forward back
  Notice how stiff and sore your RIGHT LOW BACK was just now
  Rate the irritation on a 1-10 scale, 10 being the worst (R)_____
  Notice how stiff the LEFT LOW BACK was just now
  Rate the irritation on a 1-10 scale, 10 being the worst (L)_____

You are about to repeat the same test again holding various substances one at a time in your left palm.

When you repeat these tests notice if you feel:

Better

Worse

The same (no change)

Continuing on, put three green grapes in your left hand and repeat the steps above (while still holding the three grapes).

Did you notice a change?

Were you?

- Better
- Worse
- The same (no change)

Continue testing yourself holding different substances; hold one at a time (in the left hand), while doing the flexing moves above. Keep this up until you are sure that you know what happens when the body comes in contact with a beneficial substance.

You may choose your own items to hold while testing as well.

At some point, test the items that are listed below:

ITEMS TO BE HELD (one at a time)

Sugar	Bread
Water	Chocolate
Soup Mix	Nail polish / or a solvent
Salt	Water
Tomato	Vitamins
Alcohol	A formula for the kidneys

Repeat this test as often as you like against symptoms of your choosing.

Now assess your body. Is some muscle, joint, tendon, ligament etc, sore? If so quickly check earlier in this chapter to determine if it is a liver or kidney problem.

RIGHT HAND = LIVER DOMINATED problem
LEFT HAND= KIDNEY DOMINATED problem

Once you know if your problem is a liver or kidney issue, you can continue on. Have you tested your current herbals and medicines? Did they make your symptoms go away by holding them? If not, those items are of very little value to you.

To test these phenomena, look at the **KIDNEY LIST** from this chapter.

SHORT LIVER TEST

- Turn your head from the left to the right
  Notice how stiff and sore the RIGHT SIDE of your NECK was just now
  Rate the irritation on a 1-10 scale, 10 being the worst_____

- Move your RIGHT SHOULDER in a rotating motion
  Notice how stiff and sore the RIGHT SHOULDER was just now
  Rate the irritation on a 1-10 scale, 10 being the worst_____

- Flex your RIGHT BICEP round, twist it and torque it
  Notice how stiff and sore the RIGHT BICEP was just now
  Rate the irritation on a 1-10 scale, 10 being the worst_____

- Flex your RIGHT BICEP & TRICEPS
  Notice how stiff and sore your RIGHT TRICEPS are just now
  Rate the irritation on a 1-10 scale, 10 being the worst _____

- Take a deep breath and notice your lung's capacity
  Notice how much air you were able to get in your lungs just now
  Rate the irritation on a 10 best and 1 being the worst_____

(Energy can be tested; vision, emotional state, clarity of thought etc.)

Follow the same procedure that you followed for testing the kidneys. Substitute tomatoes, citrus, water or herbal formulas to evaluate how your body adjusts.

Test again.

Once you feel comfortable with this, use the technique all the time. You can even evaluate what to eat for lunch. You may appear rather interesting testing yourself (to others), but you will have certainty, regarding what you are about to eat.

Remember your body is a machine and is restricted by the same natural laws or physics that govern all machinery.

All machines:

  React to stimuli

  Need fuel

  Need to be cleaned

  Follow programs (or sequences of actions) no matter how rudimentary.

Roger Bezanis

The body is systematic in its execution of its mechanical/life sustaining schedule. Think of this schedule as the combination numbers used to unlock a padlock. Numbers that when correctly entered, create a change. In the human body, the correct sequence can produce energy or reduce pain, etc.

A Master Lock Pad Lock will not open until the numbers are "dialed in" in the correct sequence. The right numbers "dialed in", in the wrong sequence, will leave the lock closed. This whole technique is designed to unlock your body every time it is locked up.

Your body will always want the following:

Every-body (all human bodies) needs Oxygen, Food and Water. From this we derive energy or life force. All bodies must produce energy to survive.

All bodies have the exact same numbers in their programming (the sequencing does change)

1). WATER (Always # 1 or 2 in testing)
2). FOOD (= Protein or Fresh Fruit)
3). REMEDY (a formula/herb or herb mixture / multiple mixtures as needed)
4). SOME COMBINATION OF THE ABOVE 3 POINTS.

The only variable in this whole equation is the order in which it wants these items. Often you can improve symptoms without the need of Protein or Fruit. The minimum you need to successfully reduce or eliminate any symptom is water (H2O).

The role of the Transverse Colon (TC): Do not negate the influence of digestion on your liver and kidneys. As the TC stretches across the abdomen, in front of the kidneys and below the liver/gallbladder, it can play havoc on all three.

A stressed TC can push up on the liver/gallbladder and back on the kidneys causing all manner of symptoms. When symptoms persist, always check water, remedy, protein, and transverse colon (one at a time, stopping when there is an improvement).

If you are not making the headway you want, introduce a colon herb, formula or citrus to the RIGHT hand, and while holding the other items you were testing test again. Again, a simple colon herb, formula, tangerine or orange in the right hand is all that is needed to repeat this test again.

This simple maneuver can produce miraculous results. Upwards of 98% of all humans suffer with constipation or a bowel problem; therefore, check the Transverse Colon as necessary. If you are having problems with this technique, your doctor can help or you can always call me.

Man's environment requires he interact with it via touch. This being the case, it explains why this technique is so basic. Man must in a moment's notice quickly evaluate cold, hot, sharp, dull, soft or hard, etc.

This sense is so refined it has dominated our being. Yet, this is an ancient protection mechanism that has been neglected. It has taken me decades of testing to re-establish this technique. I am giving it to you here.

Use it. Use it often.

Anyone who has ever seen me work at a convention or do weekend training is amazed at how adept I am at EBT. Doctors stare in wonder as doctor after patient walks away from me feeling better and not fully knowing why.

EBT is not Kinesiology. Do not make that mistake. Quantum physics deals in mass and energy. Problems of the body are either out of balance mass or energy. When the body contacts anything containing energy the body will either balance mass, energy, or both.

Muscle testing or Kinesiology involves the use of touching or holding something to the body while another person (the practitioner) tests the strength of the body. This reveals whether the item being tested is good for the body or not.

The last paragraph explained just why I do not do kinesiology or any of its offspring. That type of testing requires one energized being (YOU) being in contact with another energized being (THE TESTER).

This kind of test is inherently faulty as there is an energy exchange between the tester and the testee. Unless you intend to live the rest of your life touching the tester (the other individual), the energy exchange between the two of you skews the test completely.

The EBT is, by its purity, 100% accurate. The only factor being, the creativity awareness and detective work of the tester to unravel what they are working with.

Do not be fooled

Should the person you are interviewing try to take control and jump ahead or starts telling you "Nothing hurts", "I'm fine", "This is silly" or some other variation of arguing, tell this person,

"Thank you, but if you are not going to cooperate, I am going to stop and we will be done. If you want my help, I need you to help me. If you do not want my help, tell me now so that I can stop."

If you are working with someone who has an expanded / descended abdomen and who insists that they do not have issues of their colon or intestines, stop. When this same person insists that they are not constipated (less than 1 elimination per meal eaten) stop. You cannot help this person, as they do not really want help. If that same person claims to never have been constipated, stop. See the chapter later on HELP.

In order to do face reading and EBT, you must be brave / confident and persistent. Do not get discouraged if you get a couple of no answers.

Remember, the EBT questions do not treat anything. It is up to you to use the right formula or herbs that will alleviate these symptoms. If you use the right formula or herbs, you can expect to see an immediate change in these symptoms. Note: an improved diet will also alleviate these symptoms, as diet is the most destructive aspect of our lives aside from drugs and surgery.

Accurate Strength Testing

While I discourage you from doing muscle testing with another person, I am including a test that involves testing strength, which you can do by yourself.

You are going to test yourself against dead weight.

1) Establish which side / hand is your strongest (left or right).
2) Use a full 3-5 gallon closed bottle of water or dumbbell (5-30 lbs.).
3) Place it directly next to the outside (not in front or behind) of your knee (4-6 inches away).
4) Using your less dominant hand, hold a substance to the center of your chest.
5) Squat down (at the knees) and grasp the neck of the water bottle or the dumbbell handle.
6) While gripping the bottle or handle, slowly stand up.
7) Notice how heavy the bottle or dumbbell appears.

Repeat the above 7 steps while holding nothing to your chest and then again while holding the substance to your chest. Notice that your strength is altered by what you hold to your chest.

This test reveals the invisible effects of quantum physics on the body. Certain substances will make the body stronger by unlocking energy. While others will interrupt this energy flow and the body will be weaker.

IMPORTANT NOTES IN STRENGTH TESTING

- First establish WHICH is your dominant side, right or left (stronger side of your body).
- Pick an item to test sugar, candy, cookie, supplement, fruit, vegetable, etc.
- Hold the item to your chest with your weaker hand.
- With the closed water bottle or dumbbell on your stronger side (next to the side of your leg).
- Bend down once or twice and lift the bottle or dumbbell without holding a substance to your chest.
- Repeat the above step while holding bread, corn chips, sugar or a cookie, etc., to your chest.

Was the heaviness of the bottle or dumbbell affected by what you were holding? You are experiencing the simplest of communications from your body.

These tests reveal what your body wants and are otherwise (weakened) harmed by.

Repeat this test until you are certain of how it works. Test with the items below. Simple tests like this will uncover foods and chemicals that make the body stronger or weaker.

Your body never lies. Learn to trust its signals and you will be healthier.

Phase 1: acquire the following items:

A) 1 closed 5-gallon bottle of water (like for a water cooler)

B) 1 candy bar made of chocolate, unopened

C) 1 small bottle of tomato juice or vegetable juice

D) 1 lemon

E) 1 apple

F) 1 packet of artificial sweetener

G) 1 packet of sugar

With the seven items listed above, do not unwrap, open or eat any of the items you are going to test with. Leave the items closed and undisturbed.

Phase 2: next, with all of your items a few feet away, do the following:

1) Stand next to your 5 Gallon bottle of water on your dominant side.

2) Bend at the knees and grasp the bottle comfortably around the neck with your

dominant hand.

3) Using your knees, stand up erect and notice how heavy your water bottle appears to you.

4) Notice how easy or hard it was to pick up the bottle a few inches off the floor.

Phase 3: Pick up an item like the candy bar and hold it to your chest with your weaker hand. Stand next to your water bottle and repeat the above 4 steps.

Repeat this test over and over again with different items held to your chest. Frequently do this test with nothing in your hand and notice how it affects your strength. Notice if your grip is weakened by what you are holding. Continue to test with various items, noticing what makes you weak or strong or has no effect.

Dr. Wayne Dwyer recommends use of this type of test to demonstrate that negative thoughts make your body weak.

This is a very pure way to test the body and supplements. It is far better than Kinesiology, Muscle Testing and Resistance Testing. If it is utilized, it will give you amazing information.

37 Fingernail, Hand and Finger Analysis
The fingernails display the state of the body as regulated by the kidneys.

Every organ system of the body is dependent on fluid for its survival. Therefore, each fingernail displays the water table / circulation / energy level of the systems of the body.

There are hundreds of techniques for healing and detecting the health of the body. I have focused this book on giving you tools you can utilize and get very good at. Fingernail analysis is an extremely good tool that can be used with the other techniques to further validate and cement your earlier findings.

Like my face reading technique, my fingernail analysis method is not exactly like other practices heretofore found. Yet all techniques attempt to give you a window to your health.

Fingernail analysis has been with us for almost 4000 years. Each finger of your hand has a story to tell. Before I tell you the story of your fingernails, I should mention that every problem of the body has three similar factors: lack of oxygen / lack of circulation and lack of energy. This is why supporting your energy is akin to supporting your life. Think of these factors as life support for the body.

If an organ or area of the body is oxygen starved, then bacteria will spread and the body will falter even further. Again oxygen / circulation and energy are the answer.

When there is a broken bone, if not enough oxygen reaches that area, it will take an extended period of time to heal. Therefore, if oxygen consistently saturates an area of the body, the body will be more resistant to so-called disease, and when problems do occur, the body will heal quickly.

One of the best herbs that can be used to increase circulation is cayenne. Cayenne stimulates circulation and has a very distinct effect on healing.

Your nails should not:

Easily split	Have bumps
Easily chip	Be yellow
Have ridges	

Revamping of your lifestyle and diet is a sure way to start correcting any condition of the body. Here is what each fingernail represents.

Thumbnails: Represent the colon and intestinal tract.

Index Fingers: Represent the state of the liver and gallbladder and therefore represent your emotional well-being.

Middle Fingers: Heart, lungs, circulation.

Ring Fingers: Kidneys, adrenal glands, pancreas, sex drive and reproduction.

Pinky Fingers: Represent the lymphatic system, endocrine system, spleen, the brain and spine; all influenced by the kidneys.

What the nails should look like or WHAT IS A MOON:

At the back of your fingernail, NEAR YOUR FIRST FINGER JOINT, is a white (or light colored) half moon shaped area. All of your fingers should have a moon except the pinky finger. The moon represents the circulation as related to the organ associated to that finger.

All fingers should have moons except the pinky fingers.
If you have a black or partially black tongue combined with no moons on any **fingers except your pinky**, this can portend a very toxic condition.

Roger Bezanis

Not a death sentence, yet if this condition persists, a very oxygen-depleted condition can spread in the body. The condition is often called cancer. Remember quantum physics states that a blockage is caused by little or no energy, circulation or oxygen. Repairing these factors repairs this condition.

When healthy, the moons should progress biggest to smallest from thumbs to ring fingers.

1) Thumb = Largest moon

2) Index finger = Second largest moon

3) Middle finger = Third largest moon

4) Ring fingers = Fourth largest or smallest moon

5) Pinky fingers = No moon at all

Beware of moons that take up almost the entire nail, as this can be indicative of severe liver problems. Memory problems are often present when there are less than four moons per hand. The other accompanying problems often presented are poor circulation and cold hands. Low energy is also very likely.

No Moons At All on Any Fingers or Thumb
This is indicative of very poor circulation. The kidney and liver and therefore the entire system are under attack. This is the result of heavy toxicity in the system that if left unchecked could lead to cancer. The person will have most, if not all, of the liver and kidney symptoms listed in the liver and kidney chapters.

TONGUE NOTE: Look at the tongue. At this point examine the edges of the tongue. Have the person open their mouth and flop or lay their tongue out of the mouth relaxed without strain. It should just lay relaxed out of the mouth.

Look to see if there are tooth indentations on the sides of the tongue; if there are, this combined with the lack of moons can signal heavy toxicity in the system or even cancer.

Two Large Moons On the Pinky Fingers
This condition indicates an overworked heart / endocrine system and possibly high blood pressure. The kidneys will normally be severely overloaded. Look at the face. Are the eyes puffy or dark? If so, you will also find low back pain, stiffness or soreness as well as sore muscles. This can include a thyroid problem / endocrine problem, which again has bad kidneys at its base. **TONGUE NOTE:** Have the person stick out their tongue; if, when the tongue is relaxed, it is pointy and red tipped this validates a heart problem.

Short Wide Reddish Nails/Short Wide Nails
This condition indicates a cardiovascular issue (i.e. heart condition), high blood pressure and problems of the arteries. The moons on fingers and thumbs may have a "halo" of white silhouetting or separating the moon from the rest of the fingernail.

This just further validates the condition of heart.

Dark Spot on the Ring Finger of the Right Hand
If you notice a black oval spot on the right hand ring finger, this can indicate a liver problem that can even indicate liver cancer.

Arched Nail That Rolls Down Over the Tip of the Finger
A nail with this condition indicates that the kidneys are not processing protein. The individual may suffer with low energy throughout the day. They may be on a kidney-irritating high protein diet. This individual may be taking iron that is not being processed. This individual has kidney issues and needs to clear their kidneys and open up the channels.

A Flat Nail with No Curvature
This indicates that there are digestive disturbances or possibly an inflamed chronic stomach condition. This also includes nails that are blackish or yellow in tone.

A Spoon Shaped Nail That Dips in the Middle and Grows Up at the Tip
This is a red flag and indicates the presence of parasites and possible growths in the system. The nail may also have a hazy look or be unclear. You may feel fatigued and crave sugar. All of this signals parasites. Those labeled with cancer may also have nails that meet this description.

White Spots under the Nails
Should you develop white spots underneath your nails, it indicates you are dealing with excess hormones. You may also see white horizontal lines on the nail. These lines further indicate kidney issues. They are not caused by protein or calcium as is commonly believed. There is one cause for these spots and one cause only, but where are these hormones coming from?
(See the HORMONE WARNING AT THE END OF THIS CHAPTER)

Red Spots
If the middle finger has a red spot on it, this can indicate a heart condition.

Nails That Split or Are Easily Broken
Nails in this condition are lacking nutrients, as are the systems the nails represent. Normally, all nails will be in this condition but isolated chipping, breaking and splitting do occur. This is always indicative of kidney challenges. Vitamin B-complex could be being eroded by parasites or just not getting into the system due to toxicity in the kidney. Alcohol consumption, caffeine intake, drug use and excessive protein may cause the same condition.

Slow Growing Thick and Hard Nails
This again is a kidney issue regardless of the nail or nails involved. Tobacco use, heavy industrial chemical exposure, which directly leads to endocrine system overload, also crafts this challenge.

Yellow Nails
Often comes with years of smoking. The lungs are very overwhelmed and oxygen is not reaching the cells at a sufficient rate. The person may have a chronic cough and digestive tribulations. Yellow nails can occur due to years of chemical exposure as these compounds have settled in the lungs. The liver supports the lungs; therefore anything that can be done to improve liver and lung function will be a benefit. Other common symptoms will include insomnia, poor energy, itchy skin, irritated eyes and extreme poor moods. Again, this condition is greatly aided by simply improving liver / lung and kidneys as these dynamos are in a weakened state.

Vertical Black Lines under the Nails
Indicates internal bleeding associated with the organ that corresponds to that finger. This is also an excellent test for parasites as parasites ingest quantities of blood. Often this condition is facilitated by a diet high in sugar, breads, manmade starches, caffeine, unhandled stress and constipation.

Black Splotches on the Nails
If a black spot is seen on the nail that does not move with nail growth this can mean cancer. Examine the tongue for color (should not be black). Notice the presence of the fingernail moons (no pinky moon) and look to see if the tongue has teeth marks on the edges, when it is relaxed and laying out of the mouth.

HORMONE WARNING: The two hormones that show up under our nails can be either testosterone or estrogen or faux versions of either one.

We live in a chemical happy "life better through science" society. Business needs to get every dollar it can from its products. The thrust in the poultry, beef, fish and dairy industry has been to deliver product to market that arrives faster and is more profitable. In the last 40 years hormones have been increasingly used to "plump up" the average animal targeted for slaughter. If the average meat yield is increased by just 3 percent per animal, this is worth hundreds of millions of dollars in profit annually.

Added Hormone (steroids) Impact on Society
- The average age for a first period is now 12?, up from age 14 in 1900.
- Teenage breast size has increased at an alarming (1.3 cup size) rate in the last 20 years.
- The number of breast cancer cases reported annually approached 900,000 in 1997, up from 572,000 in 1980.

- Juvenile diabetes (virtually unheard of 40 years ago) is on a steady rise.
- Male muscle mass is increasing while scalp hair is decreasing. Hair replacement has become a billion dollar a year industry in the last 30 years.
- Since the advent of hormone infusion into the food supply, the average height of humans has jumped by more than 4%.

How this has happened.

The answer is both alarming and maddening: beef, poultry, fish, chocolate and dairy products are your culprits. Earlier I mentioned that our meat and dairy is infused with hormones to make it bigger, meatier and therefore more valuable. Money is the answer.

Steroids are pumped into our food supply not for our benefit but the benefit of the seller.

These hormones are much like seeing a doctor and getting steroid injections. We are participating in a chemical experiment at this very moment. The only permission you gave was based on what you chose to put in your mouth.

Another source of hormones is from chocolate. Chocolate mimics both testosterone and estrogen hormones in the body and offers a double dose when you consume milk chocolate. Have you ever wondered why you feel so good when you eat chocolate? If so, the chocolate confectioners of the planet would prefer you did not mention the next paragraph.

Chemistry class 101

Chocolate creates noticeable euphoria when consumed due to hormone mimicry.

On contact with the system, chocolate quickly converts to synthetic estrogen and testosterone. Your body starts to react to this chemical cocktail. The body goes into the reproductive and growth cycle. Suddenly we are swept up in a chemically induced cloud of aphrodisiac sensation. Blood flow increases as temperature rises. Breathing quickens, as does the pulse.

The euphoria derived from chocolate has been well known by Valentine's Day marketers for decades. Did you think it was love? Did you think you had found your soul mate? Perhaps you did, but you were also drugged in the process and didn't know it.

Whenever you eat chocolate you will feel some degree of euphoria, sexual urges, and brief but quick burning energy. Long consistent exposure causes kidney / endocrine and liver failure. Now that you know where the bodies are buried, there is no hiding from it.

Unless you change, you are giving your tacit compliance to participate in an experiment where the long-range results are not known. The choice is yours. To prevent hormone overload and the resulting failure of your system, eliminate chocolate, dairy and eat only free-range meat and poultry from your health food store. Not heeding this warning your body (via steroids) will take on mass (height / breast size / muscle) and mutate in ways that cannot be predicted. Imagine your heart swelling in size, or masses growing in your brain or vital organs. These conditions are under your control but if not controlled by you, you may start living a nightmare every day.

Free-range
adj. 1 a: Of, relating to, or produced by animals, especially poultry, that range freely for food, rather than being confined in an enclosure: free-range chickens.

verb 2 a: The raising of livestock and domestic poultry; permitted to graze or forage rather than being confined to a feedlot
Synonym: unenclosed

A Word or Two on Your Fingers

Another way to detect INHERITED kidney issues (and there are many) is to look at finger length.

INDEX FINGER——-	1st finger closest to the thumb
MIDDLE FINGER—-	2nd finger (the bird flipping finger)
RING FINGER——-	3rd finger (where a wedding ring goes)

Your ring finger (3rd finger) of your dominant hand should be longer than your index finger (1st finger) of the same hand.

If it is not, there is an inherited kidney issue. A predisposition to a kidney problem (or any problem) does not have to manifest. If you are aware of potential problems, potential problems can remain potential.

Now a Word on Your Hands

Another way to check for current kidney challenges is demonstrated on this test.

Do the following.

- Stand in front of a mirror and close your eyes.
- Now lightly shake out your arms and let them fall to their full length and dangle at your sides.

- Without moving your hands or arms, open your eyes and look (in the mirror) at where your palms are facing.

Are they facing?

A) Behind you?

B) Toward your thighs?

C) More forward toward the mirror?

(Right hand = Right Kidney / Left hand = Left kidney)

A = Weak - low energy kidney on that side of the body

B = Indicates the kidneys are healthy and running well

C = Indicates hyper-condition as the kidneys are running hot

You may also notice that the hand that is facing more directly behind you is on the side where your kidney is worse today. The results of this test change on a daily basis as your kidneys run better or worse.

To further validate your findings, compare the bag or dark circle under the eye to the hand that is more directly angled behind you or in front of you.

Did you notice that your eyes agree with your hands in this test? Did you also notice other kidney symptoms such as low back pain, kidneys that feel warm (even slightly)? These tests are simple yet very useful.

38 About The Tongue

The tongue does not get much attention in western medicine, yet it speaks volumes about your health. Usually it is just in the way during dental work and examining the tonsils. In the early 1900s the tongue was far more important in diagnoses. Today it is still accepted that a white coating indicates immune system activity.

Tongue basics

Tongue Cracking

Should the tongue have cracks in it, it is due to a kidney problem. Regardless of anything else you know or that might come up, at the basis of it is a kidney problem. If the cracking is very deep then the stomach is also involved. Regardless, digestion and kidneys are at the source of this issue.

Red Spots On The Tip Of The Tongue
Indicates heart issues; the denser the spots are, the worse the condition. Compare this with other tools from earlier chapters. Read the chapter on ear piercing, as this section reveals much data. If the tongue is pointy at the tip, this is also an indication of heart issues.

Stinging Tongue (Burning Mouth Syndrome)
The totality of this problem is a liver running hot. The sensation can spread all over the mouth. The diet is at issue. Eliminate oils, spicy foods and salty food. Eat citrus, use a good liver formula (without milk thistle), drink more water and avoid caffeine. Like most problems of the body, BMS is the result of an ineffective / poor diet.

A Slightly Black Tongue
This is the forerunner to serious oxygen depletion in the body. The endocrine system, liver, kidneys, etc, are overloaded. There is never a kidney problem that does not include a liver problem; both need support. Remove sugar from the diet as well as sodium and correct the problem. See your health care practitioner and with his or her help, you can improve this situation.

A Predominantly Black Tongue
When the tongue is predominantly black, this is very serious as the system is in a shut down mode. The kidneys and liver are in very great trouble and since they support and regulate the entire system, the system is under great stress as well. Poor circulation will make the hands, feet, legs and arms cold. In later stages the body will become very hot as the immune system struggles forward. The person may have a dull, constant headache, labored breathing, dizziness and confusion. This is not a death sentence; it indicates that much must be done to immediately increase CIRCULATION / OXYGEN and ENERGY to the body.

They may be manifesting all the symptoms of kidney and liver overwhelm. If this condition is allowed to continue, the body will get weaker and show more signs of shutting down. This condition does not have to signal the end. It just indicates that to reverse the condition it will take a lot of time and work. Again, repair CIRCULATION / OXYGEN and ENERGY to the body and, of course, eliminate all manmade sugar and as many processed foods as possible.

A Pink Clear Healthy Looking Tongue Without Spots or Teeth Marks
Everything is fine and the system is working properly. If you had conditions of the tongue and they have changed, beware that the condition may return. Therefore you must be diligent. The healing of the system, and the corresponding tongue changes do not necessarily occur gradually. The tongue will improve its look as unhealthy conditions reduce and the body gets stronger. The body may feel better on contact with certain remedies and stimuli, but chronic conditions will take time to fully heal themselves.

About Your Hair

Hair gets a lot of attention in our society but for all the wrong reasons. Sure it looks great and can be colored, dyed, made curly or chopped off. More importantly, it reflects the health of our kidneys. When the kidneys are running well, the nails and hair are strong.

Hair that is thin and getting thinner indicates that the kidneys are in trouble. If the hair has thinned but has stabilized, then kidneys were a problem and have also stabilized. Graying hair is indicative of kidney weakness. It is true that we inherit our health tendencies from our parents; yet, it is what we do with these tendencies that matters.

Repeating, hair **should** keep its color; if it does not, it is due to weak kidneys. The door of health swings both ways. Hair that grays overnight or over a few days is directly due to overwhelmed kidneys. But the hair can return to its natural color if the problem is caught early enough.

I have corrected my own hair color twice (at this printing). Others are working on the same target.

The mechanics of it work this way. Due to kidney blockage or overwhelm, the kidneys are not getting or are not processing B-complex and other nutrients (which supports kidney function and hair color). When this occurs, the hair loses its color. The hair can also start falling out.

The other factors are of course decreased oxygen, circulation and energy. Repair all three and kidney function and any condition can change even hair color.

Correct any problem of the body with the same 5 steps:

1). Determine what you are being exposed to that is facilitating the problem (this is the stimulus).
2). Eliminate the stimuli causing the problem.
3). Strengthen or clean via detoxification the organ affected by the stimuli.
4). Don't re-introduce the stimuli that caused the problem.
5). Repair circulation, oxygen and energy flow in the body.

39 Iridology and Face Reading, The Dream Team

Iridology is pronounced: Eye-ri-dology

Definition: Iridology is the dynamic visual system of analysis of iris structures to establish the strength, weakness and tendencies of all the tissues and vital organs of the human body. An auxiliary aspect of iridology is the detailed study of the white part of the eye called the sclera. Surrounding the iris the sclera gives another detailed picture to study the body with. Sometimes sclera study is referred to Sclerology. It is important to note that iridology is not used for diagnosis. Rather, it is used as a means of assessment for conditions and levels of health.

It has been my privilege to study with some of the great minds of our time. One man that is head and shoulders above the rest is Dr. David J. Pesek. He is the President of the International College of Iridology. His care and loving of all who he comes in contact with is legendary.

Dr. Pesek is on the faculty of several institutions that teach natural and integrative medicine. Over the past three decades, his pioneering work is bringing about the renaissance of natural healthcare through his dedication. When you get a chance to study with Dr. David, you should do it without question, as the experience is always enlightening and rewarding.

Respected by many as the leading Iridologist in the world his honesty and passion for healing is beyond compare. It is because of Dr. Pesek that I have been fortunate to learn so much about iridology. Whether you have a working basic understanding of the modality or you are an expert and use it in a professional practice, iridology is a fantastic tool.

The history of man, body and especially the eyes tell a remarkable story. Ancient texts revere the eyes as a link between the physical and spiritual universe. This is why a full understanding of them is of supreme interest to anyone who wants to study the healing of mankind.

The belief in the power of the eye for all manner of learning and spirituality is not new. Studying the historic record reveals details that are missed by many. It is generally accepted that iridology dates back to Mesopotamia (Central Asia). Texts exist indicating that some form of iris study was done in this region as early as 3,000 years ago (1000 BC).

Long before man took to cutting and dissecting flesh to comprehend what made his fellow man tick, he was doing visual analysis for clues to mortality. Men had to observe and insightfully use their five senses to comprehend the complexities of the human body.

The old time Egyptologist will insist that Isis and Osiris were Gods. Yet literal translation of the words reveals that they were not gods but "states of being." Just as Christ and Moses are different from "blessed" and "saved," Osiris and Isis are different from "knowledge" and "soul."

"The eyes are the window to the soul" is credited by scholars to have been taken from the bible in Mathew 6:22-23.

Other sources simply state that it is an old English or Arab proverb. When we reflect on Egyptology the saying becomes less murky as to where this translucent statement and eye emphasis derived from and what they mean.

Etymologists know that life can be understood if we know the words. Therefore a pure translation of this saying "the eyes are the window to the soul" would be "The eyes are the soul."

For man to experience and sense life he must be able to view it with his soul. His soul, not being of the physical universe, must take shape in the physical being. This is what the eyes are as per expert Egyptologist David Cintron and others. They are the physical embodiment of the soul that allows man to experience and take into his being the totality of life itself.

Ask any doctor who has witnessed death. When the eyes fade the body is dead. When the soul starts to leave the body, the patient can no longer see until he is free from his Earthly vessel.

Thus iridology is actually the study of the soul of man as it interfaces with the body. This one statement brings all of the previous and later emphasis on the eye together under one umbrella. This is not a quantum leap in understanding but a simple lining up of truths and then following them back to their natural source.

With the aforementioned in mind consider:

Isis means spiritual knowledge and Osiris means "Seat of the eye," "Place of the eye" or "Throne of the eye." The question then becomes: what does "the eye" mean?

The focal point of the eye is the Iris.

The name Isis means "Spiritual knowledge"

The name Osiris meant "Seat of the eye," "Place of the eye" or "Throne of the eye."

The first religion found on Earth was Osirianism (circa 2991 BC Pre-Dynastic Egypt).

Osirianism was the "pursuit of the afterlife through the pursuit of knowledge." This statement explains religions that are focused on the understanding of God and thus manifesting him in ones heart via one's own deeds and understanding.

In a nutshell, Egyptology teaches that man (Horace) was trying to be one with Osiris (his soul). Once he achieved this goal he attained spiritual knowledge (Isis). After death, if he embraced the spiritual knowledge, he attained Sokar (spiritual freedom) to be reborn.

The festival of Sokar in 3150 BC is then also explained as it was "The festival celebrating rebirth."

In essence, early Egyptians were attaining salvation of the soul via the eye which they believed to be the physical embodiment of the soul. Again iridology is actually the study of the soul of man as it interfaces with the body.

Take a moment and think of "eye quotes" and write them down. Replace the word eye with soul. Read them again. "An eye for an eye" would become "A soul for a soul" etc. Simple quotes take on much deeper meanings, don't they?

In iridology and, to a lesser extent, other modalities we study the eyes. The bridge between the spiritual, mental, emotional and physical aspects of our human nature is experienced via the eyes.

It is logical to study the look of the face and the iris of the eye as it is directly connected to the brain, sympathetic nervous system and spinal cord. Therefore nerve signals from the entire body are collected and sent to the eyes. The eyes literally "see" the whole body.

The optic tract extends to the thalamus area of the brain. This creates a close association with the hypothalamus, pituitary and pineal glands. These endocrine glands, within the brain, are major control and processing centers for the entire body.

Because of this anatomy and physiology, the eyes are in direct contact with the biochemical, hormonal, structural and metabolic processes of the body via the nerves, blood vessels, lymph and connective tissue.

When a yogi closes his eyes and looks through his body for a problem, he is in a pure sense, "looking" with his optic nerve along sheaths that connect the entire body. The window to the soul leads all the way to the soles of the feet if the road is traveled.

The eyes reflect the state of the following organs and systems:

Brain	Lymphatic system
Bowel / Colon	Pineal glands
Digestive system	Pituitary glands
Immune system	Hypothalamus
Circulatory system	Spine
Skin	Central nervous system
Heart	Musculature
Lungs	Bone structure
Liver	Reproductive system
Gall bladder	Respiratory system
Kidneys	Appendix
Pancreas	Vocal expression
Adrenal glands	Five senses and more
Thyroid gland	
Parathyroid gland	

Face reading and Iridology were the first two great studies of the nature of the man.

Born on the island of Kos, south of the mainland of Greece, in 460 BC, Hippocrates is credited as the "Father of Medicine." He is believed to be the first "western" practitioner to do both face reading and iridology.

His own words express as much.

He said, "Inquiries are to be made and symptoms are to be noted, those in the whole countenance (face), those on the body and those in the eyes." He was regarded as the greatest physician of his time. Many patients were lucky to have him as their physician as his observational skill was exceptional.

Also from the bible, St. Luke (11:34-36) writes that Christ said, "The lamp of your body is the eye. When your eyes are sound, you have light for the whole body, but when your eyes are bad, you are in darkness."

Again the body and spirit are seen as one in the eyes. Therefore the maintenance of and observation of the eyes and face are paramount for anyone attempting to understand the body and its workings.

Iridologists all over the world know that having modalities of equal magnitude in their tool box makes the job much easier. Competently using face reading and Iridology, one can easily see the tendencies, strengths and weakness of the body.

Iridology gives an amazing snap shot of the body at birth, as does face reading. Yet iridology is very deep as it is possible to detect exactly what system is affected at the exact point of affliction. Face reading gives a slightly more general assessment, but with the Energy Balancing Technique™, it is possible to get more defined.

Face reading is very much a "now modality" as the face changes rapidly and reflects challenges being experienced at the present moment. The changes seen in Iridology manifest an assessment of the body up to about 2-4 months prior. These detailed cross-sections are of laser precision. Commingled the two "understanding via observation techniques," you have readouts so good that an MRI (Magnetic Resonance Imagining) specialist would be jealous.

That is why whenever there is a chance to learn both Iridology and face reading it is important to jump at the chance. More and more, colon hydrotherapists, Chiropractors, Naturopaths, Nutritionists and other "grounded" excellent traditional medicine practitioners use both modalities / tools.

Iridology is infinitely workable as health changes dramatically follow how a person eats, drinks, feels, thinks and lives.

Iris analysis and face reading can uncover hereditary predispositions to degenerative conditions and early pathogenesis decades before symptoms occur or diagnostic testing reveals them. Thus, it is a valuable asset for preventive healthcare.

During the first half of the 20th century, IRIDIAGNOSIS (as it was called then) was utilized here in the USA primarily by medical doctors. The following is a quote taken from a text by Henry Lindlahr, M.D. circa 1919.

"The 'regular' school of medicine (allopathic), as a body, has ignored and will ignore this science (of iridology), because it discloses the fallacy of their favorite theories and practices and because it reveals unmistakable the direful results of chronic drug poisoning (pharmaceuticals) and ill advised operations / surgeries."

Due to increasing political and economic pressure upon medical schools by the emerging pharmaceutical industry, the teaching of iridology was removed from the curriculum. Eventually this art and science was lost within the allopathic medical practice.

An advanced system of iris analysis, called Holistic Iridology®, researched and developed by David J. Pesek, Ph.D., includes and travels beyond the traditional physical assessment. Through this leading edge system it is possible to understand the "whole" person. Mental / emotional and spiritual aspects can also be interpreted along with the physical.

Each eye gives us different information. The left eye correlates with the left side of our body and feminine aspects while the right eye correlates to the right side of our body and masculine aspects.

RELATIVE STRENGTH OF THE BODY'S CONSTITUTION AS DEMONSTRATED VIA THE IRIS

STRONG

WEAK

GOOD

POOR

FAIR

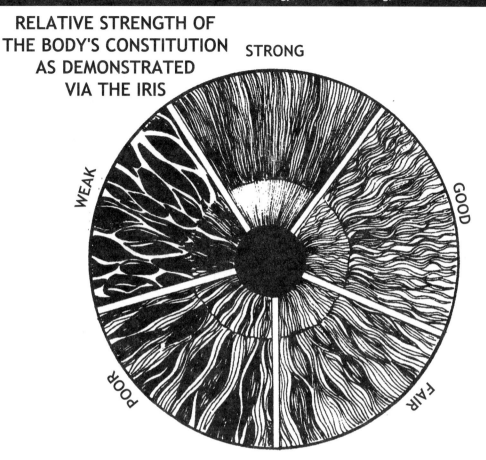

The fiber structure of the iris and its density (see above) gives the relative strength of a person's inherited genetics going back generations. This genetic constitution is our ability to withstand stress on all levels, i.e. physical, emotional, mental and spiritual. These iris fiber structures indicate not only organs, glands and other tissue strengths; they also reveal conscious and subconscious thought and emotional patterns.

Overall the constitution is a significant factor because it gives an indication of the strength of the entire body. People with weak constitutions require more care and nurturing for their body. The channels of elimination and detoxification tend to become congested more easily. Nutrients are required at a higher level to feed the organs, glands, nervous system, bones, etc. Greater attention to what they eat, how they exercise, where they live and the type of work they do are considerations.

On the other end of the scale, we see the strong constitution. Individuals with this type of body tend to have greater resistance to illness and disease and a higher stamina emotionally and mentally. Some people with this make-up tend to abuse themselves and not feel the effects as much as the person with the weak constitution. However, abuse of the physical body will have a cumulative effect upon anyone, be they weak or strong in constitution.

Roger Bezanis

Brain Reflex Areas of
HOLISTIC IRIDOLOGY®

© 2000 David J. Pesek, Ph.D.
Revised © 2002

12

11

1

CONSCIOUSNESS / VITALITY

SENSORY MOVEMENT

EXPERIENTIAL / PERCEPTION
(PSYCHOLOGICAL)

SEXUAL EXPRESSION

SURVIVAL

FIVE SENSES

SELF - ESTEEM

VERBAL EXPRESSION

LOGICAL INTELLECT

(TEMPLE FOREHEAD)

H.   PIT.   P.

RIGHT IRIS BRAIN AREAS
Right Side of Body - Masculine Aspect - Polarity is Positive
THOUGHT / EMOTION CORRELATION

CONSCIOUSNESS / VITALITY
One's vitality and enthusiasm for being rational, logical and
energetic; integration of spiritual, mental, emotional and
physical aspects.

SENSORY MOVEMENT
One's feelings of movement; getting started in the
rational world; expressing thoughts through
bodily movement.

FIVE SENSES
All thoughts and actions as beliefs and experiences related
to and integrated with visual, tactile, auditory, olfactory
and gustatory senses; and correlated with linear/rational
thought, outgoing actions and the masculine nature.

EXPERIENTIAL / PERCEPTION
(PSYCHOLOGICAL)
One's perceptions and experiences of what was or
was not received from the environment, from father,
or from primary masculine figures while growing up.

SELF-ESTEEM
Concern about what someone else thinks or feels about
one's actions, thoughts, words or the masculine aspects;
self image.

SEXUAL EXPRESSION
Possible sexual trauma, confusion, compulsion or
suppression of sex drive, either experientially or
genetically, from the masculine aspect.

VERBAL EXPRESSION
Organizing one's thoughts, experiences and perceptions
into words, then clearly expressing them, in writing or
speech, from a logical perspective.

SURVIVAL
Birth trauma, breathing difficulties, resistance to
inspiration from the rational/logical aspects; concern
about survival in career, education, financial matters
and business relationships.

LOGICAL INTELLECT
The aspect of utilizing one's mental ability to
express outwardly to the world what one knows
one's logical/rational, mental capabilities are.

ABBREVIATIONS

H.   HYPOTHALAMUS
P.   PINEAL GLAND
PIT.   PITUITARY GLAND

International
Institute of
Iridology.

375 PARADISE LANE
WAYNESVILLE, NORTH CAROLINA
28785 USA
TEL: 828-926-6100
e-mail: drpesek@holisticiridology.com
www.holisticiridology.com

DIAGNOSTIC Face Reading and Holistic Healing

Brain Reflex Areas of
HOLISTIC IRIDOLOGY®

© 2000 David J. Pesek, Ph.D.
Revised © 2002

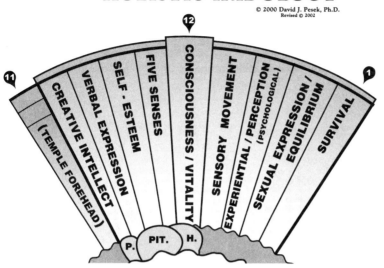

LEFT IRIS BRAIN AREAS
Left Side of Body - Feminine Aspect - Polarity is Negative

THOUGHT / EMOTION CORRELATION

CONSCIOUSNESS / VITALITY
One's vitality and enthusiasm for being creative and loving;
integration of spiritual, mental, emotional and
physical aspects.

FIVE SENSES
All feelings and emotions as beliefs and experiences related
to and integrated with visual, tactile, auditory, olfactory
and gustatory senses; and correlated with creativity,
intuition, spatial perceptions and the feminine nature.

SENSORY MOVEMENT
One's feelings of movement; getting started in the
creative world; expressing emotions through
bodily movement.

SELF-ESTEEM
Concern about what someone else thinks or feels
about one's creativity, emotions or the feminine aspects;
self image.

EXPERIENTIAL / PERCEPTION
(PSYCHOLOGICAL)
One's perceptions and experiences of what was or
was not received from the environment, from mother,
or from primary feminine figures while growing up.

VERBAL EXPRESSION
Organizing one's feelings, experiences and perceptions
into words, then clearly expressing them, in
writing or speech, from an emotional level.

SEXUAL EXPRESSION / EQUILIBRIUM
Possible head injury or blocked, intense memory. Possible
past genetic epileptic center. Possible sexual trauma, either
experientially or genetically, from the feminine aspect.

CREATIVE INTELLECT
The aspect of utilizing one's mental ability to express
outwardly to the world what one knows one's
creative, mental capabilities are.

SURVIVAL
Birth trauma, breathing difficulties, resistance to
inspiration from the creative/emotional aspects;
concern about survival in emotional/love relationships.

ABBREVIATIONS

H.	HYPOTHALAMUS
P.	PINEAL GLAND
PIT.	PITUITARY GLAND

International
Institute of
Iridology®

375 PARADISE LANE
WAYNESVILLE, NORTH CAROLINA
28785 USA
TEL: 828-926-6100
e-mail: drpesek@holisticiridology.com
www.holisticiridology.com

Roger Bezanis

Iris analysis is most effectively done by imaging both eyes with a specialized microscope and digital camera. The pictures are then enlarged and carefully examined by a qualified iridologist who possesses the highest skills and standards.

The topographic map that is produced has representations and locations of structures of the body like those listed earlier. This map or chart bears a correlation to the embryological development of the human fetus to present day.

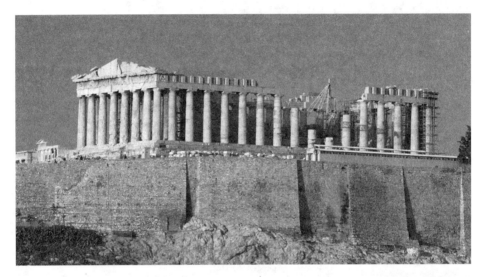

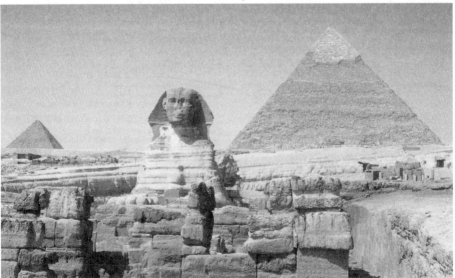

DIAGNOSTIC Face Reading and Holistic Healing

HOLISTIC IRIDOLOGY®

© 1999 David J. Pesek, Ph.D.
Revised © 2004

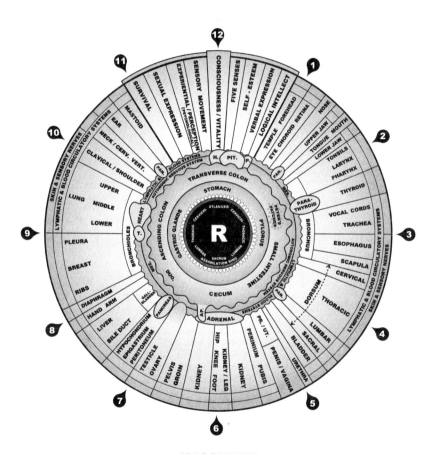

MASCULINE

ABBREVIATIONS

A.	AORTA	P.	PINEAL GLAND
AP.	APPENDIX	PAN.	PANCREAS
CERV. VERT.	CERVICAL VERTEBRAE	PIT.	PITUITARY GLAND
DUO.	DUODENUM	PR.	PROSTATE GLAND
H.	HYPOTHALAMUS	T.	THYMUS GLAND
MES.	MESENTARY	UT.	UTERUS

International
Institute of
Iridology®

375 PARADISE LANE
WAYNESVILLE, NORTH CAROLINA
28785 USA
TEL: 828-926-6100
e-mail: drpesek@holisticiridology.com
www.holisticiridology.com

Roger Bezanis

Chart of
HOLISTIC IRIDOLOGY®

© 1999 David J. Pesek, Ph.D.

Revised © 2004

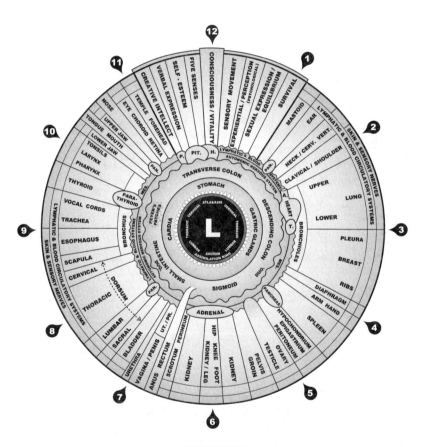

FEMININE

ABBREVIATIONS

A.	AORTA	P.	PINEAL GLAND	
AP.	APPENDIX	PAN.	PANCREAS	
CERV. VERT.	CERVICAL VERTEBRAE	PIT.	PITUITARY GLAND	
DUO.	DUODENUM	PR.	PROSTATE GLAND	
H.	HYPOTHALAMUS	T.	THYMUS GLAND	
MES.	MESENTARY	UT.	UTERUS	

International Institute of Iridology®

375 PARADISE LANE
WAYNESVILLE, NORTH CAROLINA
28785 USA
TEL: 828-926-6100
e-mail: drpesek@holisticiridology.com
www.holisticiridology.com

DIAGNOSTIC Face Reading and Holistic Healing

The iridologist should be certified through the International Institute of Iridology® in Holistic Iridology®. This advanced approach to iris analysis, which is now being used worldwide, encompasses various systems that are integrated into a truly holistic model.

I have examined almost every modality for the understanding of the body. Other than face reading I have never seen a technique that offers the kind of concrete results that Holistic Iridology® does. In a pinch a cursory look of the eyes can be done with a strong flash light and good eyesight.

For a full proper assessment that reveals the true aspect of the conditions of the body, find an iridologist trained with use of the digital camera and microscope. Attend workshops and training courses and learn iridology for yourself.

Practitioners are needed all over the country. Anyone who heals needs to know the workings of Holistic Iridology® as it is a prime technique based on history and science. No practitioner ever has enough good gear in his health tool kit.

Remember that an investment in yourself and your knowledge carries with it rewards beyond measure.

This 3,000 year old art and science may seem new and different to you. It is not different at all. It is different from what "other people" are doing and believe. You are a maverick and that is why you are reading this book.

In this chapter you have learned much about yourself and where we came from. You even have an understanding of Egyptology most Egyptologist do not have and never considered. I only bring you the very best information and advances. These advances, like face reading, are not new. They are time tested and sage in their wisdom.

I encourage you to explore the possibilities that can be realized by combining face reading with time tested and revealing Holistic Iridology®. The future is waiting for you to look closely at it and tell it what you see.

See yourself happy, healthy and in full charge of your life. Use both face reading and iridology.

Your friend,
Roger Bezanis

40 The Hidden Keys to Weight Loss and Body Repair

The true epic struggle of understanding food, the body and where we came from

The future of mankind, while seemingly a chance operation, has been a scripted event. In manufacturing, imposed obsolescence, built-in antiquity or break down of machinery is common place. This practice is not openly discussed yet; it is part of every business plan and model. Production schedules are dependent on such predictability. This is witnessed in the manufacturing of automobiles, washing machines, computers, TVs, etc.

Imagine what would happen if a machine was adaptable / upgradable and therefore lasted for 100, 200 or 300 years? If hardware never wears out and shows no appreciable or noticeable wear or tear, the financial results are disastrous. This would spell financial losses and changes in manufacturing that would threaten world economies.

Because man has involved himself in commerce, the pressure and need to sell new items and advancements has changed the way we interact with each other. It may have even changed our very lives and shortened them.

Man's longevity is cited again and again in one of the oldest texts on the planet, the bible. Are reports of 800 years of life exaggerations? As extreme as this seems, it may be 100% accurate. Make no mistake; this book will not attempt to enter a theological / science debate. That is not the purpose of this work.

The fact is that these incredible reports / stories exist of man's extreme life span and are reported over and over again. If nothing else, even the casual observer will find his curiosity at a peak in such a discussion.

What happened to man to reduce his longevity? What secret plan or gross error in human body maintenance facilitated this awful change in his fortunes?

That is the purpose of this chapter. In it I am giving you data and empirical conclusions that cannot be refuted.

Weight loss is the most controversial subject on the planet less religion. There are more theories on weight loss than countries on Earth.

Certain things are taboo: telling someone they a have gained weight, look older, have body odor, practice the wrong religion or have the wrong diet.

We are all very sensitive about our bodies. These vessels of life are our shrines. We decorate them with tattoos, piercings, colorings and clothes. We abuse them with foods, chemicals and physical stresses. Given that they are ours, we feel it is our right to treat them the way we see fit. Regardless of what we do to them or think about them, they are always with us.

Shockingly, with so much familiarity about them, they never cease to amaze and tantalize our minds. This is due to pressures and enormous confusions regarding how they actually work. If you put two people together (doctor or laymen), and ask them about body function, there is likely to be an intense argument.

The next several pages explain much about man's history and his decisions that have consequently shaped your life. Man's colloquial traditions and habits are ingrained in all of us and are affecting you right now.

Consider that there is a history of man in every one of us. In it is the vast panorama of right and wrong decisions. Included are the ancient habits that compose our present time tendencies and quirks which order our day.

First, let us examine what the human body is. Simply, it is a mobile, hollow skeleton, soft skinned carbon / oxygen burning machine. It uses fuel and produces waste.

Like a computer, it runs on a set of programs that are designed to compute the best possible solution to any given problem. It is also programmed to run a certain schedule of activities that are based on principals handed down from one generation to the other.

If this programming is supported, it is possible to lead a very active and pain-free life.

Its programming allows it to go for long periods of time without food, a shorter amount of time without water and little time without oxygen.

Its life span is between circa 80 to circa 100 years.

At full maturity the human frame can expand between 80 to 350 pounds. It can sustain weight up to 1235 pounds. It can weigh as little as 50 pounds as it dances on the slicing edge of death.

Weight above 325 pounds is very unhealthy unless the individual is a professional athlete. The general rule is that the more one weighs the shorter the life span. A lean man stands a better chance at longevity than an obese man. Every five pounds that an individual is overweight causes a 1 - 5 percent decline in health. This can be graphed via high blood pressure, etc. Excess weight directly impacts health and well-being.

Hypertension, diabetes, heart attacks, hardening of the arteries, stroke, sexual dysfunction, cancer and more are linked directly to obesity or excess weight.

Interestingly, it is a mystery to most as to what causes weight gain. Some will claim with a mouthful of taco, hotdog, pizza or hamburger smothered in onions that they have no idea why they are overweight.

Even with these confusions, most will agree that food and eating do have something to do with gaining weight. We all have theories on diet.

If we collected all the printed works on weight loss and diet it would fill, from top to bottom, a one bedroom apartment.

If you want to get into a fist fight, argue with anyone who is happy with their weight loss plan, no matter how backward it is or appears to be.

I personally know someone who lost 40 pounds in his late twenties eating just Kentucky Fried Chicken and plain M&M's. This was a bombastic and stupid thing to do. How do I know this? I was the guy who did it.

Yes, your humble author has been there and done it. I have done things you would never even consider. Medical science practices experimentation on rats, cats, dogs, mice and college students in need of cash. What college student does not need cash? For me and my work possible life changing testing is out of the question unless the test subject and the tester are the same person. I have always been my own guinea pig.

In the next several paragraphs you will finally have the answer to weight gain and weight loss. These answers have been with us but have been ignored, neglected and or scattered about for the better part of three hundred years.

We sit in our quiet times and wonder about such questions, waiting for divine inspiration to lead us to the answers. I have been actively compiling these answers for ten years.

These answers are sought after, and DO EXIST IN PLAIN SIGHT, but they are occluded or convoluted by advertising and marketing of the perfect lifestyle.

The following description of a food-based Utopian existence is based on gluttony and the pursuit of hedonism (pursuit of pleasure to the exclusion of all else).

When you read this you will understand who has sold us this "pie in the sky" dream. They would be fast food companies, desert companies and restaurant chains trying to make a living.

DIRECT FROM THE WALL STREET
MARKETING MACHINE ON IDEAL LIVING

I GIVE YOU

*****THE PERFECT LIFESTYLE*****

1)   Eat often
2)   Eat anything
3)   Eat at midnight or later
4)   Eat everything new and tasty
5)   Eat for taste and pleasure not health
6)   Never worry about getting fat or consequences.
7)   Eating pleasure is more important than relationships!!
8)   You must eat what others eat or risk not fitting in and being ostracized.

The above 8 points may seem scary. They are and we swallow them every day. They are promoted in commercials and there are slogans devoted to their repetitive power. They pervade the psyche of every consumer on the planet.

Since weight is altered by what we eat and how often it is eaten, let us look at the definition of the word "dinner."

Archeologists dig up bones, mummies, scribing and pottery all to piece together a world long gone. Etymologists do the same thing with words and their fragments. From this these grammatical detectives trace their origins. It is an indisputable fact that men change as their words change.

"Neat-o" became "keen", became "cool", became "hot" which led to "bitchin" twisting into "way cool" morphing into "sweet" and then "nice". Words tell a story every day and every minute.

Definitions give us a trail to follow to understand the reasons behind life as we know it. Earnestly grasping the language of definitions, we can fully comprehend who we are and where we came from. Motives and actions begin to make sense as well as mysteries that we otherwise could know.

Esoteric terms and usages might only be known to a few. Examined and then compared to the known data, these data begin to spin a tale. Suddenly a subject is full and alive and an entirely new picture is painted. Without this kind of work we are left in the haze of mystery. Understandings that could change existence remain lost.

UNRAVELING THE MYSTERY OF EATING

There are four meals that have been woven into human existence in so called civilized society.
- Breakfast
- Lunch
- Supper
- Dinner

How did we end up with all of these meals in our lives? We will now look at the definitions of each meal.

DINNER: The main meal of the day, formerly eaten in the morning now eaten in the early or late evening derived from disner, Latin: 8th century (800 BC).

Breakfast: 15th Century (1500 AD) The first meal of the day, especially taken in the morning.

LUNCH: Date 1812 (as early as 1708) A usually light meal or snack; especially one taken in the middle of the day.

SUPPER: A late evening snack derived from Old French soper.

Supper: (a light evening meal; served in early evening, if dinner is served at midday or served late in the evening at bedtime).

Supper: (a social gathering where a light evening meal is served)

Passover- supper – Seder: (Judaism) The ceremonial dinner on the first or both nights of Passover.

Supper is the oldest recorded word referring to a meal of any type. Passover is a yearly celebration and Passover Supper was observed as part of this observance.

Now reflect on the word **DINNER.**

DINNER: The main meal of the day, formerly eaten in the morning, now eaten in the early or late evening

(The following are not my words, they were found in:)

The American Heritage Dictionary of the English Language: Fourth Edition. 2000.

Word History: Eating foods such as pizza and ice cream for breakfast may be justified etymologically. In Middle English, dinner meant "breakfast," as did the Old French word disner, or diner, which was the source of our word.

The Old French word came from the Vulgar Latin word *disi n re, meaning "to break one's fast; that is, to eat one's first meal," a notion also contained in our word breakfast.

The Vulgar Latin word was derived from an earlier word, *disi i n re, the Latin elements of which are dis-, denoting reversal, and i i nium, "fast." Middle English diner not only meant "breakfast" but, echoing usage of the Old French word diner, more commonly meant "the first big meal of the day, usually eaten between 9 a.m. and noon."

Customs change, however, and over the years we have let the chief meal become the last meal of the day, by which time we have broken our fast more than once.

STOP! Consider the Earth-quaking magnitude of what you have just read! The history of mankind has just been laid out before you. You are the result of changing definitions! The size of your waistline and state of your health were predestined and influenced long before you were born.

Words have formed you!

The Latin origins of Dinner date back to the 8th century or 800 BC.
Again, reflect on the depth of what you have just read.

Breakfast: Is a relatively new idea and became common 500 years ago. Its origins were correct in being the first meal of the day. Its flaw was in the fact that dinner (also meaning breakfast or break-the-fast) was never removed from the meal schedule.

Lunch: It is a relatively new meal that comes into common verbal usage only 196 – 300 years ago. The term derives from the Spanish word lonja (a slice of ham). The Oxford English Dictionary indicates that the word means small snack of the size that fits in ones hand. This snack was often eaten in the field in the middle of the workday and sometimes called nunchin.

The word nunchin is where a new word luncheon derives from. Dr. Samuel Johnson wrote what is believed to be the first dictionary of the English language ever scribed. Johnson defines luncheon this way; "Luncheon: as much food as one's hand can hold." The former indicates that when lunch was eaten, it was a hurried snack-like affair including several bites of sustenance before resuming work.

Again lunch is all based on the evolution of man's workday and his ability to carry food while working. Lunch / snacking were not intended to alter our lifestyle. They were meant as a treat. Why? The answer will become obvious later.

Supper: Is a ceremonial meal that dates back 3458 years.

Dinner: Was breakfast and was first noted circa 2808 years ago.

Reading forward you will begin to understand the old adage of "Breakfast like a king, lunch like a prince and dine (dinner) like a pauper." Such little reminders and sayings will take on a new meaning as you unravel the mysteries of the body and our practices feeding it.

CHRONOLOGICAL ADDITIONS OF MEALS TO OUR LIVES:

Supper (3458 years ago)

Dinner (2808 years ago)

Breakfast (500 years ago)

Lunch (250 to 300 years ago)

Why did we change our eating habits? Clearly Dinner was the only meal of the day for thousands of years. The word history above makes this abundantly clear. Dinner means "to break- the-fast."

The fast occurred from breakfast to breakfast.

This piece of data explains why someone later coined the phrase "Breakfast is the most important meal of the day."

It turns out it was the only meal of the day. Consequently its importance is beyond compare for someone not immersed in a week or month-long fast. But even in the statement there is an enigma. What was the other meal?

Breakfast is the most important MEAL of the day.

Investigation reveals that this statement is actually nothing more than a reminder. The statement is just a command to break -the-fast with a meal every morning. In other words, this was a repeated maxim, credo or reminder of proper health. Such as "an apple a day keeps the doctor away."

Later when you are reading how the digestive tract works the idea of dinner being the first and only meal of the day will become crystal clear and irrefutable.

In the last 2000 years man's understanding and or misunderstanding of food has continued to advance or decline depending on your point of view.

In the field of food preservation, not only did we learn to preserve meats with salt, we developed the ice box. We started selling food to those who were now domesticated as farm life ceased to be the norm.

Farms were and are self-sufficient eco-systems. The need for a restaurant to a farmer is laughable. The old country saying "as useful as teats on a bull" springs to mind as apropos when considering these two incongruent thoughts restaurant and farm. Farmers probably mused "Who in their right mind would go to a sit-down restaurant, when there is good eating at home?" The answer is; the former and newly domesticated farmer. Progress and industrialization has made us a needy crowd.

Settling into cities meant that the large amounts of public became dependent on a few to supply their needs. Lacking access to fresh produce and live stock facilitated the need for the local eatery. Suddenly we were no longer independent. We were dependent on the hands of others to feed us our meals.

With these new eating facilities, domesticated man had easy access to food whenever he wanted it as it could be served to him 16 hours a day. After the ice box and later the refrigerator were created, the country store was firmly established. It was now possible to eat around the clock.

For a business to survive it must sell its wares. A restaurant sells no muss, no fuss dining experiences 16 hours a day. Eating out at the eatery for breakfast, lunch and dinner were off shoots of marketing.

Yes, houses have always had the traditional meeting place and focal point of the family: the fireplace. Here stories were told, bodies warmed, food cooked, information exchanged, etc. Growing hamlets beget townships and eventually cities all saw the increase in size of the fireplace.

Eventually, the fireplace or fire pits led to the common day hearth. The hearth was the foundation that served to cement the home as a permanent fixture and springboard for the city. Where there is warmth there is growth.

Man was accumulating in large numbers at focal points where water and food were plentiful. All archeologists know that the presence of the hearth is the determining factor that separates a home from just a building.

Now localized, socializing man struck out to meet his fellows in larger numbers which led to the town meeting hall. Where man congregates, food is always present. Hence we had the beginnings of the eatery and the restaurant.

Looking at these facts and understanding the natural progression of any business or venture one would also conclude that profit is necessary. Consequently it is not surprising that the proliferation of the restaurants / pubs / eateries coincided with adding meals to our lives. A business that is limited to three to four hours of operation a day is a business dancing on the razors edge of failure.

Anyone who sells anything needs to promote to his market or his business becomes a memory, not a legacy. Business seldom supports our morays or traditions. On the contrary, businesses mold and rebuild the very fabric of our lives without regard for good health or need.

The financing of culinary commerce influences our lives today just as it did 600 years ago. Most agree that sugar is a detriment to human health. Yet, check the menu at any restaurant. The dessert menu is almost as large as the entrée menu. Dessert is very lucrative and that is why it is pushed.

The old adage, that "if you build it, they will come" also translates to restaurants, "if you serve it they will eat it."

Translation: Via so called progress, pressure and changing lifestyles we have abandoned the time proven ingrained eating habits of our forefathers.

Today's dinner which used to be called supper, was an OPTIONAL light smattering of fresh juices and or light juice-filled fruit.

Citrus is well known as a tonic and aid to digestion. This is the reason that orange is served at the conclusion of traditional Japanese cuisine. The acid kills parasites (if they are present) and improves digestion to a marked degree.

Regardless of the fireplace and hearth for family gatherings, our ancestors would not and did not eat the largest meal of the day in the evening.

Clearly based on our own language and later (in these pages) based on bodily functions, it is detrimental to consume food past a certain hour. To do so would have invited sickness and exhaustion.

An exhausted body would be of little use to a man needing to forage for food and hunt for game. Our personal habits ensured the future of mankind and were not self serving. There was no time for thinking of oneself when part of an interlinked chain based on survival. Exhaustion invites death at all times of history regardless of the activity.

Our forefathers were sage. They knew how to heal the body via the time clock of the body. They knew that eating correctly prevented disease and catapulted the group forward into the future. Survival meant being healthy and useful to the group that depended on its members for their future wherewithal.

MEAL SUMMATION:

1) Supper was a yearly ceremonial meal that later became a "sometimes" treat or occasional light snack in the early evening.

2) Dinner was the morning meal from Latin meaning "To break the fast." This was THE meal of the day.

3) Breakfast was added to our meals in addition to dinner. We now had two BREAK-THE-FAST meals. The second meal was a complete aberration based on commerce. In essence we had just added a second break-the-fast to our lives. Buying into this notion, we added calories to our bodies without adding more activity or a longer day to sustain such an increase in food.

4) Lunch was an occasional snack served at midday and was intended to be a light treat. Advancing forward through history we are alerted to the fact that formal lunch was added not as an aid to survival but a result of business savvy and entrepreneurship.

5) History indicates that the addition of BREAKFAST, LUNCH AND SUPPER were the direct result of the masses relocating to cities.

In fundamental nature, our habits came under attack by those who we allowed to be our judge and jury. When you watch a commercial for the latest product and you are told to go purchase it, this is what has happened. This is not to say that all advertising is bad, far from it.

When we allow our values and life sustaining habits to be eroded without proper investigation to the validity of the advertisement, it is folly.

For example, I am being very persuasive in these pages petitioning you to take control of your life.

My only request is that you do not listen to me and follow me blindly without personal inspection. Your results will dictate the rightness of what I am writing herein. By adopting the tenets of this chapter, you can not only lose weight, you can redress long standing physical conditions.

Roger Bezanis

When once independent ranchers, farmers, mountain men and country folk gave up "that life" for a life in the city, there was no inspection only awe.

Lost was the man who had life habits that worked. Suddenly he was increasingly dependent on the skill of others to provide food. This led to the butcher shop, bakery, dairy, country store, grocery store, eatery, eventually the restaurant and finally fast food.

Our meal times have been modified further by our work schedules, which have little or nothing to do with the feeding, care or health and healing of the body.

Dinner which meant "To break the fast," was now served twice a day, including a lunch and now a supper meal. The care and healing of the land was replaced with the care and feeding of the palate.

What is fasting and what does it have to do with the morning meal? Before we immerse ourselves in this question, ask yourself, why the morning meal was called "DINNER."

Remember, dinner means "To Break the Fast."

Fasting can last from a few hours to a few weeks depending on the purpose.

Definition of fasting: Fasting is voluntarily not eating food for varying lengths of time. Fasting is used as a medical therapy for many conditions. It is also a spiritual practice in many religions.

Why were our forefathers eating a huge morning meal and then FASTING the rest of the day? They were fasting all day and night and ONLY EATING IN THE MORNING.

For what purpose was this habit practiced?

Our forefathers ate to achieve the best possible survival for themselves and the group that they supported. The above data is obvious and empirical.

PERSONAL HEALTH WAS A GROUP DIRECTIVE

500 years ago and earlier, adherence to the group dynamic was the fabric that ensured survival and the furthering of life and prodigy. The individuals had a personal responsibility to his group. Your group is composed of the people you work with. When someone does not show up, it puts a strain on the rest of the group.

In antiquity, the importance of the group was beyond parallel. Each member had a specific job to produce meals, find food, maintain the young, protect the group from attack, maintain and repair the living quarters and shelter and create and maintain the material worn to cover the body.

All groups rely on individual contribution for hunting, gathering, etc. In a small to medium sized group, the dropping of one's hat is an offense that is punishable by death. The survival of the group is senior to the survival of its parts.

Therefore, being out of shape, sick, overeating and over sleeping can also appear to be capital offenses.

Examining the bible and the tablets brought down from Mt. Sinai speak loudly of group protection. The last six of the 10 commandments are commands or edicts that protect the assemblage and its survival.

5) Respect your father and mother. In practice this keeps the group sound by not upsetting it with cries for change. A focused one leader group is a harmonious group. Where there is desertion there is mutiny.

6) You must not kill. Aside from the spiritual and moral implications of this commandment it also dictates something else. This commandment indicates that death of a group member will not be tolerated as the now weakened group is the eventual actual victim.

7) You must not commit adultery. Again the spiritual and moral implications are obvious. Regarding the group it is again in disharmony and weakened.

8) You must not steal. If any group is feasting on itself for whatever reason it is a group that is in turmoil and is easy to topple. Should a day's hunt be dispatched with it could spell doom or at least famine to a group barely making it.

9) You must not give false evidence against your neighbor. When the honesty of a group is in question the group is no longer cohesive and will fracture.

10) You must not be envious of your neighbor's goods. You shall not be envious of his wife nor anything that belongs to your neighbor. When this symptom arises it is due to a greater problem that needs to be addressed. The group has begun to falter on an individual basis. Why else would a group that shared its wealth be jealous of equal wealth?

Harmony in any group spells strength. Early man knew this and we know this today yet today man has become more solitary, not depending on his neighbor.

Early man had a responsibility to be the best he could be as the group needed his contribution. This supposition has stood up to historic scrutiny and offers a sad yet accurate explanation of how man has changed.

We have individuated from our interdependent groups. Work is not seen the way it once was. The unemployed are boosted up with government aid. This relaxed and stunningly cavalier attitude influences not only our eating habits but the way man lives. Survival and the loss of the group dynamic has cost us our eating habits and affected our health.

The game of survival has been so watered down that man has made it an occupation to eat. The group dynamics that motivated man 500 years ago have diminished to a self serving pursuit of tasty cuisine.

Business and the need to fight for and hunt for food have further morphed the individual into a working pawn versus fighting forager. No group to support and be a part of again changed man to his detriment.

What was germane to prehistoric man, serfs, settlers, ranch hands, farmers and homesteaders is not considered important today. Man can eat for pleasure and eat as often as he wants. Our group determined values have drastically change.

----READ ON----

WE ALL HAVE HEARD AND CAN RECITE:

**BREAKFAST IS THE MOST IMPORTANT MEAL OF THE DAY
THIS STATEMENT IS 100 PERCENT ACCURATE**

Considering our FLIP FLOPPED eating style, is it any wonder why we crash at 3:00 p.m.? By then, our bodies are exhausted from our self imposed dietary punishment.

Two to four hours after we gorge ourselves on sweet rolls, coffee, cereal, crispy bacon and other breakfast treats, we pump ourselves up again. This time we gulp down more bread and imitation meats with soda and who knows what else. When 3:00 p.m. rolls around we feel terrible and drink coffee which makes us feel worse. Soon we are home or a restaurant for dinner and we eat our biggest meal of the day. Finally we eat a snack and go to bed on a full stomach.

The drama that unfolded above is common to most everyone on the planet to one degree or the other. It is also the single most debilitating and damaging habit any of us can have.

Attempting to sleep when the body is loaded with a full belly is a proven digestive and restorative challenge that cannot be won. It can be tolerated but the stress induced by a full stomach is never conquered.

It is impossible to heal the body during the sleep cycle if the body is made to digest a new meal.

Noun, singular: dinner; plural: dinners
1. The main meal of the day often eaten in the evening...

It should be very obvious that we have reversed our meal schedule, and due to this, attempted to alter our body function. Based on the soaring rate of obesity, it is not working.

SNAPSHOT: THE VALUE OF MAKING DINNER THE MORNING MEAL

The body is an organism that runs the exact same way that a business does. Businesses want deliveries in the morning so that they can be processed throughout the day.

Shipments arriving late in the day interfere with productivity and cause the staff to work overtime. Staffs that are not allowed to go home, eat and rest are less effective the next day. Sleep is supposed to recharge and replenish the body. This will become much clearer later.

WHAT IS DIGESTION?

Digestion is the multistage process of chewing food (mastication), extracting its nutrients via chemical process and optimally evacuating the residue from the body 24 hours after ingestion. If this process is interrupted the least that will take place is weight gain.

Chewing is seldom discussed in any depth as it seems so simple and innocuous. The fact is that unless our food is fully chewed we cannot digest it. The body cannot digest what is not pulverized by the teeth. Once we swallow we have no other way to grind down our meals. Ancient and sage health disciplines encourage intense chewing prior to swallowing. It is a great plan to employ up to 100 jaw presses pull bite before swallowing.

Digestion starts from the moment you place your food in your mouth. Your saliva produces an enzyme called amylase. All the simple starches in your food are broken down by this enzyme and rapidly ingested by your body. So powerful is this process that these nutrients are carried directly into the bloodstream once they are mixed. The more you chew your food, the more completely this digestive process takes place. Chewing also cleans your food before it hits your stomach - saliva is antibacterial.

Chewing sends messages to your stomach about the nature and amount of food that is about to be digested. If your stomach knows ahead of time that there is an apple, piece of beef or tangerine slice, it can better prepare the right amount of acid to help digest your food choice.

If the stomach acids are not working sufficiently — which is often the case in those almost all "Western diets" or if food is gobbled on the run this too interrupts digestion. In your stomach there the food will remain for hours undigested. Hitting the intestines and finally the colon we have the makings of a rotting, festering compost bin all creating ill health. Make no mistake about chewing; work your teeth and save your health.

Anyone who can chew can their way to better and happier health.

SNAPSHOT: AFFECT OF DAILY MEALS

- An early large meal consumed by 9:00 a.m. is of course digested all day and leaves no stress on the digestive tract at night. BREAKFAST

- A midday large meal consumed at 12:00 noon is digested but is starting to impinge on the restful sleep that is needed to rejuvenate the body. LUNCH

- An afternoon large meal 3:00 p.m. if eaten will without question put strain on the digestive tract thus impacting sleep. **SUPPER**

- An evening large meal 5-7:00 p.m. when consumed completely turns sleep into a stressful digestive job. It robs the body of its restorative cycle. **DINNER**

Under ideal conditions the aforementioned meals are digested and evacuated from the body 24 hours after consumption. Why? Because a new meal is about to replace it. Remember the analogy of the business and shipping department.

If your shipping department spends hours trying to unravel what has just been received or it is a multistage shipment full of confusing parts, the result is storage for later use and overwork.

When orders are delivered at the correct time, the work is easy.

Because these meals were eaten at the correct time, by evening (9:00 p.m.) they will have escaped the upper digestive tract. They will be just entering the lower digestive tract and then eliminated after the morning meal in 12 hours.

The body deposits meals eaten in the morning in ascending colon at 9:00 p.m. in the evening. This begins the last stage of digestion. From there it takes 12 hours to travel the last 5-6 feet of colon to exit the body at 9:00 a.m. the next morning.

Meals eaten late are left undigested in the upper digestive tract splitting the bodies' resources and taxing the entire system. This plays havoc with the entire system and interrupts sleep.

A late large meal is an irritant and magnet for energy consumption as it sits in the digestive tract. Because so much energy is being expended on this misplaced meal, sleep is compromised and rough.

Sleep is vital to the health and healing of the body. It cannot be interrupted or the body will suffer with all manner of aches pains and illnesses. Stressing the upper gastro-intestinal tract or any system of the body is harmful unless it is done for via physical exercise.

Overworked by a late night or evening meal, you wake up exhausted sore and stiff. If you have experienced this it is unmistakably obvious that there is something wrong.

Interrupted sleep is the single worst contributor to poor health or declining health worldwide. Of course if you sell mattresses your mattress is the answer. For those selling sleeping pills your product is the answer. Look at the all the mattress stores pushing you to get rid of your lumpy old mattress. Perhaps you too need a sleep number bed.

The above words on mattresses are not an advertisement but to call attention to how far astray your quest for a good night's sleep can go. When you hear about the latest sleep aid, now you know where the real culprit is hiding. It is in what you put in your mouth and when you put it there. You hold the key to restful sleep in your hand every time you choose to eat.

Sleep is the only real time when the body can fully recharge and realign itself.

Weight gain and weight loss are modified by when we eat. Correct eating times facilitate proper sleep. They balance the body's ability to burn mass and convert it to energy. Your choices are the hinge or pendulum swing that dictates whether you are getting healthier or sicker. You are the key to these important results.

MANY OF YOU ARE NODDING YOUR HEAD,
THINKING "YES, THIS IS ALL TRUE, I KNEW THAT"
IF YOU KNOW THIS,

THEN MORE THAN NOD YOUR HEAD.
NOD YOUR HEAD WHEN YOU ARE TALKING WITH SOMEONE.
TO BENEFIT FROM THIS INFORMATION,
YOU NEED TO DO MORE THAN NOD YOUR HEAD.

THIS CHAPTER IS ABOUT ACTION. IT IS NOT AN INTELLECTUAL DISCUSSION OVER TEA AND COOKIES.

The body runs on energy and is made of mass. It needs food to replace the mass that it routinely burns. If a body was starved of mass (food) it would continue burning its own stores / reserves until it had no more mass to burn. When the body was depleted of mass (to create energy) it would die.

TRUTH: ABSENCE OF MASS = DEATH

TRUTH: ABSENCE OF ENERGY = DEATH

TRUTH: TOO MUCH ENERGY = DEATH

TRUTH: TOO MUCH MASS = DEATH

TRUTH: EQUAL MASS AND ENERGY = HARMONY / BALANCE

When mass and energy are not cohabiting in a structure at equal levels we have either stillness or death. The more a body is overwhelmed by one or the other element the slower it will move until if finally collapses under the strain. Of course there are other symptoms that would accompany this breakdown that I will not cover here as they are covered completely in other chapters.

SIMPLE BASICS

Weight loss = Mass burning faster than it can be replaced.

Weight gain = New mass added faster than it can be burned.

The above two lines sum up the basics of body sculpting. It can get more complicated, but these basics are the root of the activity.

24 HOUR MACHINE (OUR BODY)

Like the Earth, the human body runs on a 24 hour cycle. Every organ in the body runs on the same 24 hour routine regardless of its function or location in the body. When the body changes its locality to a different Earth time zone it still maintains the same 24 cycle.

Each organ and system has a specific time that it repairs itself. For purposes of this study, I am not going to list all of the body repair times. These times are detailed in depth in other chapters. This work only focuses on digestion and feeding the body.

Every day the human body performs the exact same functions. While these events vary in frequency they do not deviate in performance as they are paramount to life on Earth.

EVERY DAY THE BODY
Pumps blood **
Takes in food
Converts food to energy **
Collects waste **
Eliminates waste **
Rests IN THE EVENING UNTIL MORNING

NEXT DAY THE BODY
Pumps blood **
Takes in food
Converts food to energy **
Collects waste **
Eliminates waste **
Rests IN THE EVENING UNTIL MORNING
(** denotes procedures performed throughout the 24 hour day)

The above six points we will call this the HUMAN CYCLE

These six functions, while seemingly simple, elucidate what the body must do every day if it is to survive beyond a few minutes or hours. If any part of the HUMAN CYCLE is interrupted, the body will either gain or lose weight.

The list below is repeated again later as these symptoms are germane to all body breakdowns.

Switching off or suppressing the Human Cycle can cause:

Faster Aging	Building degeneration of tissue	Tumors
General toxicity	Interrupted sleep	Poor skin
Poor hair	Poor nails	Poor teeth
Poor eyesight	Brittle bones	Poor joint health
Poor hearing	Vertigo	Poor liver function
Poor gallbladder function	Kidney malfunction	Adrenal gland weakness
Easily sick	Poor digestion	Constipation
Exhaustion	Bad skin	Nightmares
Hemorrhoids	Organ weaknes	Bad moods
Lethargy	Cancer	Sexual malfunction
Can't confront life	Poor sleep	Poor libido
Isomnia	Weight gain	IBS
Diabetes	Hypo/Hyperthyroidism	Fibromyalgia

AXIOMS AND LAWS OF HEALTH AND DIGESTION

AXIOM 1) Sleeping is for resting not digesting

AXIOM 2) Digesting is reducing 24 hour activity

AXIOM 3) The evening is the time to lubricate and rest the body for sleep.

LAW 1) FOOD EATEN AND DIGESTED IN 24 HOURS CAUSES NO WEIGHT GAIN

LAW 2) FOOD EATEN AND NOT DIGESTED IN 24 HOURS WILL CAUSE WEIGHT GAIN

LAW 3) FLUIDS MUST BE PRESENT FOR THE BODY TO DIGEST, HEAL AND REST

LAW 4) AN OVERWORKED AND UNDER-IRRIGATED BODY / DIGESTIVE TRACT WILL CAUSE WEIGHT GAIN

TRUTH: Our condensed schedules and social lives all contribute to weight gain.

With the previous list in mind, consider again exactly what is the importance of digestion.

WHAT IS DIGESTION?

Digestion is the multistage process of chewing food (mastication), extracting its nutrients via chemical process and optimally evacuating the residue from the body 24 hours after ingestion.

THE COMPONENT PARTS OF DIGESTION:

Step 1: INFUSION of chemicals and extraction of prepared compounds.

Step 2: RECLAIMING of the remaining chemicals and compounds.

+++ Mouth
+++ Stomach
+++ Gallbladder
+++ Pancreas
+++ Duodenum (first part of the small intestines)
+++ Jejunum (second part of the small intestines)
+++ Ileum (third part of the small intestines)
+++ Caecum (an onion size pocket just above the right hip and at the base of the ascending colon. It connects the small intestines to the ascending colon. At the bottom of the Caecum is the Appendix).
+++ Appendix
~~~ Ascending Colon
~~~ Transverse Colon
~~~ Descending Colon
~~~ Rectum

Our digestive tract is made up of the following.

Stomach

The **Small intestines** are 25 feet of coiled tubing sitting behind the skin of the abdomen and layer of fat just below that. It coils down to just above the right hip where it attaches via the Ileocecal valve to the ascending colon.

Caecum, as mentioned above, is an onion-sized pocket that is the warehouse where flora is produced in the appendix, mixed with food matter and dispersed into the colon.

The **Colon** is 5 feet long and breaks up into 3 parts.

The **Ascending Colon** is a wide digestive tube that starts just above your right hip and ends just below your right rib cage. It attaches to the right side of the Transverse Colon.

The **Transverse Colon** is a wide digestive tube that starts just under your right ribcage. It travels from right to left across the top of the abdomen to just below the left rib cage. It attaches to the top of the Descending Colon.

The **Descending Colon** is a wide digestive tube that starts just under your left ribcage. It travels down your left abdomen down to your rectum.

To not interrupt sleep and weaken the body, the digestive system must have either no food in its confines or near fully digested matter. Otherwise sleep will be rough or not restful.

All parts of the digestive tract—COLON, INTESTINAL TRACT AND STOMACH—nourish and repair themselves in our nighttime sleep.

Human digestion breaks down into two distinctly different parts or functions. Carefully study the following paragraphs. Fully duplicating / understanding the functions listed below will concrete and supplement your awareness of what and why your body does what it does.

Without question, awareness of this data ties together and is the glue of this chapter. Read it as many times as necessary to ensure that you have a full grasp of what I am writing.

Review the list above marked with +++ and ~~~ and now again study it.

The organs marked with +++ above all chiefly infuse chemicals into the food passing before them. They also excrete compounds, but the emphasis is on INFUSION. When food is ingested it must be addressed by the body before it can be used. The body uses acids and salts to prepare these foods and substances for digestion and nutrient extraction.

---ALL OF THESE ORGANS INFUSE CHEMICALS INTO FOOD MATTER TO PREPARE IT FOR TIMELY DIGESTION---

These fluids aid the later organs in breaking down and extracting nutrients from what was consumed. This process must be left undisturbed. Outside fluids (excess water) and or other digestive stresses slow down and delay these actions. They act to dilute or diffuse the body's ability to perform these actions in a timely manner.

The performing of these actions are chiefly imperative to life on Earth.

The organs marked with ~~~ above all solely reclaim fluids passing before them. This aspect of digestion is so important that there is an entire field of medical science focused only on understanding its function.

The reason this final process is so important is that the body absorbs available matter presented to it. Therefore, if this step is slowed by the rerouting of resources to handle a newly ingested meal, the absorption time is lengthened.

Lengthening the absorption time guarantees the assimilation of bacteria and elements not meant for amalgamation. These factors spell disaster for a body needing nutrients. Very quickly the liver is overwhelmed and the body experiences pressures and headaches.

If these dietary insults are allowed to perpetuate, the body will break down in the manner or points listed above. It has been said that "death starts in the colon." No doubt you can now see the wisdom of this statement.

---ALL OF THESE ORGANS RECLAIM CHEMICALS AND FLUIDS FROM THE FOOD MATTER TO PREPARE IT FOR TIMELY DIGESTION---

Proper colon function will gather two thirds of the fluid available in the material passing through it. Reclaiming these fluids is vital for the body to function properly. Some of these RECOUPED FLUIDS are then utilized by the INFUSING ORGANS of the body to perform their actions again. Once taken in, they act to resupply, feed, safeguard and heal these vital organs. You can now see that the body, to a great degree, is a mobile ecosystem that utilizes its own waste product attributes to perform its delicate functions.

These processes are simultaneously being performed. It has been said that "a butterfly flapping its wings in China affects the whole planet." This may seem incomprehensible. But we are interconnected not just on a dietary, group and family level; we are connected to and affected by every function of our body.

Finally, once this fluid reclamation process is complete, the body will expel the refuse. he only question being, how long will the food / waste matter be in contact with the colon before it is expelled? If your food choices and eating times are all over the map, the body and its resources will be stretched.

The result is constipation.

If you are suddenly thinking that I am suggesting that constipation is a direct indicator of digestive disorder brought on by operator input error, that is exactly what I am suggesting. Constipation is defined as less than one bowel movement per meal eaten. Meals do not collect and rush out of your body all at once like a football team running down a tunnel at a homecoming game. They fester and sit until the body masses the energy necessary to push the food (or by now decrepit rubbish) out of the system.

MAPPING THE PLAYING FIELD OF DIGESTION

Ideally, a meal eaten in the morning at 9:00 a.m. will reach the junction of the intestines and Caecum at approximately 9:00 p.m.

The rest of its journey through the ascending colon, transverse colon and descending colon to expulsion will take the remaining 12 hours to accomplish.

The body can do this job correctly if this job of digestion is left undisturbed.

Again the initial components of the digestive tract all infuse fluid. The last segment of this system reclaims water or fluid.

The requisite item that must be present at all stages of digestion is water. But ingesting water with a meal interrupts and diffuses the acids and salts infused by the body.

For that reason alone, make the ingestion of water or any mealtime drink a separate activity. Make it a policy to not consume any fluids within a half hour of eating.

Yes, make it a policy to not consume any fluids within a half hour of eating. The elongating of the initial digestive process is just as harmful as elongating or dragging out the later or last process. Slow digestion creates a compost bin in your stomach.

THE IMPORTANCE OF WATER TO LIFE

Water is the vital building block and wild card unifying element that is behind all body processes, fluids and chemistry.

With no H2O present the body cannot make:

- Enzymes (made in the pancreas)
- Blood platelets (made in the spleen)
- Flora (made in the appendix)
- Bile (made in the gallbladder)
- Mucus (created by all hollow organs)
- Lactic acid (the result of muscle exertion)
- Hydrochloric acid (made in the stomach)
- Uric acid (the result of joint activity)

The body's need for water will vary depending on its activity level (exercise), climate located on Earth, diet consumed, stress level and level of current health.

Bodies getting more and more congested will need more and more water to satiate its needs to complete its processes.

Consequently, if there is NO fluid present, there is no digestion. With no water made into other chemicals and salts, harmful matter remains intact and food is left to compost in the stomach.

THE HUMAN CYCLE OF REPAIR CANNOT CONTINUE WITHOUT WATER

Bodies rich with available water can nourish and repair each organ at the appropriate times without delay.

Correcting body wear and tear is 100% dependent on water being present for these jobs to be executed. Depending on climate, diet and activity level, it may take as many as 128 ounces of water a day to heal the body.

Due to eating at the wrong times (late, for example) the body will not completely perform its repair PROGRAMS or HUMAN CYCLE. This process can be retarded by as long as 24 hours.

When the body is made to digest food late, it shuts down. It reroutes fluid away from where it is needed and on to the new meal just eaten.

The normal repair of the body is made second to new digestion. Remember the shipping and receiving analogy? This is the process that you are dealing with on a daily basis, like it or not. From 11 p.m. until 9 a.m. the organs being rested and repaired are the upper and lower digestive organs. When food is in the upper digestive tract, the organs being rested are the lower digestive organs (see below).

REPAIR TIMES OF THE DIGESTIVE TRACT

11 p.m.-1 a.m. ASCENDING COLON
1-3 a.m. TRANSVERSE COLON
3-5 a.m. DESCENDING COLON
5-7 a.m. INTESTINES
7-9 a.m. STOMACH
FROM 9 p.m. UNTIL 5 a.m., THE ORGANS BEING RESTED AND REPAIRED ARE THE DIGESTIVE ORGANS.

If anything interferes with this cycle the body will gain weight as waste will not be processed and the digestive system will not be properly serviced.

All late meals suck water and energy away from the repair cycle and route it back to the upper digestive tract where water and energy is expended not collected.

What you the operator put into your body today must be digested and through your system in 24 hours or less. If not, you will gain weight and start the process to body breakdown.

Like the Earth, the human body runs on a 24 hour cycle. Every organ in the body runs on the same 24 hour routine regardless of its function. Even if the body moves from one location on Earth to another the body still maintains the same 24 hour cycle of repair. Each organ and system has a specific time that it repairs itself.

When we eat; the initial organs involved in digestion all infuse our meals with fluids that cause digestion to be possible. When this process is finished the body then reabsorbs the fluids previously used in digestion. This is a form of conservation of energy and resources. The final step in digestion includes this extraction process and lasts 12 hours in total. It begins at 9:00 p.m. and concludes at 9:00 a.m.

When we eat at the proper times our meals enter the ascending colon at 9:00 p.m.. This food matter ideally leaves the ascending colon prior to 11:00 p.m. when it starts its nightly repair cycle. This routine repeats itself with the transverse colon, the descending colon, small intestines and finally the stomach. For the body to be optimally healthy this protocol must be repeated without interruption every 24 hours.

Again recall the old adage "death begins in the colon." It is more relevant to you now than most people that have ever heard that statement. Make no mistake: what you are reading in this chapter has never been explained in this fashion in recorded history.

You are the keepers of knowledge that was hitherto lost, ignored or not known. Refer to these pages often until you learn it and can live it.

Undigested food is a symptom of poor digestion and gross operator input error.

UNDIGESTED FOOD TABLE AND THE SCALE

Undigested food routinely left in the digestive tract multiplied over the course of a year, will cause the body to gain weight at the following rates:

3 ounces a day X 365 days = 68.44 pounds a year
2 ounces a day X 365 days = 45.63 pounds a year
1 ounce a day X 365 days = 22.81 pounds a year
1/2 ounce a day X 365 days = 11.41 pounds a year

Undigested food does not just magically disappear. Scales clearly demonstrate that this is not true. A person trying to control their weight that does not own and use a scale, will run into trouble.

The non use of a scale is like attempting to do brain surgery on a four day delay. In other words, the information you are getting is too old to be of any use as it no longer represents your present state.

This type of individual "allows their clothes tell them how much weight they have gained or lost." You may have noticed that clothes do not think. Clothes stretch and are forgiving. They are not designed to accurately do anything but cover your frame. Some people try to monitor their weight by how they look in the mirror. Again this promotes folly. The body has gained weight even if it is just two tenths of a pound.

Even the most skilled body contour specialist finds it nearly impossible to "see" less than three pounds of weight gain.

Fat is dispersed over the entire frame of the body. Some is placed in strategic areas like the buttocks, hips and stomach, yet it is distributed everywhere. For this reason alone it is hard to "see" a change.

Even when fat "seems" to only build up in one area, a 6 ounce mass increase is impossible to visually detect.

If this "visual" or "feel" weight gain technique is your approach, throw it out.

A scale tells you on a daily basis exactly what your weight is. If you eat more fruit one day and drop eight tenths of a pound, you need to know this. Scales measure the rightness or wrongness of your food choices and dietary habits.

They do not care how great or bad you look, they just report the facts.

PROPER USE OF A SCALE TO MONITOR AND

INCREASE HEALTH

- Get a good scale
- Place it in your bathroom or on a solid surface for easy access
- Get up at the same time to weigh yourself every day
- Do not eat or drink anything before you weigh
- Evacuate your bladder and colon if necessary
- Take off all of your clothes including underwear and jewelry
- Step on the scale and record what your weight is exactly
- The next morning repeat this process. Continually record your weight and compare one day to the next. Your weight will dictate the rightness or wrongness of your dietary decisions the day before.
- If you weigh less than you did the day before (and were trying to lose weight) you have done something right.
- If you are the same weight as the day before you are treading water.
- If you weigh more the next day (and you were not trying to gain weight) you have made an error.

If you are trying to lose weight, the most that can be taken off in one day is two and a half pounds (2 ½ pounds). Conversely, one can gain seven to ten pounds in one day if they eat enough.

If you follow the routine above you can master your health and weight. To further monitor your health use urine PH strips to evaluate your acid alkaline level.

PH URINE LEVEL INDICATOR

- 7.2 ideal
- 6.8 TO 8.2 healthy
- 5.0 to 6.6 weak kidneys
- 8.4 to 9.0 weak kidneys and liver

Urine ph strips can be found on the internet and some pharmacies. The odor of your urine speaks volumes about your health.

If you want to immediately balance your ph balance eat a thumb size piece of raw beef. Chew it very well before swallowing it perhaps 40-100 chews. In two one to two hours, make another check of your urine ph. You will notice that your ph rose considerably. Do not be surprise at the spike in this reading.

URINE ODOR INDICATOR

- No odor neutral
- Ammonia = weak kidneys and liver
- Fruity = weak kidneys
- Nutty = strong healthy kidneys and liver

If you use these indicators along with tracking your weight, health maintenance becomes child's play.

Every moment of the day and night the body is entwined with the HUMAN CYCLE. For proper health every organ of the body must be routinely being repaired and be nourished.

This HUMAN CYCLE of maintenance lasts between two to four hours. At this time the body focuses a tremendous amount of energy and resources on the organ or system that is to be serviced.

If that organ or system is made to work during its HUMAN CYCLE, it THROWS THE WHOLE BODY OFF SCHEDULE. Without fail the body becomes stressed and will retain undigested matter. That matter will lay undisturbed until the next day.

A body that is behind in its schedule is a body retaining more and more weight.

Now consider our meals.

We are taught that breakfast is the most important meal of the day. You the reader now know that the morning meal is paramount to survival.

The next question becomes what is the sequence or steps to follow to assist the body in following its inherently ingrained routine?

BREATHING AND SLEEP

Consider the affects of sleep and breathing. While we sleep we are of course, breathing. If we have eaten correctly we are dehydrating at every exhalation. Dehydration is not a problem, it is expected and needed. The water that you are exhaling is waste water released during the final moments of the human cycle.

The reason that dehydration at night is so important in regard to eating is simple. Late meals force your body to divert water resources to digestion rather than repair, dehydration and the making of urine. It will frantically be trying to utilize the available water to move and digest your meal.

Your liver uses a tremendous amount of water during the night while in its own repair cycle. Late meals interrupt your liver repair cycle as well. I will explain this later in this chapter. Therefore your upper digestive tract should be extraordinarily dry as you wake in the morning. Consider just what your body needs are based on the repair times of the body.

REPAIR TIMES OF THE DIGESTIVE TRACT

11 p.m. - 1 a.m. ASCENDING COLON
1 - 3 a.m. TRANSVERSE COLON
3 - 5 a.m. DESCENDING COLON
5 - 7 a.m. INTESTINES
7 - 9 a.m. STOMACH

Water and fresh squeezed citrus juices are just what the body ordered to fulfill its needs after a long nights sleep.

For the first time the body will have the opportunity to receive the life giving lubricant that it has been expelling all night long. Six to eight hours have passed since you last had it and that is just what the body needs BEFORE IT RECEIVES ANY FOOD.

Just as a field of growing green produce needs to be irrigated, so does the body. After you have weighed yourself make an effort in ingest 8-20 ounces of:

• Water is the "stuff" of life the lubricating blood of the body. This water must be of good quality not the popular "constructed" water. I recommend reverse osmosis water not fluoridated and polluted tap water.

• Fresh squeezed citrus juice. All forms of citrus are a tonic and restorer for the liver and digestive tract. Eating citrus after every meal is also an amazing tonic and digestive aid anytime that they are used.

THE HIDDEN WILD CARD THE LIVER

In the past several pages I have been indoctrinating you with a sledgehammer regarding the correct times to eat based on body function. The evidence has taken 20 years to congeal and is irrefutable. I am now going to add the final piece that makes this picture complete.

The liver and gallbladder routinely repair themselves during the hours of 11:00 p.m. and 3:00 a.m.. The fluid that is being reclaimed from the colon is then utilized by the liver for this process.

You have no doubt eaten late and awakened in the morning feeling exhausted. The reason you woke up feeling so poorly is because your liver and gallbladder were not allowed to repair themselves. They were trumped by the needs of your upper digestive tract.

When the body is fed correctly, upon bedtime, there is no need for upper digestive activity as there is no need to digest a new meal. New meals require large amounts of digestive fluids.

The correct state for the body to be in at bedtime is "hunger." Your body should be preparing for a new meal the next morning.

The correct activity taking place at night involves riding the body of yesterday's morning meal. The body is recycling digestive fluids from the ascending, transverse and descending colon. These fluids can then be utilized by the liver and gallbladder to repair and flush.

The liver and gallbladder need a tremendous amount of fluid to perform their nightly activates.

The one place digestive fluids are not supposed to be located while sleeping is in the upper digestive tract.

REPAIR TIMES LIVER / GALLBLADDER

11:00 p.m. - 1 a.m.   GALLBLADDER
1:00 a.m. - 3 a.m.   LIVER

If the liver and gallbladder are not allowed to flush and repair correctly the results can be rough sleep, nightmares, insomnia, restlessness and sore muscles. There is another huge problem that occurs when meals are eaten late. The predicament is lack of weight loss.

During your sleep you should be burning between; 1/10 to 3/10's of a pound of water per hour until you wake in the morning. The first thing that you do every morning is unburden your bladder. This is the result of the waste water created during the liver and gallbladder repair cycle. It also consists of waste water filtered from the colon during its repair process.

None of the above processes can take place if the vital fluid of your system is diverted to digesting a meal or meals eaten late in the day.

If digestion is interfered with; water will be utilized in the initial stages of digestion rather than being reclaimed and excreted from the body.

If you understand the previous paragraphs then you have the hidden keys to weight loss solidly in your grasp.

The body is always forced out of balance by late meals which de-harmonize the entire system. The aforementioned is an accurate. Remember that during the repair times of the digestive tract the liver and gallbladder are also being repaired.

You now fully understand the complex balancing act that is performed by your body on a nightly basis. The failure of this process to be executed is the most influential factor in weight gain today.

Read this section and entire chapter as many times as needed to ensure complete comprehension. Please revisit this chapter often.

EMPIRICAL LESSONS FROM OUR FOREFATHERS

Sage, time tested or learned behavior became such due to direct observation or empirical study. It is empirical that touching a hot stove causes burns. In the arena of health, direct observation is available, but since large results (such as growths and organ stoppage) takes longer to manifest, the cause and effect relationship can go unnoticed for centuries.

That is why sayings were developed. Prior to mass literacy the spoken word was the only way to pass on information to large publics. The town crier is an example of this. His words were meant to convey alerts or to be a quick reminder that could be repeated encouraging proper behavior. This type of information is in the fabric of our everyday lives. Sayings have persisted through time due to their truth and workability.

The erudite few were warning and educating the common man of consequence resulting from actions or failed actions. Some common examples of empirical sayings are:

- Never eat swine.
- Don't eat before swimming.
- Never go to bed on a full stomach.
- Feed a cold and starve a fever.
- Let the food be your medicine and the medicine be your food.
- A stitch in time saves nine.

- Never eat raw pork.
- Never eat raw fowl.
- Wash your hands after using the bathroom or restroom.
- Cover your mouth when you sneeze.
- Wash your hands before eating.
- To lengthen thy life, lessen thy meals (Benjamin Franklin, 1755)
- A man too busy to take care of his health is like a mechanic too busy to take care of his tools. (Spanish proverb)
- The way to keep your health is to eat what you don't want, drink what you don't like and do what you'd rather not. (Mark Twain 1835-1910)
- To feel "fit as a fiddle" you must tone down your middle.
- Those who think they have not time for the bodily exercises will sooner or later have to find time for illness.
- Refuse to be ill. Never tell people you are ill; never own it to yourself. Illness is one of those things which man should resist on principle at the onset. (Edward G. Bulwer-Lytton, British poet, politician and critic 1803-1873)
- The pursuit of good health is unnecessary if you do not give it away first.

Consider the above list and ask yourself how many of these sayings do you really understand. Why do you feed a cold and starve a fever?

The answer is simple. When the body is cold or has a cold it is asking for fuel to battle the invader. In the case of a fever, all of the body's resources are now at work fighting the invader. A fever says "hands off this immunes system is working!"

A cold says "I am in need of help send for the reserves."

How many of these verbal reminders really make sense? Are they still valid?

The verbal passing on of knowledge takes a circuitous route as it heads to oblivion. Wherever knowledge is not recorded or the recordings have been lost, it is not long before memory is also skewed.

Observable technical data handed down verbally, follows exact stages as its message is watered down or lost. Which is why this book needs to be read not quoted unless you are quoting right from the book. What is not written down mutates and becomes weaker or nonexistent as time marches forward.

HOW KNOWLEDGE DRIFTS INTO UNCONSCIOUSNESS AND OBLIVION.

Man learns via observation and repetition as a supplement for language and conceptual understanding. Animals in the wild learn successful and unsuccessful habits from their mothers. The unsuccessful are weeded out as success breeds reward.

We are not the authors of our health as our bodies were handed to us without a manual. This chapter brings you up out the morass of confusion known as "Life on Earth and feeding the body." With these pages you should be operating at the top rung of the list below. The lower one is on the ladder of understanding, the more they will be victim of their body.

- Understanding based on knowing why, can adjust based on circumstance.
- Understanding based on observation of the example set by others
- Understanding something practiced with no foundation as to why (rote behavior).
- Rote behavior is practiced without understanding any purpose.
- A saying is established attempting to enforce rote behavior.
- Not understood the saying is altered.
- The saying disappears from the historic record only to be discovered later by archeologists.
- Knowledge rediscovered and analyzed.

Everyday our lives are influenced by media which attempts to reprogram our thinking. Peers do the same thing as do societal constraints, traditions and other influences. If we are to take back our health, we must readopt, understand and know the simple lessons learned here regarding body function and food input. By doing so, it is arguably possible to heal even the worst body conditions.

THE ULTIMATE PLAN FOR HEALTH ACHIEVED THROUGH EATING

The following are rules that, if followed, make retooling your body easy. This section can be copied and placed on your refrigerator, bathroom mirror and at your office. By making these rules your own you will be free of the need for constant doctor visits and eventual disease.

- **Waking:** Upon waking and weighing yourself drink 8-20 ounces of water or fresh squeezed citrus juice.
- **Morning:** When the clock strikes 9:00 a.m. eat your breakfast / dinner meal. This is the largest meal you will eat.

- **Noon:** Noon is the time if, you choose to eat at all it is advisable to eat grapes, tomatoes, berries or any fresh fruit.
- **Afternoon:** Afternoon (3:00 p.m.), like supper this is an optional snack. Should you take part in it, it is best to eat fresh juicy fruit, nothing heavy.
- **Dinner:** Dinner or the late meal known as dinner is best to not eat at all. If you do, drink fresh squeezed citrus juice, eat citrus or drink water.

EVERY DAY THE ROUTINE SHOULD BE THE SAME

Adopting a routine of any type is a lesson "self discipline." The routine becomes easy as it dictates your behavior. Following it is nearly effortless as you can now count on something that is bigger than yourself.

STEP 1: ALWAYS IRRIGATE WITH 8-20 OUNCES OF WATER OR FRESH SQUEEZED CITRUS JUICE. WATER OR FRESH SQUEEZED CITRUS JUICE IS VITAL TO IRRIGATE THE DIGESTIVE TRACT. THIS IS THE PRIORITY EVERY MORNING.

STEP 2: MAIN MEAL OF THE DAY 9:00 AM. THIS IS THE TIME TO CONSUME THE MAIN MEAL OF THE DAY. MAKE THIS AN IMPORTANT MEAL AS IT SHOULD LAST YOU THE WHOLE DAY.

STEP 3: OPTIONAL LIGHT JUICY MEAL OF FRUIT.
STEP 4: ABSTINENCE OR LIGHT JUICE FRUIT OR FRESH CITRUS JUICE.

The above are repeated here again to ingrain them in you. These four steps, while simple, are life changing. In a nutshell, they work. Remember, the best time to start lunch / dinner is 9:00 a.m., because this gives the body the most time to digest and be ready for bed.

Now consider our meals. We are taught and now FULLY KNOW that breakfast is the most important meal of the day. You, the reader, now know that the morning meal is paramount to survival. So important is this meal and routine that, if it is off, the whole day may be consumed in righting this wrong.

You have seen how angry a dog gets when someone is messing with his food? You too will fell this kind of indignation if you are not allowed to follow your HUMAN LIFE CYCLE approach to body conservation and healing.

The next question becomes: what are some of the foods that can be seized to best fit into our all important morning DINNER MEAL? We know the sequence and can recite it backwards. But what does one actually eat beyond citrus and water? The following foods are powerful healing agents and support your inherently ingrained routine. Use them at the proper times and you will soon be at your best.

Some options for BREAKFAST/DINNER are

Avocado	Sprouts	Purple cabbage
Beets	Greens	Broccoli
All onions	Garlic	Cauliflower
Tomatoes	Tomatillos	Carrots
Cucumber	Zucchini	Squash
Eggplant	Rare or raw beef	Rare or raw deer meat
Rare or raw lamb meat	Pineapple	Radishes
Kale	Chicory Root	Peppers
Apples	Oranges	Tangerines
Lemons	Limes	Grapefruit
Peaches	Guava	Blueberries
Blackberries	Strawberries	Pomegranate
Watermelon	Cantaloupe	Honeydew melons (& all melons)
Green and dark grapes	Peaches	Nectarines
Quinces	Pears	Cherries
Plum	Mango	Papaya
Coconut (the raw meat and milk)	Sushi (raw salmon, tuna etc. but not rice)	Bananas (are heavy and digest slower than all other fruit)
Leafy greens, such as romaine, arugula	Raw nuts (nuts are very dense in protein. A few go a long way.)	Salad dressing is a personal choice. Beware of soy and sodium content in dressings.

The sole purpose of learning to run your body is to invigorate and heal it. Further, you can prevent future breakdowns by being proactive in your choices of food and eating times. What you have been learning here is data that has been lost, ignored or was not previously known. You have at your fingertips the hidden keys to weight loss and body repair.

THE ROLE OF ENZYMES IN DIGESTION

Enzymes are proteins made up of amino acids. Present in all living cells they make the furthering of life possible. The job they perform is vital to all living things big or small. In order to be digested, all food requires some form or enzymatic change.

When they mix with this matter they start a chemical chain reaction or process that makes possible the conversion of food substances into usable energy.

All fresh fruit and vegetables are whole foods that are packed with natures little helpers: enzymes. Enzymes allow nature to self regulate. When an apple falls off a tree and rots on the ground, it is the enzymes that return it to nature as fertilizer.

Enzymes are very delicate just like the human body. Destroyed at very low temperatures, any cooking at all makes them useless as an aid to digestion.

Just as we will boil and die at a temperature of 106 degrees for any length of time, enzymes perish as well. Once heated to 110 degrees, these little powerhouses of energy combustion are rendered impotent.

Therefore, cooked food puts a tremendous strain on the human body. The pancreas, Caecum and appendix must now overcome the overwhelming odds to keep you healthy.

The ingestion of enzyme-free foods can triple and otherwise cripple your digestion. A process that should have taken 24 hours now takes 144 hours or 12 days.

If you feel that I am suggesting the adoption of a raw food diet you are correct. If you chose to do it that is your choice. I am a raw foodest. There are numerous studies supporting the remarkable healing benefits of adopting such a lifestyle. Later in this book I will speak to this topic directly.

But consider what would happen to you if you cut back on cooked enzyme- dead food by 60-70 percent.

It is well known that protein is destroyed when it is heated to 150-171 degrees. The protein is virtually unraveled and no longer identifiable to the human body.

Your body and conscience dictate your actions. If you are sick enough that pain is motivating your changes, it is not too late.

Roger Bezanis

Bodies that are constipated are the most susceptible to breakdown. Constipation is why we put on weight as food is backing up in the system. Calories are units of energy. Weight gain is caused by backed up food that is both calorie dense, excessive or excessive and calorie dense. This combination exceeds the body's ability to burn it off in a 24 hour period. The remaining unburned material becomes weight gain.

The formula to maintain weight is:
Mass x Heat divided by 24 hours = 0.00

The formula to lose weight is
Mass x Heat divided by 24 hours = -1.00 (or more

The formula to gain weight is:
Mass x Heat divided by 24 hours = +1.00 (or more)

Remember that constipation is defined as less than one bowel movement per meal eaten. The death of enzymes spells the end of healthy digestion if it is allowed to continue for any length of time. The longer we go without enzyme assistance, the more we risk sickness and body problems.

"Self decomposition," occurs in whole, uncooked fresh fruit, vegetables and all raw meats. Self-digestion allows the body to direct its energies to all extant body problems rather than exhausting itself trying to digest enzyme depleted foods.

I am in large part against adding enzymes to the diet in a supplement form as this indicates that the diet was poor to begin with. A fresh raw diet needs no added enzymes.

HEALTHY BACTERIA OF THE DIGESTIVE TRACT

The human body is a cacophony of noise on a subatomic level. This traffic seems to be unrelated at first glance, but it is all interwoven. The body is a storehouse of microbes inhabiting all aspects of our internal existence. For ease of future reference, we will call these microorganisms flora bacteria.

Many of these flora bacteria have never been fully mapped as to their exact function, yet most are still as mysterious as the moons of Saturn. With the limited understanding that we have, it is obvious that they are necessary in great supply to keep us healthy.

These bacteria can be found anywhere in the system. Regardless of their location, they do a myriad of jobs to keep us in good physical shape and health.

Since the digestive tract is spotlighted in this chapter, we will be focusing on the flora bacteria found in the colon and intestinal tract. The purpose of these bacteria is to aid the body in digesting your meal choices. Some of the most common flora bacteria are:

- Lactobacillus
- Bacteroides
- Clostridium
- Bifidobacterium
- Acidophilus
- S. Thermophilus
- L. Salivarius

All of the above bacterium are present in the body as well as hundreds more of a similar nature. One of the most common flora bacteria found in the human gut is the almost ubiquitous Bacteroides. This one bacterium composes approximately 30% of all floras found in the colon and intestinal tract.

The acid / alkaline balance of our digestive tract is imperative if we are to stay healthy and have proper evacuations. Colon health requires an environment that is slightly acidic: 6.4 PH. This acid temperature needs to remain constant or the result is less than optimum colon health. Obvious dietary and meal timing mistakes will of course overwhelm and burden our colon. The villain that benefits from these guffaws is the common yeast called Candida or Candida Albicans. Candida exists best in an environment that is 7.0 or above.

On this bio-drama stage, flora bacteria and Candida are in a constant life or death fight for dominance of your gut. Should one cripple the other, we will have either perpetual constipation or diarrhea.

Human equilibrium of the gut is central to the health of the body as this is the portal from which we get our nutrients and vitality. Even a slight push above 6.4 PH can spell constipation. Should we dip below 6.4 PH the result will be diarrhea. This is, in a real sense, is the equivalent of dancing on the razors edge.

When the colon is congested, so is the body. The result can be a stuffy nose or sinuses, burning or red irritated eyes, blurry vision, dark cloudy urine, insomnia, tingling skin, hot flashes, bad moods and low energy.

Reversing these symptoms to the other extreme is diarrhea and that can spell a runny nose, watery eyes, frequent urination, rapid heartbeat, sore joints, sore / stiff muscles, feeling faint, and loss of balance or hearing problems. Shockingly, these symptoms are all facilitated by the gut being out of balance.

This is also why so many people think that the remedy to healing the body is forced heavy handed colon purging. Even though the earlier paragraphs make this seem to be a viable alternative, it is not the best possible solution.

I implore you to address the body holistically and address all parts of the body not just one part at a time. The proper diet and eating schedule is always the place to start.

The body is not defenseless at all. Just above the right hip at the bottom of the ascending colon lays a worm-shaped structure called the appendix. For the better part of 5000 years its actual function has been shrouded in mystery. All that has been known about it is that it can infrequently become infected to such a degree that it must be removed.

In 2005, 321,000 Americans were hospitalized with appendicitis as per the Centers for Disease Control (CDC). Nowhere in the known historic record has there been an explanation of what this enigmatic tiny formation of human tissue function actually is.

That was until 7, October 2007 when immunologists at Duke University uncovered and published its true purpose! As per the Duke "Blue Devil" researchers the appendix is the store house and human bio-lab that creates our healthy flora on a day to day basis.

Under extreme duress the appendix will act to reboot or reseed the colon and intestinal tract with flora. Stresses such as antibiotics and high fevers can leave the colon sterile without any viable means of replacing flora bacteria.

In this type of emergency the appendix is a superman of utility as it will reboot the system allowing flora to repopulate. Think of the appendix as the "emergency medical assistant" of digestion. A healthy appendix aids the digestive system in running smoothly even in the face of antibiotics.

Nevertheless, beware of antibiotics as even brief use can sterilize the colon or cause damage to flora bacteria. If you have had a bout with antibiotics, take measures to eat from the list in the following paragraphs to reseed your colon.

Certain foods aid the appendix in doing its vital work.

The endowing building blocks FOS, GOS & XOS (Fructooligosaccharides, Galactooligosaccharides and Xylooligosaccharides all create new flora with the aid of the Appendix. These simple plant-based organic sugars are perfectly matched to the needs of the body.

We will call them the OSs. They are prebiotics or fertilizers that seed the appendix so that it can produce its life giving properties.

To be clear, prebiotics stimulate the growth of healthy flora by combining with extant elements to produce new flora bacteria. These widely available components are found in plant foods. Good sources of OSs include RAW broccoli, kale, green cabbage, onions, garlic, artichokes, jicama, bananas, oranges and chicory root. The emphasis on getting these plant-based sugars raw is vital as cooking and canning destroy their life giving properties.

Considering the above list that stimulates the OSs, I am against the adding of lactobacillus products in supplement form to the diet. If you eat a healthy diet your need for added (usually dead) flora is moot.

There is an ongoing and huge debate as to the use of flora bacteria supplements. The debate is based on the efficacy of refrigerated versus non refrigerated cultures. Flora bacteria are living organisms and quickly die if they are not kept cold and used quickly. The longer the wait from bottling to ingestion the less alive the cultures are in the bottle. The fact is that unless the bottled flora bacterium is kept below 50 degrees and above freezing the content is dying or dead.

To be as viable as possible, these supplements must be refrigerated upon manufacturing, shipped in a refrigerated truck and then put in a refrigerated display case in your health food store. The other option is to purchase via phone or online and have your order shipped to you overnight with a dry ice brick. This step takes a leap of faith that the product that you are purchasing is now and has been previously kept cold and then shipped to you.

If you purchase a supplement featuring flora bacteria that is not intended to be kept refrigerated, what you are ingesting is all window dressing. It looks good on the label, but is not viable in the bottle.

Yogurt is a poor source of flora as it is in an abhorrent dairy form. It is 70% bad and only 30% good as its delivery system is a dairy form which is known to constipate and block the system. We humans are all lactose intolerant, yet some of us have more symptoms than others. Nevertheless, we are all poisoned by it. We are the only mammals on the planet that consume dairy after infancy and the only mammals that consume it from a different species.

Highlights of this section:

• The wrong diet and poor eating times will kill off flora bacteria and make the body constipated.

- Candida keeps the colon slightly alkaline 7.0 PH. If Candida overwhelms the colon the result is constipation.
- Flora bacteria strains keep the colon slightly acidic 6.4 PH. If these bacteria overwhelm the colon the result will be explosive diarrhea.
- A healthy colon is a combination of competing Candida and flora bacteria that are living in harmony.
- The appendix is attached to the bottom of the ascending colon above the right hip. It is the body's storehouse for replenishing healthy flora after a fever or antibiotic (colon sterilizing) attack.
- FOS, GOS and XOS all reseed the appendix and allow it to again heal the body.
- The vegetables broccoli, kale, green cabbage, onions, garlic, artichokes, jicama, bananas, oranges and chicory root are all loaded with the elements FOS, GOS and XOS which feed the appendix.
- Do not add flora building supplements to your diet unless you are positive that your product is and has been refrigerated prior to you receiving it.
- Do not eat yogurt or yogurt-like products to infuse your body with flora cultures. This dairy medium does more harm than good. Your benefits are lost because the bacteria cocktail that you are ingesting is in a worthless and constipating dairy form.
- Supplementing flora building products are not necessary if you are eating a healthy diet.

Summation:

The target of this book is to help aid you, first in understanding your body and second, to own its processes, thus becoming master of your own life. The subject of flora bacteria may seem to be too small to worry about, but they are not.

You have just been introduced to the microbiology that governs the body that you seek to conquer and reclaim ownership of. From this day forth, ignorance is no longer a viable excuse should your health start to decline. I have given you the keys to repair your own life and vitality. Your choices, henceforth, will advance your health or subdue the vessel that is your body.

The sustenance that you regularly consume and the times that you ingest it influence your ability to cope with life. Such is the importance of your diet. You are constructing your life puzzle. The piece that you now hold in your hand is huge. Treat it with reverence or become a victim of your neglect.

THE ROLE OF TOXICITY ON THE BODY

You have learned that the time that we eat is the acme of the care and healing of the human body.

Toxicity is the result of a system that is blocked due to constipation caused by wrong foods eaten while the body was trying to rest. It is also caused by a diet rich in substances that do not break down or alter the system and its functions. They are:

- Caffeine
- Sugar
- Salt
- Sodium
- Processed oils
- Alcohol
- Drugs
- Junk food
- Pesticides
- Man-made chemicals (colorings, dyes, nail polish etc.)

Your Chiropractor may be very gifted in helping you to heal, as can the Colon Hydrotherapist. Getting a colonic means that water is eased into the colon and massaged up into all parts of the colon to loosen up and free old corroded waste. The results can be staggeringly amazing.

Cleaning the lower bowel with the aid of a trained professional has saved lives. Some of the most grounded, heady, clear-thinking health experts on the planet are colon hydrotherapists.

Colon hydrotherapists are trained in real world results, not esoteric propaganda delivered from the AMA, FDA or a pedantic and nearly useless university education.

Universities teach theory, biology and anatomy. Every honest medical doctor will tell you that their college education paled in comparison to what they leaned in practice in their later years after college. This is why your colon Hydrotherapist is so important and such a useful connection.

HOW TO RIGHT THE SHIP CALLED YOUR BODY

Restaurants are built on late night clientele arriving in the evening to eat a big meal. If you partake in such fare it is up to you to defend yourself and order what you want rather than what they are serving. If you go to a restaurant after 3:00 p.m., order fruit or keep your intake very light. The worst time to eat anything heavy is after 3:00 p.m. Anything heavy eaten in the evening will contribute to weight gain.

Are there solutions to weight control? Yes. It is achieved every day via exercise, diet, detox and establishing proper health routines. These points are covered in detail in other chapters. Choosing exercise will add 20 minutes to two hours to your daily routine. It is without question one of the best avenues to create lasting benefits.

Proper diet requires what some consider the most work as we are easily addicted emotionally and physically to what we eat. Correcting your diet is by far the best life-repairing and life extending approach to exacting improved health. Its power exceeds even that of exercise. Correct dietary habits are paramount to all human health endeavors.

Detox can stand alone or commingle with either of the above approaches. Commonly used herbal combinations do a fantastic job to reset the body as do sauna sweat programs. Detoxification is grounded in all cellular activity. The body is performing detoxification tasks to a greater or lesser degree every moment of the day.

Diet and exercise, when properly executed, are intense and life-changing forms of detoxification. Yet the diet and lifestyle routines printed in this chapter unaided are so important that they alone will allow you to reshape and heal your body.

Skipping meals to allow the body to catch up on its work is a very bad choice. If done often enough, the body goes into starvation mode and will lose weight at a very slow pace or seemingly not at all.

Remember the body is a self perpetuating organism and is programmed to take the best action to achieve the longest possible survival. Should you stop eating, for whatever reason, the body reacts. It does not stop burning fuel stores. What does happen is that all of the body's processes are lowered to minimal survival ratios. Therefore starvation-based dieting does not work as the body resists it from head to toe.

The body computes the best possible solution to the conditions it encounters. It will start to ration its food stores (fat and eventually the muscle) until life is untenable and the organism dies of starvation.

Regardless of the diet being exercised, under no circumstances can sleep be interrupted by food in the upper digestive tract. These channels must rest to repair and heal themselves. Attempting to rest the body while involved with a recent meal in the upper digestive tract is a promise of disaster. Sleep must be a sacred and uninterrupted activity or we risk organ and system interruptions up and down the line.

The following list has been borrowed from where it was printed earlier in this chapter. It bears reading again as the body always breaks down in the same ways when it gets sick or it is poisoned.

Mixing food and sleep leads to:

Faster Aging	Building degeneration of tissue	Tumors
General toxicity	Interrupted sleep	Poor skin
Poor hair	Poor nails	Poor teeth
Poor eyesight	Brittle bones	Poor joint health
Poor hearing	Vertigo	Poor liver function
Weak gallbladder	Kidney malfunction	Adrenal gland weakness
Easily sick	Poor digestion	Constipation
Exhaustion	Bad skin	Nightmares
Hemorrhoids	Organ weakness	Bad moods
Lethargy	Cancer	Sexual malfunction
Can't confront life	Poor sleep	Poor libido
Insomnia	Weight gain	IBS
Diabetes	Hypo/Hyperthyroidism	Fibromyalgia

If we are to take back our health, we must readopt, understand and know the simple lessons learned here regarding body function and food input. By doing so, it is arguably possible to heal even the worst body conditions.

Pre Step one: Understand what your body is trying to do.

Pre Step two: Understand what history has taught us about food intake schedules.

Schedule step one: Wake up and get out of bed at roughly the same time every day.

Schedule step two: Urinate (and evacuate your colon if you need to).

Schedule step three: Weigh yourself (record this for easy reference the next day)

Schedule step four: Upon rising ingest water or fresh juice (this lubricates and activates the digestive tract as it has dehydrated during your sleep)

Schedule step five: Around 9:00 a.m., ingest hearty foods such as meats, vegetables and fruits.

Beware of man-made foods from cans, cartons, bags and mills such as breads, pasta, cereal, oatmeal etc.

Schedule step six: From 12:00 p.m. until bedtime, limit food intake to only fresh juices and or fresh fruit. Citrus is best eaten after each meal as a tonic for digestion and sleep aid.

After you have reached your ideal weight and level of health all you have to do is maintain it. Can you goof off and occasionally eat something that is not healthful? You can, but you risk falling into bad habits again. Your lifestyle must be modified to meet your own discipline level.

If you start goofing off and feel terrible and again gain weight, the problem is based on your imposed mistakes. You have the power to correct your guffaws.

These changes may not be easy but they do not have to be hard. As I write these words I can report to you that a friend of mine who is 42 years old has dropped from 134.8 to 111.4 in three weeks by approaching food and eating habits as laid out on these pages. She is of course thrilled with her results. After seven and a half weeks she was 96 lbs. She is very petite and has dropped from a size 8 to a size 1.

Being a size one is not possible for all women. Most body structures do not support such a diminutive size. We all need to find the size that is healthy for us as individuals, not based on some esoteric standard.

With a little work these changes all become second nature. You can do this, just as our forefathers did. You can do this just as I have and thousands of others that I have taught have. The door is open all you have to do is walk through into a new world.

In upcoming chapters, I will lay out for you specific diets that can be followed. My diet is of great interest as I am the living breathing poster boy for all parts of this book.

CONSIDER THE LESSONS OF THIS CHAPTER

We have abandoned our time tested eating habits due to advertising, misinformation, peer pressure and the hazing of our traditions. What was once based on the common good is now based on individual whim as the group dynamic has been buried by the dust of time.

- Lives have been confused by the changing definitions of dinner, breakfast, lunch and supper.
- Industrialization has helped to distort our group values and responsibilities while robbing us of our need to support something bigger than ourselves and our family.
- Moving to cities we have become sedentary and charged with the headlong pursuit of

hedonistic palate pleasing food and oral stimuli.

- Our body continues to run on the exact same repair LIFE CYCLE program that it ran 20,000 years ago. Regardless of what we intend or want our bodies to do it continues to inflict its will 24 hours a day. Our approach to food must take this into account.

- Cooking habits / food preparation have destroyed our food and left us to stand naked against the ever changing landscape of culinary whim.

- We alone have the responsibility to take back our health and stand up to those who would seek to control and poison us.

- Toxicity continues to plague us with untold poisons that break down every channel and system of the body. Toxicity must be challenged and reduced.

- For most, it is necessary to do a full body detox as part of your body correction plan.

- Do you have to be perfect to control your weight? No. If you employ the listed behaviors on this page, you can't help but control your weight.

- It is common to lose 1 - 2 ½ pounds a day when on the right schedule.

- On the wrong schedule it is possible to gain 3 - 6 pounds a day or more.

Summation:

Your skin color, hair density, size, temperament and general health were passed down to you by your parents and their forefathers. How you played the hand dictated the condition that you find yourself in right now.

Blaming the medical establishment, your parents, spouse, advertisers, friends or yourself is not productive. When the ship is sinking, pointing fingers at those who should have fixed the holes does not bail water.

Ultimately we are all culpable for not paying attention and fighting against the onslaught of misinformation that we have bought into.

Reading these pages you have concluded that little in the field of health has ever made more sense. The reason is because these are the bare bone basics. The application of the basics that you have learned in this chapter can be the spring board to feeling better tomorrow.

The prose on these pages is not some esoteric ivory tower blather designed to leave you a babbling servile sycophant automaton. The purpose here is just the opposite. I want you alive, awake and fighting for your life. Take a few minutes to reflect on this chapter and reread anything that caught your attention.

Roger Bezanis

Neither this chapter nor anything in my work is written to make you wrong. It is here to empower you to achieve the goals and targets that you set for yourself.

Every day you are being lied to and made to doubt the validity of your decisions regarding personal health. We are buried in a waterfall of propaganda insisting that we change the way we eat and live, thus modifying our lives to fit a sales model established in an office meeting. The TV, radio and computer intrusively spew a programming blitz designed to create self doubt and drug / doctor dependence. A constant disinformation flow is all that is necessary to change or reprogram thought processes, minds and habits.

You might think that I am selling you something. You would be one hundred percent correct. I am promoting that you take possession of a commodity of incalculable value. Your independence, awareness and will power have been savagely and systematically ripped away from you. These pages are written to give you those gifts back. I AM selling you your own lost, given-away and stolen independence, awareness and will power.

With these gifts back in your control, you can make the changes necessary to heal yourself. Honestly, you can't buy these gifts. You have to decide to take and own these presents. Taking control of your body and therefore your life starts the moment that you decide to seize the moment and take the plunge.

It is easy to get on track.

Tomorrow morning get up, urinate and weigh yourself! Take pleasure in taking the steps that will forever free you from your nutritional oppression. What comes next has been burnt into your memory. Remember that you can always refer to these pages again and again. You do not have to be an expert. You just need to get on track.

Remember the diet and lifestyle routines printed in this chapter unaided are so important that they alone will allow you to reshape and heal your body. The chapters surrounding these words are also vital to read and combine with this section. Everything in this tome when applied creates results. It is up to you and your tenacity to apply these chapters and benefit from the dynamic health domino effect that follows.

Your friends do not have this information available to them. I strongly suggest that you show them. The power of this chapter is unlimited. Your use of it is paramount to your future health. Remember this is completely doable!!! Earlier you read about a friend of mine; as she dropped from a size 8 to a size 1 in 7 ½ weeks. All she was applying was the reliable data contained in this chapter.

She was 134.8 pounds and has now nine weeks later evened out between 96 -100 tight shapely pounds. Keep in mind that not every woman can or will be a size 1. This is not a target for every woman as some frames can never be a size 1. My friend happens to be very petite. No amount of the correct diet and lifestyle will change a large frame to a petite one.

Correctly altering your diet and lifestyle will aid you in achieving your best size for your frame. Consequently her health has immensely improved. Previous arthritic symptoms are now gone. Her skin glows. She now sleeps through the night. Her hair is growing at a tremendous rate and is stronger and not brittle. She claims to have not felt this good physically and emotionally since high school.

A surgically repaired right shoulder (car accident) is now flexible and robust. Her frequent migraine headaches are a thing of the past. Periods are light and easy.

By all accounts she is healthy and happy and takes great joy in the task of purchasing new clothes. An auto mechanic friend of mine has wrestled off 12 ½ pounds in 2 ½ weeks following this simple plan.

Previously you read how much weight can accrue if just a few ounces of food are left undigested day after day in the digestive tract. Computed over a year the amount of weight gain from such a small error is mind-bending and startling. Miscalculations that are routinely compounded by time equals a snowballing disaster of magnitude.

Just as Einstein said circumstance and point of view dictates relative pleasure or pain. To a man speaking to a beautiful woman an hour seems like a minute. The same man with his hand on a hot stove will tell you that a few seconds feels like a lifetime.

It only takes a few bad meals over a day or two to add significant weight. When one understands and adapts this chapter; weight loss is significant and almost effortless.

The question that everyone wants answered is how much weight can be lost in one day. All of my work with 1000's of others including myself indicate that the answer is two and a half pounds a day (2 ½ pounds a day).

Reflecting on the last paragraph I reiterated that as much as 2 ½ pounds a day can be lost via correct diet and eating times. Notice that nowhere in that paragraph did I say that you would be a failure if you lost less than 2 ½ pounds a day.

If you are trying to lose excess weight and lose 1/10 of a pound in a 24 hour period, you have still lost weight. The scale is your friend and never lies to you. It just gives you information. Do not take weight readings from different scales. To do so is inviting all manner of emotional panic into your life. Suddenly you will be thinking that something is wrong when it is only the scale you are using.

It is also very important to note that if you currently are of the correct weight; you will lose no weight at all by use of the data in this chapter. What would occur is the revival of lost levels of health. Do not be misled by the title of this rolling jaunt through body workings. The ultimate goal of this chapter and this book is the attainment of perfect health. For those who need weight loss to accomplish that end a scale is mandatory.

Correct pound estimation includes weighing yourself 24 hours apart in the same location on the same scale. If you normally weigh yourself in the bathroom and then weigh yourself in the bedroom you are likely to get a different reading. Scales are not evil or bad they just are devices that we attach significance too often far beyond their structural limits.

Once you have started using a weighing estimation device; use THAT scale or you will drive yourself to distraction with worry over what is wrong with you.

I have heard reports of as much as five pounds in a day being lost but I have never seen it personally. I suspect it did happen yet it had to be a fluke as that kind of weight loss is not common and should not be expected.

This chapter does not take into account how much your weight will alter via exercise or body wraps and exercise. Day spas usually offer body contouring that includes body wraps and sauna or steam bath use. These methods are found to be affective for weight loss especially when used with a diet and lifestyle approach such as what I have offered here.

Regardless of the approach you take in addition to this chapter, you are heading in the right direction. Be it two and a half pounds or 1/10 of a pound, you will see weight dropping off when you apply these principals. When all of the above rules are followed, miracles do happen. If you monitor your heart rate and blood pressure, they are two areas that show positive change rapidly when this approach is taken.

Do not fear that you are going to waste away to nothing as your mother warned you when you did not clean your plate. Remember you are eating highly nutritious food on a regular basis. Simple accounting principles and the same mathematics that you learned in the third grade tell you that as long as you are eating you will eventually plateau and not lose any more weight beyond that point.

If necessary, remind your friends, spouse, mother-in-law (she probably did not approve of you anyway) and mother that you are remodeling your body and retaining a level of health that you have lost. You are retraining your emotions, habits, behaviors and organs to serve your best interests, thus enhancing your life and increasing your long term survival. Bad habits are like bad relationships. They once gave you pleasure and now they are just an anvil around your neck. Good habits flow with you and allow you to flourish on all planes of existence.

Having achieved your ideal weight your poundage will gradually fluctuate in a tight range. This is to be expected and is healthy. Nothing stays the same but if you understand the mechanisms that make change possible you can manage that change. With that in mind, you can choose your weight and keep it in a range that suits you. Fluctuations from plus seven pounds to minus four pounds from your ideal weight is normal.

If you consistently weigh 153 pounds, you will occasionally get down to 149 pounds and later climb as high as 160 until resettling back at 153 pounds. This is fully normal and is just your body going through its normal balancing processes.

Make no mistake: this chapter is not meant to be a short fix only to return to bad habits. Some of you may take years to fully integrate these lessons into the core of who you are. These are lifestyle and life changing tools. I fully want you to adopt these lessons not for a day or a week but for the rest of your life.

I do not get a brownie or a new toaster if you take these words and weave them into the fabric of your being. I am not in an ivory tower somewhere getting my jollies knowing that you are eating a huge breakfast and then eating fruit for the rest of the day. Do not even consider the idea that I am slovenly choking down Twinkies, hot dogs and Häagen-Dazs Cherry Garcia ice cream covered in gallons of ketchup or Beluga caviar while I torture you with my whimsical words. These principals work and I am living the same life that I am encouraging you to follow. My payoff is fully knowing that you are forever better and therefore making the lives of all that you contact better as a natural result. These changes, which are your changes, affect the planet. The world is a better place if you are happier and healthier in it. That is what I want for you and this planet.

The power of this chapter is truly without limit; less the restrictions that you place upon yourself. It is easy to make excuses as to why use of this data will be hard or too difficult to apply. Perhaps peer pressure will be an issue.

Your peers do not live in your skin, nor do they feel your aches and pains. They are not up with you when you have heartburn at midnight. They are not with you when you look in the mirror and not like what it is you are looking at. They are not there as another diet plan fails.

You are your best friend and must remain so. This chapter puts you in charge of your own life. There is much in the world that may seem out of your control. But what and when you feed yourself is your right; a right that you need to protect and fight for.

Leaders lead and followers follow. The mere fact that you are reading this book proves that you are a leader. You are the person who can and does influence others. Your example matters. Bulimics and anorexics can greatly benefit from this chapter as well. Early editions of this section have circulated around and reached many in these groups and received great approval and fanfare. Do not forget to read and employ my life changing chapter that follows this one "Diet for a New Century." With use of both of these compendiums you give yourself the best chance at building a new you.

We all need guidance and a workable plan to follow regarding how and when to eat. Without question every word of this episode of text works and offers fantastic gains if applied. Get started. The world is counting on you to be the best that you can be and so am I.

Be good to yourself
Your friend,
Roger Bezanis

41 Diet for a New Century

There has been much curiosity, consternation, contemplation, trepidation, resignation and other "ion's" regarding what I eat. Being the central focus of a self created vortex of dietary mystery leaves me with a stack of requests for my wisdom on a daily basis.

The following dissertation is not just a rundown of how I eat and guidance for you the reader, but more so an effort to save mankind from my many form letters.

The questions I get range from "what do I eat? To do I cheat". My answers may surprise you, but I am no different than most people. I just strictly enforce a meal plan.

This chapter is devoted to explaining these queries in detail and giving you the inspiration to tackle your challenges with a of blanket confidence.
Don't be too surprised, bewildered or dismissive of what you read here. My food approach has been adapted from great minds before me and, like all of my work, is based on results and science.

Before I explain how I have changed the lives of so many with what I preach, you need to know why I do it. There are many reasons. In my chapter on obsessive personalities you will get more details and understanding into the minds of those who lead others.

Without question I am an obsessive personality. This means that I live life to extremes. Where many have more restraint, obsessive personalities know "about" restraint. They have many or at least one area of their lives where restraint seems to be missing. Some see this as incredible talent. Talent without drive or obsession is potential not realized.

Note there are basically five different kinds of obsessions.

1) Self abasement (drugs, bulimia, anorexia, etc.)

2) Self enhancement (exercise, cleanliness, etc.)

3) Collecting (toys, records, odd little items)

4) Creating (art, etc.)

5) Production; which is a variation of self enhancement.

Here are more details about me:

- I was bulimic.
- I was anorexic.
- All bulimics and anorexics are frustrated nutritionists needing guidance.
- Due to my eating extremes I was in physical pain. It hurt to eat junk food and a processed food diet.
- I am extremely vain (an obsession about looking the best I possibly can) and was gaining weight at such a mad rate, I was vilely repugnant to myself.

This was the springboard that vaulted me into my new obsession of learning how my body worked and correcting my health. Objective one was mastery of me. The following are some of first observations and future steps that I took in rebuilding my body.

- Bread and pasta were no longer viable eating options. They caused instant bloating, huge sugar crashes within minutes of eating and severe indigestion at midnight. So did hot dogs, potato chips, bagels, ice cream, chocolate, pizza, burritos, hamburgers, pickles, rice, cheese, black tea, French fries, etc.
- Due to the above I was waking up with sore joints, constipation, digestive warfare and urinating all night long.
- Next I became obsessed with herbs treatments and formulas.
- I used everything I could including vitamins and recorded my findings.
- I read (obsessively) on the subject and used myself as the guinea pig to validate the results. This, too, I wrote down for later reference. Everything I tested had to stand the test of real world scrutiny. The values of these texts were only adjudicated to be so if they produced real

world results. My future road was being paved with building blocks that were foreseen by no one, yet valuable to everyone.

- My face (via face reading, a new study back then) indicated my body was in terrible shape, yet starting to show positive changes.

Make no mistake: I had no choice but to make these changes.

I was backed into a corner and had only two ways to go. I could get worse and die or pull myself up from my bootstraps and conquer my demons.

I had to channel my obsessions or die because of them.

I was in a boxing match with myself. I had backed into a corner and was beating myself to a pulp. I was my own corner man as I trusted no one to help me. Winning this fight meant that I had to become an expert on the subject of me or continue to remain a victim of my body blows. I had no idea that my life / dietary trials and tribulations would ever be of interest to anyone. I am an example of what can be achieved and is now achieved on a daily basis.

The following is a rundown of what I have eaten on a regular basis for some years now. While reading the details of my routine, please make note that this is not set in stone. You must adapt these habits to your own lifestyle.

Take notice that the closer you come to matching these standards, the better you will feel. Human endeavor at every level seeks to control and predict outcomes prior to somersaulting in. This sort of prognostication is so valuable that careers have been won and lost on its very existence.

Human bodies and the structure of mankind respond very favorably to the happiness we garner from adapting to routines. Effects that we can count on we cherish and revere.

RAW FOOD

I am an advocate and promoter a 100% raw food diet! The eating of processed foods has been proven time and time again to cause serious health issues. Whole uncooked foods do not suffer the insult and torment of man killing them only to be reconstructed in some culinary Frankenstein experiment gone badly.

When I see mega chefs Rachel Ray, Guy Fieri, Alton Brown, Paula Deen, Bobby Flay or Emeril Lagasse, I see rabid mad scientists swooning audiences with addictive smells and tastes. Cooked food is so addicting and ingrained in our genetic past, it is like a built-in cocaine habit just waiting to be discovered.

So powerful are the physical responses to cooked food that the mere mention of it affects the salivary glands. Notice how your mouth waters when you consider a big, perfectly prepared, delicious steak. Imagine further that the plate is garnished in your favorite vegetables. Look closer at the steak. Is it smothered in southern gravy or roasted onions? Are you salivating like Pavlov's Dog? Cooked food is addicting.

Chefs tend to be a bit on the heavy side because it is nearly impossible to be around cooked food and not partake in it. Over time the body expands. Rachel Ray works hard to keep her shape.

Trying to lose weight via exercise while eating a cooked diet causes your workout to be 70% less affective as your diet is working against you. In other words, you must exert 70% more effort to achieve the same results that can be found if you were ingesting a raw food diet. On a raw food diet the weight comes off rapidly, whether or not you include a physical workout.

Working out and consuming a cooked diet is the equivalent of exercising with a 25 pound weight around your neck. Imagine getting the same benefit in ¾ less time at the gym. Further imagine getting ¾ more benefit in a workout of the original cooked food diet length. Amazing is it not?

What is raw food and what are raw foodists?

Meats and plant-based foods in their original un-heated and uncooked form are the materials that raw foodists routinely ingest to heal and sustain their bodies. Many raw foodists include a wide variety of fruits, nuts, vegetables, seeds, sprouts, certain meats, legumes, seaweed and fresh squeezed juices in their diets.

Live, raw foods contain a wide variety of vital life enhancing vitamins, minerals, amino acids, fresh whole enzymes and oxygen. The benefits of raw foods have been validated again and again in research for the last 70 plus years. No doubt one day an archeologist will unearth a stone or papyrus manuscript written in cuneiform that explains the virtues and handling of the "normal" raw food diet. Yes, cooking food is a learned aberration. History has taught us that we have learned to eat far differently than we used to.

Cooked food was the equivalent of a "treat" that was partaken in once or twice a month. In the days before cooking was "the way of life," a cooked meal was a reward for hard work or celebration. Much like having a special evening would be today.

The body knows the difference between pseudo "Frankenstein Food" and whole food. Whole uncooked food needs no digestion. It decomposes in the body entirely on its own. Meaning that all of the body's resources can now be fully commissioned to heal and strengthen the body rather than protecting it from being poisoned from food.

The raw food diet is so threatening and dangerous that it alone could topple the world economy. This is no joke. If tomorrow everyone on the Earth had an epiphany and switched over to a raw food diet it would cause a worldwide depression. Suddenly 100 million people or more would be unemployed.

Farmers would be transformed into overnight billionaires. Earth's economy would now be controlled by men in blue denim overalls and boots. The hard working dirt under his fingernails farmer would be an oil sheik or more accurately a food sheik. Fresh produce would cost more that oil, gold and so on.

Grocery stores would have to reorganize or go out of business as 70% of its floor and shelf space would be empty. Imagine overnight the following would disappear: canned goods, frozen foods, dairy products (except eggs), boxed foods, bagged foods, bread, cookies, baked goods and more, all gone.

The last three paragraphs spell out the depths of the morbid fear that the RAW FOOD MONSTER represents to the economy of Earth. A complete switch to raw food would be the equivalent of an atomic economic explosion.

For those who cannot fully make the switch to raw food, there would be the pusher selling well-done steak in darkened back alleys or food hooch dens. Argentina would supplant Columbia as the world leader in illegal goods as it would export coveted lamb chops and gravy to cooked food addicts.

If you really look at every successful diet, it features some measure of raw food. The 90/10 diet is a silly mix of 90% so-called good foods and 10% bad. On further inspection, it turns out to be far worse than what it claims to be. Nevertheless, it does feature enough raw food that weight loss does occur.

But not everyone needs to lose weight. The raw food diet corrects the body's ability to heal itself, therefore allowing the body's immune system to be fully armed and fully on! Nothing could be better than having your body working with you toward radiant health versus being the bane of your worry and concern.

Quietly, celebrities have made it known that they are raw foodists including Demi Moore, Tool Time Star Taran Noah Smith and tennis great Martina Navratilova. Juliano Brotman is chef and owner of the Santa Monica based raw food restaurant RAW and has been very vocal in this movement. He has several illustrated books on the subject and is much respected.

David Wolfe is a leader in the raw community as he co-wrote the book *Nature's First Law: The Raw Food Diet*. Doctor Ted Morter wrote the now out of print *Your Health Your Choice* which was (in my opinion) the medical version of David Wolfe's book.

The China Syndrome is another landmark book on the subject. The non-profit Price Pottenger Nutrition Foundation in Lemon Grove, California, has been studying the effects of nutrition and agriculture on health for almost 60 years. The books *Pottengers Cats* by Francis M. Pottenger, Jr. MD and *Nutrition and Physical Degeneration* by Weston A. Price, DDS (dentist) are so profound that they are required reading by many certified professional alternative health college education programs.

Price and Pottenger are two of the great nutritional pioneers of our time.

The volume of data supporting a raw food conversion is gargantuan. For the greatest part of man's existence on Earth we were raw foodists. It is up to your good sense and desire to return to the roots from which you came that will propel you to radiant health. The wall of data is so imposing regarding the detrimental effects of a cooked diet on the human body that it is no wonder that we are all finding our way home.

Be a leader and "go raw." You will be shocked by the positive changes that you will rapidly experience.

MY ROUTINE

Every day I eat the following:

8:00 a.m.-8:45 a.m.
I drink 20-52 ounces of fresh squeezed orange juice or tangerine juice. I eat nothing until this juice is ingested. Adherence to this practice is extremely tough when I go on the road which means I must arrive early to go shopping and stock my in-room refrigerator.

9:00 a.m.
Option 1: I eat a big salad (or two) that consist of Romaine lettuce, tomatoes, onion, cucumber and 1000 Island or Caesar dressing.

I will (perhaps 3 times a week) add in a thumb-sized piece (about a 2-4 ounce piece) of raw beef or raw salmon with my salad.

**Raw beef, raw salmon, raw deer meat or raw lamb meat (these meats need to be grown without pesticides or steroids) are points of curiosity in my diet. I will write about this at the end of this chapter. For those of you who can't wait, go look at this data right now.

Optional salad ingredients include: Avocado, broccoli, radishes, carrot, cilantro, basil, cabbage, celery and bell pepper.

NOTE: I always say that if salad dressing is the worst thing that you eat, so-be-it. On the other hand, if you are in pain due to your dressing choices, make your own fresh dressing.

Option 2: I will eat eight to ten ounces of pear or cherry tomatoes or tomato wedges with 1000 island or Caesar dressing.

11:00 a.m.-3:00 p.m.
I snack on either cherry / plum tomatoes, grapes, tangerines, apple, blueberries or all of the above. I do vary these fruits but not very often as my results are excellent.

Some may ask how I can eat the same thing every day. The answer can be seen in nature. What do Elephants eat on a daily basis or other animals? They do not have junk food or choices. They eat for survival, not taste.

3:00 p.m. until BED TIME
I might eat some cherry or plum tomatoes or drink 16 ounces of fresh squeezed tangerine or orange juice.

THE NEXT DAY I DO IT ALL AGAIN
Since grape juice is such a great tool for purging the gut and aiding the liver, I always have it on hand and in a pinch can drink 12-16 ounces. Grape juice is never found in a raw form so I will drink a good health food store brand or kosher brand from the grocery store.

Grape juice has a curious attribute of purging the colon in as little as an hour if consumed first thing in the morning if used instead of fresh juice. It rapidly leaves the system. Many who have used it this way have described the "grape juice stool" this way: it races out, smells like grape juice and is somewhat green in color.

Water is vital and I will consume 60 to 120 ounces a day depending on my other fluids that I ingest. My usual fresh juice or water intake is 90 to 160 ounces a day.

DO I CHEAT?

At the present writing of this edition, it has been months since I last cheated. Therefore it is safe to say that I very seldom cheat. The reason I cheat so infrequently is because I always want more. As a former Bulimic and 100% extremist all the time; fast foods / processed foods are very dangerous to play with for me. As an extremist, I am extremely happy not eating these things.

If, on occasion, I do cheat, it is with something simple. If I am unhappy with my health or am fighting some problem requiring perfection to beat it, I will not cheat at all. Most people do not realize that perfection (or close to it) may be necessary to beat the most severe problems.

If I do cheat it will normally be in the morning (as I then have more time to recover from this self-imposed abuse). I will cheat with something salty such as:

- A pickle
- Two bites of potato chips and then throw out the rest
- Ritz's Bits Crackers (sandwich crackers) are addicting. I must admit that I love these things but seldom eat them unless I let myself have them when I fly. If I do get them (a rarity) I will eat one or two and throw the rest out.
- I love Orville Redenbacher theatre style popcorn (served in theatres). I will occasionally order a tiny bag, eat 2-10 bites and be done with it.

I love sneaking a bottle of fresh squeezed tangerine or orange juice into the theatre and sipping that. Believe it or not this is much better than cheating on food.

Cheating is not a necessary evil to everyone. I have gone as long as 3 years without cheating without any ill effects. Cheating seems to serve the purpose of giving hope or aiding in comforting the individual.

Many people use food to comfort them. We all know that this is not a healthy attitude regarding food.

Depending on our upbringing, food can represent many things. Some see it as success, others like salvation. The best way to see it is as just food.

My mother, like most mothers and fathers who lived through the Great Depression of 1929, was completely fanatical about not wasting food. Food was so scarce that it was a luxury to some. Wasting food was not an option. This led to gluttony and hording for many who lived through this period.

Roger Bezanis

This is where the phrases like "clean your plate because there are kids in South Africa going hungry" came from. My mother was so maniacal about food that she would buy it and hide it unopened "so that it will last longer." If you are scratching your head on that one it is understandable. I was too.

The fact is that it is fine to waste food or food-like substances. If food runs your life, take your life back and make your own decisions about food.

Your choice to cheat "once and a while" is entirely up to you. If you must cheat in the beginning to keep your sanity, that is fine. Changing the way you eat and view food is quite an endeavor. Be nice to yourself. The following paragraphs can be used as often as you like.

RAW BEEF, SALMON, DEER AND LAMB

I have found great benefit, great satisfaction and healing power in the eating of raw meat. Some people are terrified of parasites that can be found in raw meat. Do not eat pork or fowl of any kind raw but our larger four legged friends do supply a good protein source for those of you inclined to indulge.

Vegetarians who can exist just fine without meat as protein sources are plentiful. Trace amounts of protein exists in all fruits and vegetables, so fear not. Protein is always present in our diets.

The China Study details amazing findings regarding raw diets as does Dr. Ted Morter (*Your Health Your Choice*), David Wolff (*Nature's First Law: the Raw Food Diet*) and the Price-Pottenger Nutrition Foundation (*Pottengers Cats and Nutritional and Physical Degeneration*). Raw meats are a source of:

Amino acids: Amino acids are like the glue that holds the body together. They make up 75% of the human body. They are central to every bodily function. Every chemical reaction that takes place in your body depends on amino acids and the proteins that they build. Amino acids are critical to life, and have a variety of roles in metabolism.

Zinc: Zinc is an essential mineral, necessary for sustaining all life. It is vital for a healthy immune system and reproductive system. Those who have sexual dysfunction will find a healing friend in the use of zinc. Most men with sexual dysfunction show deficiencies in Zinc.

For optimum wound healing it is optimum take at least 15 mg of zinc a day. Lack of zinc can also lead to weak hair, nails and poor kidney function as the kidneys receive direct benefit from zinc.

Zinc is vital for metabolic function of over 300 enzymes and is considered vital for proper cell division.

Zinc Deficiency Test

Zinc levels in the body were very hard to evaluate since hair, nail and blood tests proved to be very inconstant. Until the late 1970's when the oral swish test was developed.

The prestigious *Lancet* (*The Lancet* is one of the oldest peer-reviewed medical journals in the world, published weekly by Elsevier, part of Reed Elsevier. It was founded in 1823 by Thomas Wakley) first reported a new test that involves the following:

- 1 Purchase granulated zinc sulfate at a pharmacy or health food store.
- 2 Dissolve 0.1 % zinc sulfate in a cup of distilled water.
- 3 Do not eat, drink or smoke for at least an hour before the test.
- 4 Swish a teaspoon of the solution around in your mouth for 10 seconds while noticing the flavor.
- 5 If it tastes unpleasant or metallic you are probably zinc deficient.
- 6 If the solution tastes like water, you are getting all the zinc you need.

Again results are defined as:

- 1 Unpleasant taste = ZINC DEFICIENCY
- 2 Tastes like water = NO ZINC DEFICIENCY

ZINC TOXICITY

If 80 mg or more zinc is taken a day this can be toxic. Too much zinc intake can cause other minerals to be thrown out of balance. These include iron, calcium, selenium, nickel, copper, phosphorus and Vitamins A, B1, C and more.

Consistent overdosing of zinc may also create digestive problems, hair loss, anemia, loss of libido, impotence, prostatitis, ovarian cysts, menstrual problems, depressed immune functions, muscle spasms, back trouble, kidney weakness / failure, vertigo, vomiting, liver weakness and many other issues. Since too much zinc can overwhelm the liver, cholesterol levels can also swing wildly.

The type of diet that I follow is saturated with vitamins and minerals that are instantly useable by the body as they are in an undisturbed raw form.

MY USE OF SUPPLEMENTS:

I use supplements as needed but not obsessively. What do I take? Since I am not selling anything here, the most I will say is that I am aware of my own kidney and liver weakness. Therefore I do supplement with herbs for both organs. Colon function is another one of my concerns, so I am always aware to eat citrus and supplement for the colon as needed.

Needless to say I give my body what it needs.

By definition, Raw Foodists do not cook food. These iconoclasts prepare food or just pick it up (such as a tomato) and eat it. Over the last few years I have developed several fun and tasty things to eat.

My intent is not to give you a cook / food preparation book but to give you some tasty treats that you can make and weave into your diet and life. Not one of the recipes below needs any heat to taste good.

If you follow my directions you will recreate my food choices in your own kitchen.

FOOD PREPERATION

The following salsa recipe was adopted by Larry Parkers Beverly Hills Diner in 1990 as their restaurant salsa. Alas, Larry closed his doors forever in 1997. Many celebrities ate there including: Julia Roberts, Jason Patrick, Peter Falk, John Cleese, John Travolta, Paul Williams, Muhammad Ali, Stevie Wonder, Mike Tyson, Shawn and Marlon Wayans, Jennifer Lopez, Chris Rock, Sean "Puffy" Combs, Dr. Dre, Coolio, Jamie Foxx, Denzel Washington, Wesley Snipes, Angela Bassett, Natalie Cole, Snoop Dog, LL Cool J, Eazy-E, Busta Rhymes (before he was famous) and Tone Loc.

SALT DISCLAIMER

You know that I do not recommend the use of salt as it upsets the balance of the kidneys and pushes them "off line." Salt is well known as a kidney altering substance as it interferes with their function. The movement of water/fluid in the body is under the control of the kidneys. Salt reprograms the body and redirects water to stand still in the body, radically affecting kidney function. Salt commands the body to "retain water" regardless of all previous programming.

You will notice that a few of the recipes below use a pinch of salt. For the most part salt can be substituted with WHITE VINEGAR or BALSAMIC VINIGAR depending on the recipe.

To me, if a pinch of salt once a week is your worst vice, that you have it is survivable. But if this amount of salt is causing you stress (high blood pressure, etc.) then DO NOT USE IT.

You must be the judge on this as recipes are not your judge and jury you are. Monitor your results; they will dictate your actions.

1 PICO DE GALLO / SALSA AND CUCUMBER SLICES

The following is a wonderful recipe for a delectable treat.

Directions
6 Medium to large Roma tomatoes DICED small
1 Medium white, yellow or brown onion (sweet onions work best) diced small
3 Green onions chopped up fine
¼ cup of fresh chopped cilantro
¼teaspoon of ground or powdered cumin
1 to 4 yellow peppers minced
¼ of medium bell pepper diced up small
½ tablespoon lemon juice
½ tablespoon lime juice
½ teaspoon minced garlic
A pinch of fine French sea salt

(A medium avocado can be diced up and added to the mix for those who want a protein rich Pico. But the avocado goes bad quickly and should be eaten within 12 hours).

Mix up thoroughly and place in a bowl.

Option 1 - Take one large peeled Cucumber and slice it into ⅛ to ¼ inch pieces.

Option 2- Take one to two carrots and slice them up into ⅛ to ¼ inch pieces.
Serve the cucumber or carrot slices or both with the Pico de Gallo and use the slices in the place of corn chips.

Other fruit and veggies that can be used are zucchini, squash, radishes, red onion sections, Vidalia onion sections, red cabbage leaves, tomato hulls, apple slices, pear slices, papaya and mango slices.

2 ROGER'S RAW GUZPACHO COLD SOUP

Mix together and serve cold. This is a southern European soup meant to be served cold.

4 to 5 ripe tomatoes chopped
5 cloves of garlic minced
1 large cucumber diced
1 lemon squeezed
1 lemon meat minced
1 red bell pepper diced
1 red onion chopped
3 green onions chopped
1 firm avocado peeled and diced.
8 large basil leaves chopped fine
1 small handful of cilantro leaves chopped up fine
1/8 fine ground teaspoon French Sea salt

5 tomatoes and 1 half red delicious apple liquefied in a blender mixed with 2 tablespoons of lime juice and 4 teaspoons balsamic vinegar. The result should be a watery red/pink mixture. For those of you who are not purest you can also add 3 ounces for organic ketchup to the mix. For those who want to save time, you can purchase a 16 ounce tub of fresh grocery store salsa (chunky) or Pico De Gallo. Then follow the directions above. Just play with it and you will be amazed at how good it tastes.

Optional chopped raw beef or raw salmon can be added for protein. Another tasty treat that can be added is raw corn kernels off the cob.

Mix together and serve like soup in bowls.

3 ROGER'S CORNY DIP

(in a food processor or Vita Mix blend)
1 apple
2 medium strawberries
20 pine nuts
1 clove
6 medium mushroom tops

After blending stir in:

The corn from 2 raw corn stalks
2 green onion stalks chopped fine
Serve room, as dip with tomato wedges, celery, red cabbage leaves or with a thick soup

4 ROGER'S SWASHBUCKLING ISLAND SOUP

(In a blender or Vita Mix—This can also be served as a frozen desert)

The meat of one medium sized pineapple
6 ounce of coconut juice
2 cloves
2 pinches of thyme
1 ripe banana
10 red grapes
6 large basil leaves
½ teaspoon cumin
2 mint leaves

After the final mix is completed stir in 20 pine nuts add 1 ounce of chopped green onion.

5 ROGER'S TOMATO TARAGON SOUP

(In a blender or Vita Mix)

Blend 8 Steak tomatoes
1 garlic section
15 Fresh tarragon leaves

Sprinkle 1 tablespoon of chive or chopped green onion on top and serve at room temperature.

6 ROGERS RAW MEAT FILET MIGNON

Sorry folks, this is beyond simple. For you hungry sorts get a raw piece of filet mignon about half your thumb size. Spray it with balsamic vinegar dressing (spray dressing) and eat it. If no one is looking spray it again once it is in your mouth. Yummy!

7 ROGERS GOURMET MEDALIONS OF BEEF

6 slices of raw beef cut paper thin, arrange on a plate
Sprinkle fine dusting of fresh chopped chives over it
Dust with fine black pepper flakes
Spray with a light dusting of balsamic vinegar dressing

Served chilled or at room temperature.

Any time that you are eating raw meat of any type, be sure to chew it until it is fully dissolved. This way you are getting 100% bio available protein.

8 CITRUS FILET MIGNON PATE' ALA ROGER

Blend in a Vita Mix or a good food processor until the consistency is that of putty or dough.
8 ounces of raw filet mignon
½ raw sweet onion
20 whole tarragon leaves
2 teaspoons of Spanish saffron
2 teaspoons of garlic
2 teaspoons of paprika
6 small tangerines (or three oranges)
¼ cup of raw pine nuts
2 teaspoons arrowroot
2 ounces of fresh squeezed tangerine or orange juice

Blend until pasty THEN--- STIR in the following:

20 small pear tomatoes
1/3 cup chopped sweet onion
40 raw pine nuts
2 teaspoons minced raw garlic
2 ounces finely chopped raw beef
2 teaspoons fresh chopped tarragon
3 pinches of French sea salt
Either eat as a tasty paste, a spread or dip with your favorite vegetables

9 FILET MIGNON PATE' ALA ROGER

Blend in a Vita Mix or a good food processor until the consistency is that of putty or dough.
10 ounces of raw filet mignon

1 medium sweet onion
1 large chipotle chili
½ clove fresh garlic
1 teaspoon lemon juice
1 teaspoon lime juice
2 medium Roma tomatoes
1 tablespoon coarse black pepper
¼ apple wedge
Present on a plate garnished in cilantro leaves and sprinkled with paprika over the top to make the pate' look red.

10 SMOKEY FILET MIGNON PATE'

Blend in a Vita Mix or a good food processor until the consistency is that of putty or dough.
4 ounces of raw filet mignon
4 small pearl onions
10 basil leaves
⅛ cup of raw pine nuts
½ teaspoon of yellow curry powder
Mix until paste or putty like.
Then spritz with 10 sprays of Balsamic vinegar salad spray.

Then mix again for 20 seconds.

Serve on either:
Sliced tomatoes
Bell pepper slices
Sliced cucumbers
Sweet onion slices
Celery
Any other veggie that you want to try.

11 ROGER'S SALMON PATE'

(In a Vita Mix blend)

12 ounces of RAW salmon
1 small onion
1 half a red bell pepper
1 small garlic section

3 Medium Roma tomatoes
3 inches of peeled cucumber
½ ounce lemon juice
Mix well

Scoop out into a bowl and add 2 green onions chopped and 25 capers
Serve with dipping veggies.

12 ROGER EUPHORIC SALAD

2 Large cucumbers chopped
4 Roma tomatoes chopped
3 Green onions chopped
20 large basil leaves shredded fine

Mix the above in a bowl and drench in balsamic vinegar (to taste). Sprinkle on French organic sea salt and coarse black pepper to taste.

Some people will also add chopped avocado or a tablespoon of raw pine nuts or a tablespoon of raw sliced almonds for protein.

13 ROGER'S CAESAR SALAD

2 whole romaine lettuce stalks chopped up or cut up with kitchen shears into fine small pieces.
4 green onions chopped small or one sweet onion chopped up small.
1-2 tomatoes diced
2 tablespoons thick Caesar dressing

Mix well and eat. This salad should have no croutons, no cheese or anchovies. This salad can be served with any dressing, not just Caesar.

As you can see, I eat variations of the same things often. In all of these concoctions raw beef, salmon, avocado or raw almonds can be added.

14 STUFFED TOMATO ALA ROGER

4 large tomatoes hollowed out.
4 ounces of raw salmon or raw tuna chopped.
1 ounce fresh pear, ground down in a blender. Pour off excess water.

2 ounces of raw pine nuts.
1 ounces of raw black olives chopped up small (optional)
1-2 stalks of chopped green onion.
12 large basil leaves chopped up fine.

Mix together and scoop into the hollow tomato hulls.

15 ROGER'S ROMAINE ROLL UPS

In a bowl mix up

2 ounces of chopped raw salmon
1 fresh garlic section minced
2 green onions chopped
1 ounce (one small handful) of chopped cilantro leaves
½ ripe avocado chopped
1 tablespoon raw pine nuts
2 inches of cucumber chopped up fine and blotted dry of excess moisture.

Mix well and then scoop out onto romaine lettuce leaves. Roll up and eat.

16 CUCUMBER AND ONIONS SALAD

3 large peeled or unpeeled cumbers sliced very thin
2 sweet onions sliced in half and then sliced very thin
1 loose handful of cilantro leaves

Pour 6 ounces of rice wine vinegar over the contents and mix well. Let marinate for 24 hours and serve.

17 ROGER'S WOW EM' CEVICHE

8 Roma tomatoes medium chop
3 Green onion small chop
2 medium sweet onions medium chop
2 cups of chopped cilantro leaves
1 red bell peppers medium chop
½ yellow bell pepper medium chop
½ cup cucumber medium chop

Roger Bezanis

½ cup fresh lime juice
¼ cup fresh lemon juice
⅛ cup fresh garlic small chop
Optional:
½ cup chopped raw tuna
½ cup chopped raw salmon
½ cup chopped raw yellowtail

Place the contents above in a plastic storage container. Close it tight and then shake the contents until mixed well with lime and lemon juice permeating the blend.

18 ROGER'S SPRING SALAD

3 ounces of balsamic vinegar blended with one raw egg (the egg is optional)
2 ounces fresh orange pulp

Mix the above into a gelatin-like consistency.

2 Large red bell peppers (take out the seeds) cut up into ⅛ th inch strips
1 medium pear diced up
3 large broccoli tops chopped up small
12 large basil leaves sliced up into thin strips
1 ounce raw shaved almonds can substitute raw walnuts

Pour the gel-like solution over the above ingredients and toss.
Mix well in a bowl. Can be eaten as a salad or put over a bowl of Romaine lettuce or Arugula.

For those of you who like sushi...

19 THE ROGER ROLL (cut roll or hand roll give this recipe to a sushi chef)

(This roll can be made without rice)
Spicy Tuna
Kampyo
Green onion
Avocado
Cucumber
Daikon

Eel sauce on top
Spicy mayonnaise on top

20 ROGER'S SASHIMI SALAD (sushi give this receipt to a sushi chef)

On the house salad lettuce
Shredded cucumber
Green onion (chopped up fine)
Kampyo chopped up fine
Ikura (large salmon eggs) on top
This plate should be drizzled with eel sauce on top.
The plate should be garnished with spicy mayonnaise.

21 ROGER'S SHAVED CUCUMBER DELIGHT

Use the total vol. of 2 Cucumbers by shaving them down with a cheese grater
Use the total vol. of 1 pear by shaving it down with a cheese grater
Use the total vol. of ½ red peppers (no seeds) by shaving it down with a cheese grater
Use the total vol. of 2 carrots by shaving them down with a cheese grater
20 green grapes
10 strawberries chopped up medium
10 large basil leaves chopped up fine
Sprinkle with cinnamon
Sprinkle with nutmeg

Mix and serve

22 TOMATOES ON PARADE

In a blender, Vita Mix or food processor coarsely chop 2 yellow peppers, 4 radishes, 1 small onion and 1 section of garlic.

Separately
½ medium cucumber diced
Collect the raw corn from two fresh uncooked corn stalks
20 fresh raw pine nuts
Combine the pine nuts, diced cucumber and 20 pine nuts into the blend made in the first step.
Stir by hand until it is well mixed

Roger Bezanis

Next
Slice 4-6 steak tomatoes into 1 inch round pieces

Spread a ¼ inch layer of the above mix on the sliced tomatoes one at a time. Garnish with a sprinkle of finely chopped green onion tops. Serve

This spread can also be used on romaine lettuce stalks.

23 ROGER'S FINGER FOOD EXPLOSION

3 large cucumbers cut into ¼ inch slices
20 baby carrots
15 broccoli tops
4 ounces of Roger's Smokey Mayonnaise mixed with Sriracha hot sauce until pale pink.

This is veggie dip.

24 ROGER'S WILD COCONUT DIP

(In a blender or food processor mix to a paste)
13 ounces of raw pine nuts
6 ounces of coconut juice
¼ pear
2 ounces of coconut meat
2 teaspoon of cinnamon
$1/16$ teaspoon of cayenne powder
After stir in 20 small green grapes (you can add more grapes to your taste).

Serve with sliced celery or on red cabbage leaves

25 ONION GRAPE INSANITY

(In a Vita Mix, blender or food processor)

1 tablespoon Arrow Root
60 Concord grapes ground down to a gel
(This is now yummy grape preserves)

Slice two Maui or Vidalia Sweet Onions in to ¼ - ⅛ th inch slices.
Smear the grape preserves (above) on and eat.

This is a very different and tasty treat.

26 ROGER'S SILKY DRESSING

(Blend in a good food processor or Vita Mix)

1 banana
½ cup vinegar
2 tablespoon lemon juice
½ teaspoon paprika
2 tablespoon dry mustard
6 fresh basil leaves
1 teaspoon dill weed
½ teaspoon cardamom
2 cloves

27 ROGER'S HAIL CAESAR DRESSING

(Blend in a good food processor or Vita Mix)

1 ripe banana
1 garlic clove
½ half cup rice vinegar
2 raw eggs
¼ cup meat of a lemon
1 tablespoon black pepper

28 ROGER'S SMOKEY MAYONNAISE

(Blend in a good food processor or Vita Mix)

3 raw eggs
10 raw pine nuts
2 tablespoons of lemon juice
3 cloves

1 inch of ripe banana
1/8 teaspoon of fresh minced garlic
1/8 teaspoon of turmeric
Pinch of tarragon

29 JOLLY ROGER'S 1000 ISLAND DRESSING

(In a good blender)

4 raw eggs
1/8 cup vinegar
1 tarragon leaf
The meat of 2 steak tomatoes
1 tablespoon of arrowroot
1/8 teaspoon dill weed

Mix until thick and then stir in the following

2 tablespoons fresh papaya chopped fine
1 teaspoon sweet onion chopped fine

Blend in a Vita Mix on low setting or in a blender until smooth consistency is achieved.

30 PINK SPICY MAYONNAISE (Great on all raw fish)

(In a blender mix until thick)

3 tablespoons of arrowroot
3 raw eggs
4 cherry tomatoes
1/4 medium red bell pepper with seeds
1/8 teaspoon paprika
1/8 teaspoon cayenne pepper powder
1/8 teaspoon red chili powder
1 inch of dry chipotle chili

31 PINK APPLE SAUCE

(In a Vita Mix, blender or food processor)

4 peeled green apples (Granny Smith)
10 green grapes
1 half ripe pear
2 strawberries
1 teaspoon Arrow Root (for consistency)
¼ teaspoon of cinnamon
⅛ teaspoon of paprika
1 pinch of nutmeg

Blend on high for between 30 to 90 seconds or until the consistency is correct for YOUR apple sauce.

WHAT TO DRINK?

32 ROGER'S CITRUS ZEST SMOOTHIE

(In a Vita Mix or good blender always blend until smooth. Always add the ice in the last 30 seconds of blending)

1 Banana
5 Strawberries
4 Whole oranges or tangerines
1 Peach
6 ounces of fresh squeeze orange or tangerine juice
1 Kiwi
10 pieces of ice

33 ROGER'S APPLE RED BLEND

(In a Vita Mix or blender)

2 Bananas
3 Red apple slices

1 large wedge of watermelon
4 ounces of organic grape juice
6 Cherries
3 ounces of tangerine juice or orange juice
1 medium peach slice
3 Strawberries
15 Pieces of ice

34 HIGH PROTEIN BLAST

1 Avocado slice
2 Raw eggs
4 Strawberries
2 Whole oranges
6 Ounces of orange or tangerine juice
15 grapes
20 Blue berries
1 pear
2 ounces of organic grape juice
15 pieces of ice

35 CALMING SUN TEA

(In a large sun tea jar fill it up water and the contents below and let stand in the sun)

20 rose petals
3 Cinnamon sticks
3 lemon slices
3 Chamomile teabags

After 3-6 hours in the sun strain and serve.

36 ZESTY SUN TEA

(Fill a large sun tea jar with water, then add the contents below and let stand in the sun)

6 Orange Peels
4 cloves

2 Lemon peels
2 Lime slices
Step 10 pinches of cumin (in a mesh tea ball) in the tea for the last hour.

After 3-6 hours in the sun strain and serve

SNACKS

Munchies are fun things to pop into your mouth when you need a treat. All of the following are finger foods. Some you may never have thought of snacking this way.

Raw corn on the cob (very sweet)
Cherry or plum tomatoes (by themselves or with dressing of your choice)
Celery in stone ground mustard (Mustard is high in sodium this is not a great choice)
Broccoli (dipped in your favorite dressing)
Grapes (Green, purple and black)
Tangerines
Oranges
Grapefruit
Strawberries
Watermelon
Blueberries
Peaches
Pears
Apples
Cherries
Carrots
Cucumber slices
16 ounces of tangerine juice
16 ounces of orange juice
Raw fresh coconut meat
Raw fresh coconut juice

Of course there are many other treats that can be eaten. The only rule is eat it fresh and raw. If you are cognizant of what it takes to stay healthy you will know how to feed your body. Food should energize and not cause pain. You can be self regulated but you have to decide to do it yourself.

Eating is the human equivalent of giving your car the oil and gasoline it needs to run correctly. If you pour sugar and water in your gas tank, your engine will corrode. Soon you will need a new engine. If you give your car the care and maintenance recommended in your owner's manual, you will experience years of trouble free service.

Until you picked up this book, there was no manual that made the maintenance of the human body easy to follow. Make no mistake: what you put in your mouth has a profound and direct affect on your health.

Simply by reading and fully understanding and applying this chapter and the lessons of the chapter The Hidden Keys to Weight Loss and Body Repair, you can forever control your health. Eat well and be well.

42 Eyebrows

Eyebrows are not just for plucking and /or decoration. You may have noticed that eyebrow color does not always match hair color exactly.

- Darker eyebrows foretell an excellent kidneys probability factor. Your eyebrows should be darker than the hair on your head.
- If your eyebrows are naturally light in color, then it will take more work to keep your kidneys healthy.
- If the eyebrows grow sparsely and are lighter in color, this again indicates kidney challenges.
- If the eyebrow hair of either sex grows straight up and does not lie against the skin, then the liver and the kidneys are problematic.

As I said at the beginning of this chapter, the better circulation of the body, the better the health of the body will be. Do not be afraid to incorporate cayenne capsules, turmeric, cinnamon bark and wasabi japonica into your life. Take enough to create the kind of effect that you are looking for. Do not ignore your diet, as some people like to do. If diet is never addressed, your condition may return.

Summation: Oxygen must consistently saturate the body. Bodies resistant to disease are oxygen / circulation and energy rich. Utilizing the previous three factors can heal any problem.

43 Pissy Moody Kidneys

The kidneys are two bean shaped organs about the size of your fist. They are located an inch to three quarters of an inch under the muscle, flesh and the lower ribs of your back. If you are overweight they may be deeper.

They are given some protection by your lower ribcage. Because only half their mass is covered by your ribs, they are vulnerable to impact damage.

To locate your kidneys:

- Put the pointer finger of your left hand on your back at the left side of your waistline. It should be placed just above your left buttock muscle.
- Stretch your hand straight up (or vertically) so that your hand is fully spread. Your pointer finger and tip of your thumb should be stretched as far as possible away from each other.
- Having done this, the tip of your thumb will be touching roughly the center of your left kidney.

This places them for most people about 4-5 inches above their waistline.

The kidneys are vital for human survival as they monitor the entire body with regards to fluid production, movement, filtering and removal. Every action of your body requires fluid at some point in the activity.

There are many arguments as to how much water man is comprised of. Here are the statistics.

- Blood contains 95% water.
- Lean muscle tissue contains about 75% water by weight.
- Bone is composed of 22% water.
- Body fat contains 14% water
- The human body is made up of between 55-60% water

Because of the enormity of the task that the kidneys carry out every day, they are greatly affected, moment by moment ,by everything we eat or come in contact with.

The kidneys detect everything we do, good or bad. Like a mini brain they compute the best possible plan of action to sustain survival for their host.

Every organ of the human body is attempting to survive. No organ is more involved on a moment by moment basis with this task than the kidneys. Only the liver has a task equal to the kidneys.

This relationship started soon after conception. Upon the first cellular split, the two new cells became the rudimentary liver and kidneys. The importance of this split and what took place next cannot be stressed enough.

The aforementioned cell split established the beginnings of the liver and kidneys. Thus all future cell development was then dependent on these two organ systems for waste removal.

Therefore all future organs and their excreted waste products are either directly processed by the liver or kidneys. Life at any level of existence cannot expand if it is standing in its own waste. Under these conditions all life will succumb and die.

The Chinese call the kidneys the MASTER ORGAN of the BODY due to the magnitude of what they regulate. They ensure survival by providing fresh blood to the host, collecting and cleaning all muscles, joints and providing mucous wherever needed.

The kidneys regulate:

Uric acid
Lactic acid
Urine production and removal
Mucous distribution
Blood flow (i.e. blood pressure)
The heart
The ears (equilibrium)
Your fingernails
Your Hair
Most muscle groups
The reproductive system
The scalp
Fluid of the eyes
Fluid found in the colon
Waste water from the liver
Water distributed to the liver
Most joints (The liver regulates the right shoulder region down to the right elbow)
Pancreas
Lymphatic system

The liver and kidneys form two "southern" brains in the body. Our "northern" brain sits in our skull and computes information given to it by its "southern" intelligence units, the liver and kidneys.

The information sent to the brain is quickly processed (in hundredths of a second) and passed on to the body at light speed.

Literally it is the responsibility of the liver and kidneys to keep you functioning well and alive.

The liver and kidneys are constantly voting on your dietary, chemical and physical decisions, good or bad. Should the liver or kidneys detect a dietary choice that compromises your health, you are quickly made aware of it via the sensation of discomfort or pain.

Since the kidneys regulate so much of the structure of the body they may give you these sensations 12 to 30 times a day. Without question the kidneys are the moodiest, most sensitive organs that you have in your body. They are the bean shaped twins that are unparalleled in their importance to human survival.

FINGERNAIL CONNECTION

Thousands of years ago the Chinese discovered that the fingernails demonstrate the health or state of the kidneys.

Healthy kidneys are demonstrated on your fingernails by:

A smooth appearance
A bright and healthy look
Being strong and sturdy but not thick
A rapid growth rate
By straight and even growth

Unhealthy kidneys are demonstrated on your fingernails by:

Lumps, bumps and ridges
A dull appearance
A gray appearance
A yellow appearance
Cracking and splitting
An arch in the middle
Growing down over the tip of finger

For more information on fingernails please see the chapter "Fingernail, Hand and Finger Analysis.

Some medical modalities preach that "the body is enabled with innate intelligence." This statement is 100% correct.

As mentioned before, the kidneys are incredibly sensitive and react to everything you the host comes in contact with, good or bad. You may not notice their reaction but it occurs nonetheless.

They literally know where you live and like it there. This statement sounds completely absurd until you examine simple reactions that are common to 100% of mankind.

You may have noticed that when you come home from a day of work, travel, shopping, etc., and you get within two blocks of your house, suddenly you have to urinate. This reaction is universal. It is caused by your kidneys relaxing, having detected the safety of home.

Your kidneys do not like to travel.

If they could have it their way, you would never go anywhere outside of your home environment. This is a primitive, yet wholly survival based reaction. If you wander away from home where food and water is plentiful, you are risking death.

Because of that your kidneys are programmed to seek the best possible solution to the current circumstances. This includes the rationing of water usage when a new environment or situation is encountered. In this way they attempt to ensure long term survival.

The kidneys have no concept of time. Their sole focus is on the next correct action to perform. They do not have the ability to use abstract thought and thereby understand that your trip away from home is not dangerous. They have no way of knowing that you are going to the mall to try on shoes. They compute all departures from a known location as dangerous.

When you leave home, standard operating procedure is to lock-down water movement and usage. Leaving your environment, water may not be present in your new location.

Therefore your kidneys lock-up every drop and will not release more water until they are comfortable that you are safe.

Any location that you routinely frequent will eventually be labeled as "safe" providing that there is water and food at this locality.

The kidneys also react to energies emanating from other beings. Humans are an energetic organism and each has its own energy field. When you meet someone new, your kidneys are in a state of mystery as to who and what they are.

All new acquaintances are "felt out" this way. This includes a new boy or girl friend. You may have noticed that even though you are greatly attracted to a new "flame," your body could not "go" until they were gone.

This is due to the impact that the kidneys have on the colon. Without the proper lubrication of mucous, which is controlled by the kidneys, your colon will be locked-up tighter than a drum.

If you have ever had a friend that could only have bowel movements at his or her house, this was the phenomena at work.

Should you be in the vicinity of a strong electrical impulse such as a cell tower, power line, computer or even a plasma TV, you may notice the same reaction.

What the kidneys react to:

- Unfamiliar locations
- Unfamiliar people
- Unfamiliar energies

They prefer your house. They recognize the attributes of your neighborhood and identify it as home. When you leave home they begin to tighten up. They ask "where are we?" Since you do not speak kidney, you do not answer.

Leaving your house for any reason, your kidneys are puzzled and want to know:

"What's wrong?"
"Is there no more water?"
"Where are we going?"
"Are we there yet?"
"Is it safe?"

If you meet anyone new, they want to know:

"Who's the new person?"
"When will they go away?"

The kidneys would prefer to stay home and keep your same friends.

This plays havoc on the poor business traveler. This further explains why, when in a new hotel room or travel location, upon waking and looking in the mirror, you appear swollen. Of course your face looks swollen because it actually is swollen. As per your kidneys' "survival directives," you are retaining water.

On the road (traveling) you must create home in your hotel room. Scents must be the same or similar, foods must be "kidney friendly" and body abuses (via diet) must be practically nonexistent.

Roger Bezanis

RULES FOR HEALTHY TRAVEL

- Drink ⅓ more water on the road than you do at home
- Eat grapes as they are kidney friendly
- Eat tomatoes as they are pro kidney
- Eat Kiwi as the kidneys love them
- Eat romaine as it nourishes the kidneys
- Eat bell peppers as they help support the kidneys
- Eat radishes as they give the kidneys energy
- Eat blueberries as these aid the liver which supports the kidneys
- Eat citrus as it supports the digestive tract and aids with constipation
- Drink coconut water as this is a healing tonic for the whole body
- Eat raw free range beef (not everyone will do this, but it is very healthy)
- Drink fresh squeezed juices
- Bring as many items from home as you can to make the kidneys feel safe
- Do not drink alcohol as this reprograms the kidneys
- Do not eat salty or sodium rich foods as they both reprogram the kidneys
- Do not eat manmade (white) sugary foods as sugar reprograms the kidneys
- Do not consume caffeine as it reprograms the kidneys
- Do not eat breads, pasta, crackers and other processed carbohydrates
- Use a good kidney formula to aid you in traveling
- Use a good liver formula as the liver and kidneys support each other
- Use a good colon formula to aid you in eliminating built up waste
- Get plenty of sleep (6-8 hours if possible)
- Do not take drugs to mask kidney sensations
- Recognize that pain is a request for food or water, not a request for drugs
- Traveling is very traumatic to the kidneys. Please do all you can to help them

The list above is so accurate and beneficial were you to follow it in your daily life, you could heal any kidney issue.

When you go away on a trip, your poor kidneys do not fully relax until they are sure you are safe and not lost. They act like an internal mother. Sometimes it takes a day or two for your worrisome kidneys to acclimate to their new surroundings. The quicker you implement the above list, the faster your kidneys will adjust the next time you travel.

Flying note: As you might have guessed the kidneys hate to fly. Airline cabins are pressurized to 8000 feet of elevation. Unless you normally live at that altitude your kidneys will react to the pressure.

Frequent fliers often report stiff joints, sore knees, muscle soreness and even swelling while flying. This is a response to the trauma of leaving home, all the strange people, cabin pressure, airline snacks and beverages.

The airline food irritates these conditions. The supplied "air snacks" are loaded with sodium, salt and sugar. The beverages are full of sugar, caffeine and alcohol. The best solution is to bring your own water, while eating grapes or citrus while you fly.

Perhaps you have gone to the restroom while using air travel and noticed that you did not look so good. There is a very good reason why. Because of the complex superhighway of neurons, protons and synapses, etc., of the body we can actually monitor the stress of the kidneys by the look of the face. If the kidneys are stressed or in excellent health, the area (explained precisely below) will look more or less irritated.

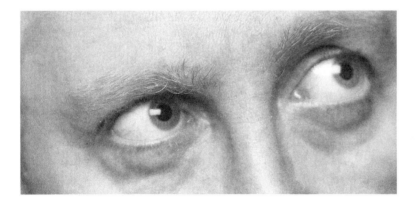

Face reading is a very old diagnostic health technique that relies on the look of the face (swellings, discolorations, redness, acne, etc.) to indicate how the body is running. Every part of the face represents a different area or organ of the body.

The half moon under each eye represents the kidney on that side of the body

- A dark circle (usually means adrenal gland fatigue)
- Puffiness (indicates the kidney is swollen)
- Discoloration (means the kidneys are not running well)

Roger Bezanis

• Growths (indicates a growth is present on the kidney)

This area should always be smooth and clear.

In the list for healthy traveling, I mentioned that certain substances reprogram the kidneys. Before that I stated that the kidneys are programmed to seek the best possible solution to the current circumstance that will ensure long term survival.

This is a statement of pure fact. The kidneys know when fluid should be released, moved, cleaned, rationed etc. Since their activities are central to the survival of the body, their care and nurturing should be paramount in our daily interests.

All substances that negatively alter, reprogram or in some fashion do not support the programming of the kidneys are dangerous.

KIDNEY LAW: All substances that negatively alter, reprogram or in some fashion do not support the programming of the kidneys and body are dangerous.

ALL SUBSTANCES THAT NEGATIVELY ALTER, REPROGRAM OR IN SOME FASHION DO NOT SUPPORT THE PROGRAMMING OF THE KIDNEYS AND BODY ARE DANGEROUS.

What we come in contact with, via food or environment, falls into one of three categories:

• Supportive: Supporting body processes
• Neutral: Neither good or bad for the body
• Toxic: Harmful to the body and its programming

What substances do this?

Caffeine: A diuretic, it auto commands the kidneys to release fluid, regardless of what the kidneys need to do next for the good of the body.

Result: The kidneys are off line for 4-6 hours.

Caffeine super heats every system of the body, races the heart, savagely increases energy (at the expense of all the other organs), increases internal organ pressure, raises blood pressure, disorients the user and creates anxiety. The rise of OCD and ADHD has been directly tied sugar and is involved in psychoses such as paranoia and other life destroying mental disorders.

Processed Sugar: A cathartic, it auto commands the kidneys to release and then suddenly hold fluid regardless of what the next actions of the kidneys should have been. The kidneys seize in a locked position.

Processed sugar also super heats the body; the body temperature actually raises as much as 2 degrees. The cathartic aspect of white sugar is powerful. It commands and shocks the body so much that the body convulses in its attempts to handle the sugar insult. The body writhes in spasms as it tries to deal with this toxic agent. It then acts as a preservative, telling the body to retain water and thus retards metabolism. Many of the same mind altering affects of caffeine are present with sugar.

Result: The immune system is suppressed by up to 95% and for as much as eight hours as per the New England Journal of Medicine.

Processed Carbohydrates: Breads, pasta, rice, cereal, grains: All convert to sugar and act as processed sugar does above.

Salt: Preservative; it makes the body retain water causing metabolism to slow.

Sodium: Preservative, acts exactly the same way salt does.

Alcohol: It depresses and commands the body to run slower. It also dehydrates the system and therefore has a diuretic affect.

It further lowers body temperature within minutes of consumption. Because of its pervasive effect it reduces hearing, vision, muscle coordination, memory and equilibrium. As more alcohol is consumed it slows breathing, blood pressure and heart rate. It reduces liver response for up to 12 hours.

Alcohol is a legal to consume poison at every level of usage.

Drugs: All reprogram the body and suppress its ability to run correctly. They act either as suppressives, accelerators, preservatives or diuretics or all four.

When presented with a toxin (all toxins reprogram the system) the body will do one or more of the following:

Increase Pain	Less heavy (**for a short time)
Decrease Pain (**for a short time)	Decrease energy
Increase stiffness	Increase energy (**for a short time)
Decrease stiffness (**for a short time)	Increase or ragged emotional response
Decrease vision	Decrease emotional response (**for a short time)

Decrease hearing	Decrease skin color
Decrease sense of touch	Dark circles or bags under the eyes
Decrease sense of taste	Increase body odor
Decrease sense of smell	Increase constipation
Increase urination	Decrease constipation (**for a short time)
Decrease urination	Decrease/Worse digestion
Decrease sexual function	Increase in internal or external growths
Increase sexual function (**for a short time)	Thinner, finer, less hair
Increase body heat	Gray or graying hair
Decrease body heat	Thick yellow fingernails
Increase heart rate	Fingernails with white spots in them
Decrease heart rate	Fingernails that have black spots in them
Tightens	Weak brittle fingernails
Loosens	Decrease longevity (life span)
More heavy (**for a short time)	Speeds the body towards death

**"For a short time above", indicates that the response listed will be short lived and then return to a weakened state.

Many of the above responses manifest quickly. Weight can adjust at a rate commensurate with the input of food matter. Yet sensations manifest immediately.

Arthritis and Gout symptoms: Uric Acid can be found all over the body, as it is a byproduct of destroyed cells. Uric acid is like spent uranium from nuclear fission in the body. Anywhere uric acid is lying stagnant, there will be irritation and some swelling. When allopathic medicine notices sore joints, they call it arthritis. It is just unmoving uric acid creating the pain and swelling. It can also crystallize causing gnarled looking joints. Gout is a severe form of the same phenomena.

Diabetes: Is an advanced kidneys issue. The last machine every diabetic is hooked up to is a kidney dialysis machine designed to replicate the function of the kidneys. If the foods listed in this chapter are eaten and the other recommendation of this chapter followed, even diabetes can be healed.

Two Rules/Facts

1) Uric acid is processed by the kidneys. This acid can be found anywhere in the body but it harbors in the joints. Once there, it causes irritation and pain. A large percentage of

diagnosed arthritis is actually due to kidney overload, as weak kidneys will have trouble sweeping the joints free of uric acid.

2) Lactic Acid is processed by the kidneys too. This acid can be found in the muscles after physical activity of any kind. Once generated, uric acid causes irritation and pain. Sore aching muscles are actually due to kidney overload and lack of processing power. Weak kidneys will have trouble sweeping the body free of lactic acid and uric acid. The moment you are labeled with "has arthritis" and you agree with it, finding the true answer becomes an unlikely prospect.

Athletes who follow the recommendations of this chapter can improve their:

• Strength

• Endurance

• Recovery time

There have been numerous cases of just this type of occurrence. For those who understand kidney function, improving ones health is fairly easy.

SOLVING KIDNEY PROBLEMS

Kidney issues are far easier to repair than most people think. Being very sensitive, even a slight change can produce dramatic results. Depending on the severity of the condition, healing the kidneys may take a few days to as long as three months to complete.

The following herbs are all fantastic in their ability to heal and support proper kidney function.

Cinnamon bark	Pygeum Bark	Borage leaves
Cedar leaves	Fenugreek	Lycci Fruit
Wild rose root	Juniper berries	Red Raspberry
Cloves	Goldenseal	Cayenne
Holly basil	Dandelion root	

The herbs mentioned above can often be found in preexisting combinations but can be used in loose form when purchased at a health food store. As mentioned earlier, depending on the severity of the condition, healing the kidneys may take a few days to as long as three months to complete. The way to take herbal combination for kidney health:

Roger Bezanis

- Three to five times a day
- With or without meals and at bedtime
- Six days a week
- Always take the seventh day off to give the body a rest.

There is much hoopla and confusion regarding the efficacy of Gastric Bypass and the Lap Band Procedure as they are touted to heal diabetes.

LAP BAND AND GASTRIC BYPASS HOAX FOR DIABETICS

Lap band surgery and Gastric Bypass surgery are touted to cure diabetes. The idea that these surgeries are a cure for anything is ridiculous.

These surgeries are like a modern day "Stone Soup." In making stone soup you start with a stone and water. Then you add six ounces of chopped lean beef, carrots, potatoes, onion, tomato etc. Stone soup has nothing to do with a stone. The name stone obscures the fact that what you are really making is beef stew.

With lap band and gastric bypass the same thing is true. Weight loss occurs not because the bowel was rerouted but because of the rules that are enforced after surgery:

Gastric Bypass and Lap Band Requirements after Surgery:

- Patient must give up junk food
- Patient must eat fresh fruit and vegetables
- Patient must exercise
- Patient must eat small portions of food (caused by the surgery)

NOTE: Numerous patients have only lost a few pounds even after surgery because they did not follow the four points above. Carnie Wilson is sadly one of them. But I have hope for her.

The above four factors are keys to ANY weight loss program. This is not a secret. It is tragic that some people require surgery to make them follow the four points above.

If we just enforced the above four points then surgery would be superfluous.

The cure for over eating and obesity is to stop making excuses and to change. Only one percent of the public are obese because they have a thyroid problem. This means the other 99% of those claiming this excuse are in denial. The problem with obesity is caused by the fork and spoon not a gland.

What the surgery does is reduce the size of the stomach by as much as 90%. Then a direct route is created extending the new small stomach directly to the second part of the intestines the jejunum. This means that $1/3$ rd of the intestines and the entire stomach is bypassed. This is where the term bypass comes from in regard to gastric bypass or stomach stapling.

The results are:

- Reduced appetite due to the new smaller stomach.
- Poor food absorption reducing calorie intake.
- Weight loss

AGAIN, WHY DOES LAP BAND AND GASTRIC BYPASS CAUSE WEIGHT LOSS?

- Patient meal size is smaller as the "new" stomach fills quickly.
- Patient food absorption is poor because there is less digestive tract to absorb with.
- Patient DIETRY CHANGE IS MANDATORY
- Patient EXERCISE IS MANDATORY
- Patient JUNK FOOD EATING IS CUT OUT

Anyone who follows the last three points above will achieve weight loss without the need for surgery.

Finally, the surgery is no guarantee of weight loss if the individual continues to gorge themselves on copious amounts of food.

I hope the above clears up any confusion that you may have with these procedures.

To recap:
1) The kidneys are a major part of the immune system in the body.

2) The kidneys regulate all fluid movement of the body.

3) The kidneys do not like to travel and prefer the home environment.

4) If the kidneys are off-line the body will come to a halt as most body functions stop.

5) All puffiness and dark circles under the eyes indicate weak and irritated kidneys.

6) The worst possible substances that you can give the kidneys and the body are sugar, salt, sodium, caffeine, alcohol and drugs.

7) A body that has received sugar can recover but it has been attacked and insulted. For some this attack may have done irreparable damage.

8) The body is equipped with innate intelligence and if given the chance can heal any problem.

9) If the kidneys don't like or are poisoned and forced off line by what you eat or come in contact with, it will get sicker and sicker until you correct your input errors.

10) Certain foods heal the kidneys.

11) Certain herbs heal the kidneys.

12) Gastric Bypass and Lap Band surgeries work because of the life changing restrictions that are enforced, not because of the surgery itself.

I am certain that if bariatric clinic gave 100 people "placebo" Gastric Bypass surgery (including a scar and stitches) the patients being convinced that surgery took place would lose weight. Of course no surgery would be administered at all. Stitches would be applied for an incision that was only made to convince the patient that surgery had been done.

Remember, unless your doctor is your partner in your health, he is your adversary. Doctors who insist that they are right regardless of what is right must be let go. If your doctor insists that you have arthritis and he will not consider other possibilities, get a new doctor.

Your choices interfere with or support your body's efforts to survive. Exactly like a computer, your body is programmed to take the exact NEXT correct action to keep you alive and in good health.

They must communicate without a voice. They can only speak to you via sensation and visual cues such as face reading. Reduction of pain (without the use of drugs) indicates that the body is improving. This always follows changes on the face, such as dark circles and puffiness under the eyes dissipating.

Increasing pain means the kidneys are rejecting a substance as it is causing stress. You can heal your kidneys and body. It just takes a little work. Some say that it is expensive to be healthy.

It is far more expensive to be sick.
If you need me I am here for you,

Your friend,
Roger Bezanis

44 Holistic Detoxification

Titling my book "Diagnostic Face Reading and Holistic Healing" has led to much peril from the world of the critic and well wisher categories of society. Diagnostic (which means to assess and understand a problem) has pitfalls of its own as it is not a warm and fuzzy word.

Holistic is another declaration full of confusions and conflict. Holistic simply means the whole entity. Therefore a holistic approach to healing does not isolate an area of the body for attack but rather encompasses the entire organism for healing.

This brings us to the point and beginning of this chapter. If we are going to use the word detoxification we first must agree on what it means.

Detoxification is a common activity carried out by the body 24 hours a day. Depending on what challenges that we are giving the body, this is an easy or very difficult and often incomplete cycle of action.

The definition of detoxification found in Webster's reads as follows:
Main Entry:
de·tox·i·fy
Pronunciation:
dē-täk-sə-fī
Function:
transitive verb
Inflected Form(s):
de·tox·i·fied; de·tox·i·fy·ing
Date: circa 1905
1 a: to remove a harmful substance (as a poison or toxin) or the effect of such from b: to render (a harmful substance) harmless

2: to free (as a drug user or an alcoholic) from an intoxicating or an addictive substance in the body or from dependence on or addiction to such a substance.

3 : neutralize

The next word for description is TOXIN as it owes its genesis to mankind understanding the nature of life and commenting on its fragility.

Webster's defines the word Toxin this way:

Main Entry:
tox·in
Pronunciation:
täk-sən
Function:
noun
Etymology:
International Scientific Vocabulary

Date: 1886
A poisonous substance that is a specific product of the metabolic activities of a living organism and is usually very unstable, notably toxic when introduced into the tissues, and typically capable of inducing antibody formation.

An antibody is a funny word meaning immune system response. This response occurs on a microscopic level. The antibody response is initiated when toxins called antigens enter the body. Antigens are irritants that, if plentiful enough, are capable of collecting and becoming a growth. These growths can only accumulate at sites in the body where circulation is reduced.

The antibody is an immune system protein that attempts to contain the toxin or antigen. Once controlled, the substance is escorted out of the body with the help of the liver, kidneys, spleen and lymphatic system. They are then pushed out of the body via the colon, skin, lungs and bladder. If you carefully follow the last three paragraphs you can see that toxicity is where all tumor growth and cancer spring from. All cancer springs from toxins that have entered the body and have not been removed. This brings us full circle back to the word detoxification.

Note: There is evidence that parasites can amass in the body creating blockages as well. The definitions that we are using encompass all of these aspects and some not hitherto appreciated or contemplated.

Detoxification simply returns balance to a system that has been overwhelmed with substances that either do not break down fast enough or do not break down at all.

Detoxification may seem to benefit only one portion of the body, yet it achieves marked improvements throughout the entire system. Because the body is a symphony of interconnected ecosystems, one positive change anywhere alters and improves the natural balance of the entire body. This is where the idea of Holistic Detoxification comes from.

Boosting man's detox process became necessary thanks to his pursuit of pleasure via toxic shortcuts. These include fast foods and drugs. His natural inclination towards speed and abundance has led him to corrupting his body in the name of hunger. Fast food is just an attempt to save time and money.

Of course we know these foods are not foods and are extremely toxic to the body. But the motivation was simply to help.

Drugs are an example of the same mechanism. The twist of evil entered when lab scientists in the early 1900's realized that drugs had a detrimental and addictive effect on the body. Faced with this realization they were in far "too deep" to quit. If they admitted failure, entire companies would fold up and they would lose their standing, savings, and lifestyle.

This is where we are today: full of drugs and preservatives as well as other human ecosystem harming toxins.

There are many avenues, including emotions that are blocked by toxins in the system. Much of today's emotional distress is caused by these irritants off-balancing the major organs including the liver.

To reiterate, the liver is the center of emotional intensity in the human body. If the liver is overloaded, emotional Armageddon may not be far behind.

The bits and pieces of food that we ingest either serve our life purposes or block them. The purpose of life is to survive. The body is programmed to calculate optimum survival based on the present circumstances encountered moment by moment. This simple statement demonstrates the totality of what the body is doing and has been doing during the entirety of biological history.

What we ingest either blocks, prevents or supports life. Energy is either expanding or contracting. Matter devoid of energy is, of course, dead. Positively charged matter infuses the body with symbiotic energy. This is where nature and its fruits and vegetables enter the picture. They are Earth-energized foods and cause a homeostasis, thus harmonizing the body with the environment it lives in.

Disharmony and disease is simply defined as a lack of harmony or lack of ease. If the body is hot while it should be cool, this is a level of disharmony or disease.

I have worked in the health industry for the past 20 years. When the word disease is mentioned people often slip into abject terror. Suddenly all confidence is lost as they have been confronted with something that knows no boundaries. Disease has the connotation of being beyond the ability of the individual to cope with on their own.

In actual fact that is not the case. People heal themselves from "so called" diseases every day.

The reason they are successful is because they have identified their problem and have devised a strategy to reverse the condition. Twenty years of healing people has taught me that the only condition that is beyond repair is death.

The nomenclature or language of the medical profession is intimidating and foreign to most people. My book and this chapter are written to dispel the confusions surrounding sickness and disharmony of the body.

The way to attack this is to wage war on the use of medical terminology. I am suggesting that we do not use it, as the use of these words spread fear.

For example, Hepatitis means the liver is inflamed. The word alone instills fear, intimidation and mystery. But saying the phrase "swollen liver" or "inflamed liver," based on survey results produces about 60% less intimidation and fear. The mystery is completely gone as the phrase describes the condition.

The other reason to boycott the use of medical terminology is that it promotes the medical profession as the only solution for healing the body.

I also surveyed the terms and phrases: AIDS, Diabetes, Fibromyalgia, Epstein Barr, and Renal Failure. The results showed that 98% of the responders could not accurately define the conditions. They also could not identify what organs were at the root of the conditions.

Disease simply means "not – ease." The medical profession has used its esoteric nomenclature to obscure the simple nature of how the body operates. The terms that the medical profession uses to describe "not-ease" mean something to doctors but not the general populace.

When people are afraid of disease it is due to the nature of the word that was just used. Cancer is an awfully big word and it only has six letters.

Disease is confused with mortality and gives the listener the idea that something has attacked the body or that the body has caught "something." Disease in the end begets death in its current form and usage. Therefore use of this word must be abandoned by any sanity-seeking individual.

Therefore, I am suggesting here and now that we forever drop the word disease and replace it with the term "physical disharmony" as this phrase is not confusing and ultimately a correct statement of being.

When a problem is stated correctly it opens the door to a correct handling. A man upset about loud noises cannot solve his problem until he identifies the source of the problem. The same man upset about the radio blasting can turn it down.

The American Cancer Association not surprisingly lists CANCER as a disease. From reading this book you have learned about our conditioning regarding the word. The public upon hearing the word, at the very least become nervous.

They know that a horrendous monster is stalking their every step.

Since disease intonates "monster on the loose," the logical response is to seek an expert in monster killing. Replete with wooden stakes, garlic and Wolfbane, he is a bonafide demon slayer. Trained at a prestigious university of higher learning, he is the oncologist and medical oncologist; "cancer's worst nightmare." He or she will assure you that a trained professional can handle your insidious and alarming condition. He may tell you to get other opinions or to research the subject yourself. Given that the vast panorama of information available is wrong the patient is often left spinning.

The patient is now living his or her own edge of your seat thriller. The problem is the life on the line is yours as the monster lurks in the dark. But what are these monsters made of?

Unequivocally the monsters are the American Cancer Association and big Pharma who create drugs and protocols to follow that "treat": their little gold mine cancer. Cancer treatment and surgery is an astronomically profitable industry. Every year millions of dollars are given to research "cancer." Cancer is not a "thing"; it is a result.

As long as the cancer "gene" is looked for, millions of dollars will be wasted and the public will remain in the dark as doctors keep treating a monster that does not exist.

The tumor growth known as cancer is such a money making proposition it will be tens of years before it stops being the focus of science.

Roger Bezanis

Our knee jerk "see a doctor" behavior is so rigid and full of rancor in our society that you can be ostracized and accused of all manner of suicidal tendencies should you opt to handle a growth without following the government medical model.

What kind of society do we live in where we are not allowed or are too afraid to heal ourselves? When it comes to health we must be our own judge and jury. We must be responsible for our own physical disharmony and take actions to correct it.

The body can repair itself if given the chance. I have witnessed dozens of people including my own mother reverse cancer tumor growth on their own. Every now and then I run into someone who claims that natural means did not work for them. In the end, we all have to make our own choices.

If we choose the medical route, oncologists are ready with chemo therapy to help you past your hurdles. Remember the dichotomy of chemo therapy. This approach is known to be toxic and works on the principal of "differential toxicity." Meaning the oncologist hopes the chemo is more toxic to "it" than it is to you.

The medical oncologist is focused on surgery and is a bit different than the oncologist you will see first upon finding a growth. Having tumors removed opens up a whole new can of worms. Mastectomies are done at an alarming rate.

Dr. Diana Zuckerman in her article "Unnecessary Mastectomies: Are Breast Cancer Patients Given Accurate Information About their Options?":

It is shocking but true: approximately one out of every two American women who have a breast removed as treatment for cancer does not need such radical surgery. Whether a woman undergoes a mastectomy or a lumpectomy (which removes the cancer but not the breast) depends less on her specific diagnosis than on other factors, such as where she lives, her income and health insurance, where she receives medical care, her age, and when her doctor was trained.

Also from her article:

Some striking research findings include:

*In some hospitals, all breast cancer patients had mastectomies, regardless of their diagnosis. In one large urban hospital serving mostly poor women in Texas, 84% of the women with early stage breast cancer had mastectomies and only 16% had lumpectomies.

*In a study of 157 hospitals, patients treated by doctors trained before 1981 were less likely to have lumpectomies or other breast-saving surgery than women who had younger doctors.

*One study indicated that women getting mastectomies were more likely to have followed their doctors' recommendations, but women getting lumpectomies were more likely to have obtained a second opinion, and felt more actively involved in making the decision.

*A study of 175 surgeons found that even doctors who know that lumpectomy is as safe as mastectomy may persuade their patients to get mastectomies by making subtly biased recommendations. Other studies showed that some women were not even told that lumpectomies were an option.

Oncologists are not bad people or inherently evil by any stretch of the imagination. Seeing an oncologist is like seeing a florist. You are expected to purchase flowers.

Deciding to be in control of your health destiny means that you have taken a step towards independence and ridding yourself of the fear of getting worse. The fear starts in the way we describe and or think of our bodies as confusing enigmas. Any subject that is complex or confusing is marbled with false information.

Modern medical science is based on only 110 years or so of what many believe to be faulty information. So confounding is this drug and surgery world of medicine that it sticks to us like glue. Ask any medical doctor that has given up their "drug them and cut them" way of life to pursue alternative medicine and they will confess the same thoughts.

One of the leading "Environmental Disease" physicians in the world, Sherry Rogers, MD, in her book "Wellness against All Odds" states:

"In the beginning, I was a simple ordinary country doctor with specialty boards in family practice and additional certification in allergy. I was happy practicing medicine like my colleagues. It wasn't until I started to develop an endless array of diseases and symptoms that nobody in medicine could cure that I started to stray from the pack."
Later she says:

"From that point on, we departed from the point of view that current medicine still embraces, namely that a headache is a Darvon deficiency"

"We departed from the world of drugs to enter the world of environmental medicine and nutritional biochemistry where the cause of symptoms can be found and real cures brought *about. Not only did we learn how to do nearly drug free medicine, but we also learned an important rule of modern medicine and that is that the patient is the keeper of the keys to wellness."*

Many openly-made statements like "I could not get people well. I was just dispensing drugs/ surgery with no end in sight" are common.

Part and parcel of the drugs and surgery approach to medicine is the basic premise that you are too unintelligent to understand the problems of your body without help. Thus highly esoteric medical jargon and exclusive university study was created, further distancing you from the truth.

To summarize, a complex esoteric theory of how to heal the body has been created. Out of control and unopposed, it is completely based in earlier confusions creating a vacuum. This black hole of complexity forces theorists to postulate more and more radical answers to deeper and deeper chasms of misunderstanding.

The resulting unintelligible babble is disseminated broadly, causing a semi-comatose state for anyone trying to understand it. Simply stated, confusion is studying confusion trying to define and correct confusion. Which leads directly and solely to where we are today in a maze of mystery.

Studies indicate that medical care-related deaths have cost approximately 1,000,000 people their lives over a 10 year period. Some of those deaths include the following:

- The Nurse Coalition credits 108,800 hospital deaths due to MALNUTRITION.
- Another study indicated hospital mishandled infections cost 88,000 people.
- HCUP reports that 37,136 people expired due to unnecessary procedures.
- Medical error accounts for 98,000 life ending mishaps.
- Advertised drug reactions have accounted for another 106,000 losing their lives.
- Hospital stay related bedsores account for 115,000 passing away.
- • 32,000 were lost during surgery as per the Agency for Healthcare Research and Quality.

Imagine how many lives would have been saved if any of these people had only had the opportunity and knowledge to take care of and heal on their own.

The deeper we dive into the devious rat hole of modern medicine, the more transfixed we become on opening a door that we cannot find with a key that we do not posses.

We are left standing in a quicksand of fear with no exit from the nightmare. Modern medicine is a virtual labyrinth of backward thinking that we must escape; otherwise we have no possible chance for health redemption.

This book gives you the basics of human life that have been misconstrued for centuries. If we are in the dark as to just how the processes of the body work we will never heal. This book is here to turn the light on brightly once and for all.

Toxicity and all cancers are the result of an accumulation of waste material collecting at a site devoid of oxygen, energy and circulation. Flood these toxic cells with circulation and the body heals. These are the simple life-supporting correct conclusions that save lives.

Holistic detoxification allows natural metabolism to return to the body so that the inhale and exhale of our cells is consistent.

Cells are little nuclear reactors that must take in fuel, throw waste off and then later be replaced by new cells. This is the proper flow that supports all life. Junk food preservatives are designed to elongate the shelf life of food to make it impervious to decay.

Those same preservatives execute an identical function of preserving our cells once they are ingested. A good label for this is cellular stagnation.

Cellular stagnation causes fat to be resistant to all manner of exercise and dietary change meaning that weight loss is a very slow process. Therefore preservatives make our cells inhuman or super human units that are practically immortal. These decay- impervious cells do not belong in the human body and actually destroy it.

Holistic detoxification is the answer to this horrific problem as these bionic super cells are the cause of many of man's miseries such as cancer.

What you have just read is one of the more vital pieces of information in this entire book. Please reread this again and again. Read it to anyone who will listen.

The fact remains that the body never "caught" anything that was not ingested in one way or the other. Even a tick bite was not the result of the magical word "caught." It was the result of a well placed and survival-programmed little bug.

Therefore we are focused on holistic or total body function and only detoxify in a fashion that opens all these channels.

Roger Bezanis

HOW OFTEN TO CLEANSE/DETOXIFY YOUR BODY

Old time wisdom states that a deep cleanse/detox should be done once a year for three solid months. In the last few years this seems to be inadequate. Today people are deeply burying themselves in new aggressive toxins at an alarmingly mad rate. Evidence now clearly indicates that a once a year schedule of detox repair is wholly inadequate to keep up with our rapidly advancing toxic menace.

The rash of new toxins from foods and the environment make it mandatory to do a full body cleanse more often than once a year. It is best to plan for performing a full three month intensive cleanse detox,s followed four months later by a one month cleanse.

Many people have great success by maintaining a yearly three month detox program. This group accounts for less than 10% of the world's population. Another much rarer faction runs famously well with a lighter cleanse schedule. Due to diet and other disciplines they comprise only 1% of the world's population.

For this group, doing any kind of lengthy detox is unheard of unless they come under some overwhelming physical disharmony. I am part of this group and have not done even a month of detox in the last 12 years.

The above may be confusing as to how anyone could seemingly be naturally healthy. There is no one who is impervious to toxicity. Eighteen years ago, I was very sick and like Dr. Sherry Rogers mentioned above, I had to heal myself.

Detoxification became my life. I became an expert on it. For six years I was performing inner cleansing and detox on myself to achieve my current level of health. If I had known what I know today, that process would have only taken three to six months.

My secret is my diet, as I spend little time exercising, yet I am 16% body fat, have few gray hairs, weigh 164 pounds, have blood pressure of 98 over 59, baby soft skin, the body of a 20 year old, a resting heart rate of 60 beats per minute and a urine ph of 6.8- 8.0 (this is excellent).

I have built my life around the chapters "The Hidden Keys to Weight Loss," and "A Diet for a New Century."

With the two chapters just mentioned, along with this one, as your standard operating procedure, you can attain fantastic levels of health at any age. You are capable of joining the 1% group that you have just read about. Adopting these chapters makes using supplements an infrequent activity. You many use them on occasion but that is up to you. I recommend using something for the liver, kidneys and colon as needed.

As mentioned before the aforementioned group (that I am part of) makes up only 1% of the world's population. Let's expand it to 10% as fast as we can.

The doors are not closed and entry is free. You must decide to be part of this group. That is the only caveat. You can achieve balance via the doorways opened to you in this book. Using the cleansing detox routines found later in this chapter will send you on the way to being healthy and nutritionally free.

Repeating: to be fully healthy, follow the "ultimate plan of health" that I lay out in the "Hidden Keys to Weight Loss" and then utilize the chapter "A Diet for a New Century." With the above tools it will only take two to four weeks to achieve a level of health that will amaze you.

Anyone needing to do a full 3 month detox, please use what follows in guiding you as to where you should start. The following questions will help you determine where to focus your inner body wash.

Regardless of where your attack is focused, detoxification always follows the same basic approach of clearing the body of unwanted elements.

Zone A

Y or N –Are you constipated (less than one-elimination per meal eaten)?

Y or N --Do you have bad breath?

Y or N --Does your sweat have a strong odor?

Y or N --Are you always tired?

Y or N --Are you exhausted after eating?

Y or N --Do you have colitis?

Y or N --Do you have diverticulitis?

Y or N --Do you have hemorrhoids?

Y or N --Do you have leaky gut syndrome?

Y or N --Do you have Candida?

Y or N --Do your stools have a strong foul odor?

Y or N --Are you always bloated?

Y or N --Do you drink tap water?

Y or N -Do you shower or bathe in unfiltered water?

Y or N --Do you use a fluoride rinse?

Y or N -Do you brush with fluoride toothpaste?

Y or N --Do you consume alcohol at least once a week?

Y or N --Do you consume milk?

Y or N -Do you consume cheese?

Y or N -Do you consume butter?

Y or N -Do you consume yogurt?

Y or N --Do you eat fast food?

Y or N --Do you eat fresh (non-frozen or canned) fruit less than once a day?

Y or N --Do you eat fresh (non-frozen or canned) vegetables less than once a day?

Y or N --Do you eat frozen dinners?

Y or N --Do you eat canned food?

Y or N --Do you salt your food?

Y or N --Do you consume caffeine?

Y or N --Do you consume energy drinks?

Y or N --Do you eat protein bars?

Y or N --Do you drink protein drinks?

Zone B

Y or N --Do you eat tuna (dangerous with mercury)?

Y or N --Do you have problems with vertigo (balance)?

Y or N -Do you have hearing problems?

Y or N -Do you have tinnitus?

Y or N -Do you have weak or numb tingling muscles?

Y or N --Do you have recurrent aches and pains?

Y or N --Has your hair suddenly turned gray?

Y or N -Does your hair grow too slowly?

Y or N --Do you have a weak bladder?

Y or N --Do you have sore joints or arthritis?

Y or N --Do you have sore or aching muscles?

Y or N –Are your nails weak?

Y or N –Are your nails brittle?

Y or N –Do your nails grow too slowly?

Y or N --Is your hair brittle?

Y or N --Is your hair weak and thin?

Y or N --Are you losing your hair?

Y or N --Do you have pancreatic problems?

Y or N --Do you have thyroid problems?

Y or N --Do you have kidney problems?

Y or N --Do you have lymphatic problems?

Y or N --Do you have adrenal problems?

Y or N --Do you have bags and dark circles under your eyes?

Y or N --Do you have high blood pressure?

Y or N --Do you have hearing problems?

Y or N --Do you have heart rhythm problems?

Y or N --Do you see floaters in your vision (small clear shapes)

Y or N --Does your urine smell like ammonia?

Y or N --Does your urine smell fruity?

Y or N --Do you have uterine issues?

Y or N --Do you have ovarian issues?

Y or N --Do you have ovarian cysts?

Y or N --Do you have uterine cysts?

Y or N --Do you have ovarian issues?

Y or N --Do you have prostate problems?

Y or N --Do you have erectile dysfunction?

Y or N --Do you have reproductive issues?

Zone C

Y or N --Do you have headaches?

Y or N --Do you suffer with allergies?

Y or N --Do you have migraines?

Y or N --Do you have liver problems?

Y or N --Do you have insomnia?

Y or N --Do you have lung issues?

Y or N --Do you have numb or tingling skin?

Y or N --Do you have dry skin?

Y or N --Do you have itchy skin?

Y or N --Do you have blotchy skin?

Y or N --Do you have acne?

Y or N --Do you have boils?

Y or N --Do you experience depression?

Y or N --Do you have strong feelings of anxiety?

Y or N --Are you always nervous?

Y or N --Are you always angry?

Y or N --Are you without emotion?

Y or N --Are you numb to the world?

Y or N --Do you have problems with mental focus?

Y or N --Do you have cloudy thinking?

Y or N --Do you have skin discolorations?

Y or N --Have you damaged your skin in the sun?

Y or N --Have you or do you have melanoma (skin cancer)?

Y or N --Are you moody?

Y or N --Do you have mood problems?

Y or N --Do you have eye problems?

Y or N --Do your eyes burn or itch?

Y or N --Do you have sinus problems?

Y or N --Do you have nerve issues?

Y or N --Do you awake in the morning exhausted?

Y or N --Do you toss and turn all night?

Y or N --Do you take antidepressants?

Y or N --Do you take medication?

Zone D

Y or N --Are you always sick?

Y or N --Are you very susceptible to being sick?

Y or N --Do you work around chemicals?

Y or N --Are you short of breath?

Y or N --Do you get sinus congestion?

Y or N --Do you get sinus headaches?

Y or N -Do you always have phlegm?

Y or N -Do you have a recurrent cough?

Y or N --Are you sedentary and get little if any exercise?

Y or N --Do you have emphysema?

Y or N --Do you have lung problems?

Y or N -Do you have asthma?

Y or N --Do you work in an office without window and ventilation?

Y or N --Do you have a long commute in traffic?

Y or N - Does your city have smokestacks from industrial plants?

Y or N - Do you live near an airport or next to a busy highway?

Y or N --Are you a smoker?

Y or N -Do you smoke pot?

Y or N --Are you around a smoker or smokers?

Y or N --Are you subject to second hand smoke?

Y or N --Do you live in a large metropolitan city?

Y or N -Do you need a nap before you go to bed?

Y or N -Are you worn out by 3:00 every day?

Y or N -Do you burn out during the day?

Zone E

Y or N –Have you or do you drink garden hose water?

Y or N –Do you crave sugar and sweets?

Y or N –Have you ever eaten raw pork?

Y or N –Do you have recurrent anal itching?

Y or N –Do you have insomnia around the full moon?

Y or N –Have you been bitten by mosquitoes?

Y or N --Do you drink stream water (directly from a stream)?

Y or N –Do you ever eat sushi?

Y or N –Do you own a dog or cat?

Y or N –Do you swim in the ocean?

Y or N –Do you walk barefoot?

Y or N –Do you get dog or cat kisses?

Y or N –Do you ever eat "non-free range" raw meat?

Y or N –Do you engage in oral sex?

Y or N --Do you change a cat box?

Y or N --Have you had parasites before?

Y or N –Have you ever had a sexually transmitted disease?

Y or N --Do you allow a dog or cat in your bed?

Y or N --Have you never done a detox before?

Y or N --Has it been some time since your last full detox?

Y or N –Have you traveled to third world countries?

Y or N –Have you eaten from a salad bar?

Y or N –Have you done a parasite detox before?

Zone F

Y or N --Do you rarely exercise?

Y or N --Have you had surgeries?

Y or N –Have you had dental work?

Y or N -Have you had a root canal?

Y or N -Do you have age spots?

Y or N -Have you been given nitrous oxide (laughing gas)

Y or N -Do you use tanning beds?

Y or N -Do you lay out in the sun often?

Y or N --Have been given general anesthesia?

Y or N --Have you had x-rays?

Y or N -Have you been given radiation for any reason?

Y or N -Do you have breast implants?

Y or N -Do you work outside in the sun?

Y or N -Do you have or have you had melanoma?

Score your yes answers below

Zone A_____

Zone B_____

Zone C_____

Zone D_____

Zone E_____

Zone F_____

The above questions are an excellent guide to determine where to start with your detoxification program. By using the scoring Zone below you will be able to formulate your plan of action to heal and maintain your health.

Zone A - Deals with GENERAL TOXICITY. Answering yes to 6 or more questions indicates a need for a full three month general system toxin eradication program. To solve and heal these issues, follow the protocol listed below und GENERAL TOXICITY AND CONSTIPATION.

Zone B - Deals with KIDNEY ISSUES. Answering yes to 10 or more of these questions indicates that the kidneys need repair. This process may take one to three months. Follow the KIDNEY PROBLEMS protocol below.

Zone C - Deals with LIVER OVERWHELM. Answering yes to 10 or more of these questions indicates that liver activation needs to be your focus. Follow the LIVER, SKIN, LUNG protocol as laid out above.

Zone D – Deals with LUNG WEAKNESS which is regulated by the liver. If you answered yes to 6 or more questions in this zone your lungs need to be supported. Follow the LIVER, SKIN, LUNG protocol as laid out above.

Zone E – Deals with the PARASITES. If you answered yes to 6 or more of these questions you need to address parasites in your body repair process.

Zone F – Deals with GENERAL TOXICITY and LIVER, SKIN, LUNG toxicity brought on by chemicals and sun radiation. The skin is regulated by the liver yet these conditions often need a special approach. Follow the GENERAL TOXICITY and LIVER, SKIN, LUNG PROTOCOL as laid out below.

GENERAL TOXICITY AND CONSTIPATION

General toxicity is caused by cellular congestion leading to constipation defined as, less than one bowel movement per meal eaten. If the body is not able to utilize fluid and expel waste, all manner of symptoms may crop up as every system of the body is affected.

All toxicity slows down or impedes body function and metabolism. This condition makes weight loss extremely difficult. Body fat absorbs and holds toxins to prevent these poisons from sickening the body. This is the same reason why fat is resistant to breaking down as our fat acts like a toxin poison prison. (Yes you are right. Saying toxin poison prison is fun.) The powerful herbs found in the list below astringe cellular waste, scrapes the colon free of putrefied matter and fecal debris.

Cellular list

Echinacea	Myrrh	Cumin
Chickweed herb	Garlic	Angelica
Irish moss	Peppermint	Astragalus
Dandelion	Elderberry	Nettle
Prickly ash bark	Peach leaves	Sarsaparilla herb
Oregon grape root	Ginger root	Bupleurum root
Barberry root	Burdock root	Cayenne fruit
Yarrow flower	Fenugreek seed	Mullein leaf
Lavender flower	Black cohosh root	

Colon List

Rhubarb root	Plum seed	Turmeric
Cascara sagrada	Aloe	Slippery elm bark
Black sesame seed	Psyllium seed	Pumpkin seed
Fennel seed	Fedegoso	Grape fruit seed
Cumin	Buckthorn bark	

Note: When purchasing a colon cleansing product, avoid Senna as it is very, very, very powerful and can cause damage.

Foods that heal and cleanse the body and colon are oranges, tangerines, lemons, grapefruit, garlic, onion, cayenne, tomatoes, bell pepper, cumin, radishes and coconut and water. Please drink at least 80-120 ounces of water a day. It is possible that you will need more water depending on the climate that you live in and your activity level.

If the above herbs are used with the correct diet, the detoxification process can be very efficient and straightforward.

The herbs mentioned above can often be found in a preexisting formula but can be used in loose form if purchased independently. As mentioned before the length of time one would be follow this protocol is three months. This book does not recommend products or companies. The research for these companies is a breeze if you use the internet.

A good company will have a track record and well known reliable product. Rooting around on the web will uncover many good companies that can help you. Also, look for a company that is well recommended. Your natural medicine doctor will be very able to help you.

The way to take this combination of herbs:

- Three times a day
- Best taken before, during or just after breakfast and dinner.
- Six days a week
- Always take the seventh day off to give the body a rest.

KIDNEY PROBLEMS

Kidney issues are far easier to repair than most people think. Being very sensitive, even a slight change can produce dramatic positive or negative results with these delicate organs. Depending on the severity of the condition it may take up to three months to complete.

The following herbs are all fantastic in their ability to heal and support proper kidney function.

Cinnamon bark	Pygeum Bark	Borage leaves
Cedar leaves	Fenugreek	Lycci Fruit
Wild rose root	Juniper berries	Red Raspberry
Cloves	Goldenseal	Cayenne
Holly basil	Dandelion root	

Foods that heal the kidneys include grapes, tomatoes, kiwi, bell peppers, romaine lettuce, raw free range beef, radishes and coconut water.

The herbs mentioned above can often be found in preexisting combinations but can be used in loose form when purchased at a health food store. As mentioned before, the length of time on this protocol may take up to three months to complete.

The way to take this combination of herbs:

• Three to five times a day
• With or without meals and at bedtime
• Six days a week
• Always take the seventh day off to give the body a rest.

LIVER/SKIN/LUNG BASED PROBLEMS

These are problems of the liver as the liver regulates the skin. Skin eruptions, skin cancer, age spots including tingling and numbness can all be corrected with the right protocol.

Niacin: This is an amazing B-vitamin that is well-known to create sunburn-like flushing on the skin. The resulting itchy sunburn-like reaction derived from niacin is caused by the opening up of capillaries and the movement of blood. In using B-3, beware that it is best to start with low levels of the vitamin at first.

As little as 50mg can create a flush that can last for 30 minutes to an hour. Niacin is extremely good for skin rejuvenation and the removal of toxins from fatty tissue.

Its other benefits include being a calmative to the central nervous system. Some people, while doing sauna treatments, will take as much as 1500 mg per day. Using niacin is of tremendous benefit but do not forget about the flush, as it will occur.

Use the following herbs with or without niacin over a three-month period and the skin can repair itself.

Bupleurum	Tangerine	Peony root
Gentian root	Irish moss	Lemon fiber
Hyssop	Yellow dock	Garlic
Cayenne	Sarsaparilla	Ginger root
Astragalus	Safflower herb	Lemon verbena
Bilberry root	Grapefruit fiber	Thyme
Dandelion root	Lime fiber	Goldenseal
Orange	Red clover	Marshmallow root

Foods that heal the liver and skin include: Blueberries, carrots, oranges, tangerines, grapefruit, lemons, limes, onion, garlic, broccoli, asparagus, red cabbage, cauliflower, green beans, tomatoes, bell peppers, romaine lettuce, apples, beets, arugula, avocado, blackberries, raspberries, ginger, radishes and strawberries. These foods practically perform miracles if eaten fresh.

Use the above herbs either in a ready-made combination or on their own. As mentioned before, the length of time one would be on this protocol is three months. Remember to use niacin sparingly as it will create a flush sensation. Never use niacinamide as it is altered in the lab. It is without much benefit and does not produce the same response that its unaltered brother niacin does.

The way to take this combination of herbs:

• Twice a day
• Before, during or after breakfast and dinner
• Six days a week
• Always take the seventh day off to give the body a rest.

PARASITE INFESTATION

Parasite infestation is one of the bleakest and most upsetting conditions known to man. Caused by as little as a tick bite (lymes disease) or from something as loving as a puppy kiss, this condition can be maddening and take a long time to handle. Murderous little pests like these are capable of mimicking every physical disharmony symptom known to man.

The fact is that 100% of us have parasites. The next question therefore has to be "if that is true, why aren't we all dead?" The answer is simple; in a healthy body and strong immune system parasites do not get a good foothold.

Therefore one can eradicate parasites via immune system strengthening or wholesale assault.

The herbs listed below fall into three categories 1) Immune system builders 2) Parasite eradication (cellular) 3) Colon and fluke (parasites in the colon) cleansing and eradication.

List 1 Immune System Builders

Astragalus	Jamaican dogwood	Cats claw
Echinacea	Hyssop	Dandelion root
Golden seal	Schazandra	Gentian root
Lavender flower	Suma	Bupleurum root

List 2 Parasite Eradication (cellular)

Black walnut hulls	Chinese Wolfbane	Garlic
Wormwood	Grapefruit seed	Cayenne
Cloves	Shield fern	
Pumpkin seed	China bark	

List 3 Colon Parasites

Fedegoso	Plum seeds	African bird peppers
Rhubarb roots	Garlic	Black sesame seeds
Aloe	Oregano	Rosemary

It is not a well-known fact that some foods prevent parasites. Foods that kill parasites in the digestive tract before they are attached or established include oranges, tangerines, lemons, grapefruit, limes, garlic, onion, ginger, wasabi, radishes and peppers.

Once parasites are ingested there are no known foods that by their use alone make the body untenable for further breeding

A full diet change can have a remarkable healing affect on the body. By completely giving up alcohol, caffeine, all manmade processed sugar (white sugar) along with foods that convert to sugar such as breads, rice, crackers, cookies, cereal and grains you can create an environment that greatly reduces parasites.

Sugar is lethal to the body but a literal fertilizer for parasites. Make no mistake, these blood-sucking vampires love white processed sugar. Whole fresh fruit and fresh vegetables which contain whole unprocessed sugars do not feed parasites. They create an alkaline environment that is not well tolerated by these micro-fiends. The more alkaline that you can make your body the less likely it is that you will have parasite related irritations.

Fresh fruit and fresh vegetables alkalize the body.

Alkalinity is abhorrent to parasites. Fruit and veggies that perform this function include fresh broccoli, blueberries, carrots, cauliflower, oranges, tangerines, grapefruit, lemons, limes, peaches, pears, kale, onion, garlic, broccoli, asparagus, red cabbage, cauliflower, green beans, tomatoes, bell peppers, romaine lettuce, apples, beets, sweet potatoes, arugula, corn, avocado, blackberries, raspberries, ginger, radishes and strawberries. These are super foods in their ability to make the body alkaline and therefore parasite and cancer resistant.

Use the above list of herbs either in a readymade combination or on their own. As mentioned earlier the length of time one would follow a parasite eradication protocol is three months. The biggest problem with parasite detoxification is not doing it long enough. Many people feel better so fast that they think that they are done and end their detoxification in only two to four weeks.

Do not make this mistake! Be sure to push yourself through the full three month process to be sure that you have finished the job that you have started.

Reminder: please do not use Vermox (a medical drug of little use) to address parasites. Finally, remember the awesome power of food to support you in your parasite detoxification process.

The way to take this combination of herbs:

• Four times a day
• Take in the morning, mid morning, early afternoon and evening
• Six days a week
• Always take the seventh day off to give the body a rest.
• Three consecutive weeks on the formula
• One week off
• Three consecutive weeks on the formula again
• One week off

Roger Bezanis

- Three consecutive weeks on the formula yet again
- You are done

Be sure to read the chapter "Parasites in Your Dinner" as it details far more background on parasites than can be included here.

The simplicity of detoxification is only mired with our own misunderstandings of just how simple it really is. With use of this chapter you can realistically disarm practically any toxicity problem that you encounter.

The alternative to holistic detoxification is the use of drugs and surgery which are barbaric and ineffective. Healing the body via herbal and dietary detoxification is the most workable and effective approach for restoring good health.

Please use this chapter to help as many people as you can who want help.

Your friend,
Roger Bezanis

45 Detox Diet Regime

All toxification of the human body begins the moment that we are exposed to a toxin in some fashion or form. Either we eat a toxic substance or we absorb it via the skin or the lungs. This material initially makes us feel strangely energized or sluggish and tired. We might itch, sneeze or cough. This is just our body attempting to reject the substance.

"Most people who think they are tired are actually toxic"
- Sherry Rogers, MD, board of Directors of the American Academy of Environmental Medicine

The end result of toxic exposure is all sorts of human body havoc. This may include feeling wired, exhaustion, poor skin, constipation, weight gain, pain, growths and eventually a general breakdown of the body. The list of what makes the body toxic is lengthy and features 1000's of substances.

The oldest form of detox is through diet. Medicines start out as food. Valium was once Valerian Root. The essence of White Willow bark is distilled down to become Aspirin. The list goes on and on.

Food is medicinal in that when it is cooked it becomes more condensed and robust. All chefs know that cooking intensifies flavor. The reason this occurs is due to molecular changes that take place during the cooking process.

The ingredients that compose chicken soup, when simmered for two days, become a gentle antibiotic. Coca leaves, if chewed, are mildly stimulating like coffee. The dark green leaves of the coca plant are rich in vitamins, protein, calcium, iron and fiber. The cocaine content of the leaves ranges from 0.1% to 0.9%.

Once they are distilled the new "white" substance, "cocaine," is lethal in its power. Cooking therefore not only increases flavor it increases the density of the medicinal or toxic value of the substance in question.

What we eat falls into three separate categories:

• Supportive

• Inert

• Harmful

A body free from toxins, excess mucous, acids, dead cells and all irritants is stronger, healthier and more vital. All harmful material ingested is irritating to the system at some level. It may be sticky and slow, the system creating an acidic environment in the body. Even inert matter such as tap water may actually be harmful.

"Study shows five glasses of tap water per day can increase the chance of miscarriage."
– Los Angeles Times, 1998

When substances absorbed or ingested resist excretion from the system, we are setting up a scenario that can lead to tumor growth, otherwise known as cancer. When indigestible matter collects in an area of the body, circulation through the region becomes strangled.

Tumors can only exist at sites of little or no circulation. Pain is the result of reduced energy flow, oxygen or circulation reaching some part of the body. It is a life supporting activity to keep these three aspects of health running at an optimum level.

The body becomes cancerous due to an exact progression. Each stage is known and can be followed as the body becomes more toxic. The sequence that all cancers follow is below:

• Toxic exposure or poor diet or both

- Poor circulation
- Toxic substances overwhelm the body's ability to remove them
- Poor liver function
- Poor kidney function
- Constipation (less than one elimination per meal eaten)
- Symptoms (aches, pains, poor skin, poor sleep, etc.)
- Weight gain (sometimes weight does not increase)
- Tumor growths

The above list can be reversed. All it takes is awareness and work on the part of the individual who intends to improve his health.

"Several government reports conclude that 60-90% of all types of cancer in the U.S. are causally related to environmental factors."
- Douglas M. Castle, U.S. Environmental Protection Agency

The solution is the rid the body of toxins and allow the body to heal. In the chapter "Holistic Detoxification," I explained what herbs and foods to eat. But I did not go into special "detox diets" that can be used to aid the process.

These diets are miraculous in their effect on the body. If you choose to use any of these diet plans I suggest using the herbs listed in "Holistic Detoxification" as well.

The diets that follow progress from the hardest to the easiest to use. Each is rated from hardest to easiest as well.

Hardest %%%%%
Hard   %%%%
Medium %%%
Mild   %%
Easy   %

All of these diets are effective, therefore choose the one that you are most comfortable with.

You will also notice that I am not pushing raw food in these diets as cooked food has medicinal value and you are performing a medicinal task by detoxing your body.

Fasting is the most difficult form of detox dieting as it involves the most discipline and the most radical departure from eating. I suggest that when you use this approach or any detox approach that you always support your liver with a good liver formula.

The formula should NOT use MILK THISTLE. Find a product that employs Bupleurum, as this is the most beneficial herb known for liver repair and support.

Fasting is based on the fact that the digestion, as well as elimination, is improved by regularly restricting food intake. Fasting does not mean the total cessation of food, although for some this can be done. Fasting is best done with fresh juices, hot water as specified and or a cocktail of water, citrus juice and herbs.

Organic Note: The use of organic produce and juices is most beneficial for all of these diet protocols. But if organic is not available use what you have at hand as you will still produce excellent results.

Headache Note: The first day or so of any dietary change increases the chance of headaches. They are always the result of liver overload. Be sure to support your liver.

DETOX FASTING %%%%% PLAN A

For 3 to 7 days do the following (this process can be followed for up to 14 days):

Breakfast: Drink 12-24 ounces of fresh squeezed orange juice

Mid morning (10:00 a.m.): Sip 10 ounces of hot water with lemon

Lunch (Noon): Drink 12-16 ounces of fresh cucumber (made in a juicer) and lemon juice, garlic with a pinch of cayenne pepper.

Mid afternoon (3:00 p.m.): Sip 10 ounces of hot water with cinnamon

Dinner (5:00): 10 ounces of white grape juice (not grape drink)

Note: Since you are not taking in any roughage you may want to test a colon formula to help move your bowels for the first day or so. But this is not absolutely needed.

DETOX FASTING %%%%% PLAN B

For 3 to 7 days do the following (this process can be followed for up to 14 days):

Breakfast: Drink 10-20 ounces of white or purple grape juice. Be aware that you may experience the GRAPE JUICE STOOL which may result in a very loose stool or diarrhea. The stool will be green in color and will smell like grape juice. You may also notice that the stool burns your rectum. This is to be expected as you are pulling acids out of your system.

Lunch (Noon): Drink 8-12 ounces of apple juice and a pinch of cayenne powder.

Dinner (5:00): Drink 8-12 ounces of fresh squeezed orange or grapefruit juice.

DETOX FASTING %%%%% PLAN C

For 3 to 7 days do the following (this process can be followed for up to 21 days):

The mix below is consumed at breakfast, lunch, dinner and whenever you want it in between. But you are only getting 64 ounces of the drink per day. If you consume all of your drink before your last sip at bedtime, you will be forced to drink water until the next day when you start the process again.

In a half gallon jug mix the following:
The juice from 2 Lemons or limes
The juice form 4 Oranges
1 teaspoon of garlic juice
3 teaspoon of dark Grade "B" dark amber maple syrup
1-10 teaspoons of cayenne pepper
1-4 pinches of cinnamon powder
Fill the rest of the jug with reverse osmosis water

You now have 64 ounces of a drink that purges the body of waste. This should be consumed gradually all day long until about 7:00 p.m. when you have completely emptied the bottle.

During this process eat no solid food of any type. You may want to use a colon formula to help move your bowels or employ the salt water flush below.

Salt Water Flush

If you are not using a colon formula as mentioned above you can dramatically flush your colon and digestive tract following the directions below:

When: First thing in the morning ON AN EMPTY STOMACH
What size: Use a quart bottle

Step one: Fill the bottle with warm water

Step two: Add two level teaspoons of sea salt to the warm water.

Step three: Shake well and drink down in 20 minutes or less

Step four: Locate yourself near a bathroom as your colon will flush rapidly.

• Do not drink more than the 32 ounces (one quart) of sea salt water as more is not better. Do not use iodized salt as it is useless to the body.

• Use only sea salt if you want this process to be effective.

• Beware that you will have several eliminations in a short period of time. This flush is best not to be used while you are on your job.

DETOX PASTE DIET %%%%

The following is one of the more unusual approaches to detox dieting that you will ever run across. It takes discipline and does work.

In a blender or Vita Mix blend the following until you have a paste.
20 blueberries
1 orange slice
1 whole banana
3 strawberries
1 half an apple (red or green)
20 raw almonds (raw walnuts can be substituted)
10 grapes
1 thin slice of onion
2 pinches of cinnamon

Make 10 ounces of the above mix. What you have just made will comprise your breakfast, lunch and dinner for one entire day. You must drink a large amount of water 80-120 ounces per for this to be fully effective.

Eat your paste at the following rates:
Breakfast: Eat 6 ounces
Lunch: Eat 3 ounces
Dinner: Eat 1 ounce

The paste should be eaten alone with nothing else. Even though the above mix is very simple the results from using it are quite impressive.

The salt water flush from "Detox Diet plan C" above may be employed as needed with this diet.

DETOX BROTH %%%

The following can be used for as long as 21 days.

In a 3 to 5 quart cooking pot add the following:
4 large tomatoes cut in half
4 whole cucumbers sliced but not chopped
3 whole asparagus stalks cut in pieces but not chopped
3 medium chopped carrots
3 medium chopped onions
2 cloves of garlic sliced but not chopped
2 medium chopped green peppers
2 medium chopped radishes
2 medium chopped potatoes
1 medium chopped cauliflower heads
1 medium chopped broccoli heads
1 medium chopped head of cabbage
1 whole beet with the tops not chopped
1 whole bunch of parsley not chopped
1 whole bunch of cilantro not chopped
¼ cup of lentils
¼ cup peas

Note: The above ingredients are more potent and healthful if they come from organic sources.

Fill the pot with the above ingredients and cover in water. Use a lid to be sure that you are not evaporating the healthful benefits of your detox broth.
Cook on high for the first 10-15 minutes

Cook on medium heat for the next 20-30 minutes
Simmer for 3 hours
Carefully drain your broth while saving every drop. Do not throw out the broth
Mash up the veggies that were just cooked
Add a half gallon of water to your mashed veggies
Cook on high for the first 10-15 minutes
Simmer for 2 hours

Drain the new broth into your first broth and drink as a nutritious tonic
Add Braggs Amino Acids to the mix on a serving by serving basis

What you have just made is vegetarian penicillin or medicine. Drink your broth as your sole form of nutrition for as long as 21 days. Whenever you are hungry have some of your broth. You will be amazed at how good you feel. Use the remaining veggies as fertilizer.

DETOX MONO DIET %%

The simplicity of this approach is beyond compare. You are eating whole food but you are only eating one type of food per meal. This allows your body to rest and repair itself as it digests your simplified meal.

You can do this diet indefinitely. Most people will do it for 3-14 days.

BREAKFAST:
Choose Only One Item to eat
10-24 ounces of fresh squeezed orange juice
4-10 oranges
4-10 tangerines
1-4 grapefruit
4-8 large tomatoes
20-40 green or red grapes
2-4 green or red apples
1-2 large slices of watermelon
20-40 blueberries
5-20 strawberries
1-5 guavas
1-5 persimmons
1-6 peaches
1-5 pears
10-40 blueberries
1-4 slices of pineapple
1-4 pomegranates

LUNCH:
Choose Only One Item to eat
1-4 Carrots
10-20 cherry or plum tomatoes
2-10 radishes

1-10 broccoli flowerets
1-10 cauliflower flowerets
1-2 Avocados
1-2 cucumbers
1-10 stalks of romaine lettuce
1 sweet Maui or Vidalia onion
2 stalks of celery
1 bell pepper
1-2 thumb size pieces of raw beef
1-2 thumb size pieces of raw salmon

DINNER:
Choose Only One Item to eat
1-2 oranges
1 slice of pineapple
1 grapefruit
1 large tomato
5-10 cherry or plum tomatoes
5-20 red or green grapes

During the day you may either have water or water with lemon or lime squeezed into it.

APPLE CIDER VINEGAR TONIC %

It is an old country tradition to cleanse the body with a tonic of apple cider, vinegar and water. Some people swear by it. I offer it here so that you may play with it yourself.

In a half gallon jug mix:
1 half cup of apple cider vinegar
⅛ cup of honey
⅛ cup of Grade "B" dark amber maple syrup
2 tablespoons of fresh lemon juice
⅛ teaspoon of powdered cinnamon
1 pinch of cayenne

Fill the rest of the jug with water
Shake
Sip throughout the day

The taste of the cider mix will take some getting used to for most. While using this tonic your diet does not have to drastically change. The better you can be with your diet the better your results will ultimately be.

As a general rule the more fresh fruit and fresh uncooked vegetables that you eat, the healthier your body will get. Do not be afraid to fast one day out of every week. This is very healthy as the body often needs the break to catch up.

No amount of healthy eating or dieting will work without water. Therefore, be sure to get at least 80 ounces of water into your system every day.

If you need me I am here for you.

Your friend
Roger Bezanis

46 What Your Body Really Needs and Wants

Albeit short, you are embarking on one of the most important chapters in this book. It unveils itself in the next several paragraphs. If you understand and apply the following data, you will almost certainly never have a weight problem again. You will be able to heal the most serious of problems. You will be almost impervious to sickness.

Imagine your body as a warehouse business. The job of a business like this is to receive goods at the receiving dock, process the items and then redirect them out the shipping door to a waiting truck. Your staff can handle 25 packages a day without too much trouble.

Your business is open from 8 to 5 p.m. daily. Processing delivered items takes 3 hours per item from delivery to shipping dock. Given that your warehouse staff needs to take breaks, lunches and go home at 5:00 p.m., it is important to make their job as simple as possible.

Otherwise, you risk them not getting home on time for dinner and thus not being rested for the next day, Should they be required to work overtime, it would be expected that they would show up for work the next day late, feeling tired or sick or all three.

With these factors in mind, when would you want your deliveries?

You would, of course, want them in the morning and no later than 2 p.m. in the afternoon. Deliveries that come late means your staff cannot go home on time. Tired workers are not effective workers.

Imagine a tired staff trying to keep up with the day's work after one, two, three or more consistent late nights of work. Imagine your order department going a little overboard with crazy or unusual items that need loads of processing just to be understood.

Delivery packages would start to stack up, your warehouse will start to have to store all of these unhandled packages.

This is the state of the human body. This analogy is accurate to how we must run our days. Eating in the morning is vital to start the day. Eating the majority of your meals no later than 3:00 p.m., while not social, is very healthy.

If you do eat in the afternoon or evening (and you can), it is best to eat fresh fruit or a light salad. You will be amazed if you adapt this approach. You will be energized and alive all day. Your body can heal itself much quicker. You will drop weight (if you need to) and look younger. Your shipping and receiving department, in order to work well, needs to handle packages that need little or no processing. It also needs those packages early.

A Short Play

Congratulations! You have just been elected to the new hamlet of Toeville. It is a sleepy little community of manicured front lawns, picket fences, bike lanes, dog walks and bouncy people. Amazingly, it is a neighborhood inside your own body.

This morning is like any other morning. The sun is up and people are happy. All of your residents (the joints, tendons and ligaments) put out their Uric Acid Trash in their tidy little cans for pick up.

Like every morning, the cans will be picked up promptly at 7:00 a.m. But unlike the other days, the UATT (Uric Acid Trash Trucks) are not going to show up. Back at the waste dump the crews must have been partying all night and are all hung-over.

The next day comes and goes. Then the next day and stills no trucks. The trashcans start to stack up. Imagine no pick up for 3 days! The crews must have passed out on a sugar high. What else can go wrong?

Trash is everywhere and the Toeville residents are so upset they are not even showering. The residents can hardly stand up without pain. They cannot take out any more trash, as they are too exhausted to move. Then the pipes in Toeville start leaking. There is sewage and water everywhere. Remember Sara Cynthia Sylvia Stout? Toeville can't take the garbage out.

Toeville is an absolute mess! The problem that was a local one has now become a statewide disaster. Everywhere in the state trash is out of control with no relief in sight.

Modern medicine would say it is a toe problem and treat the toes, never getting to the source of the problem. They would tell you that the residents need Prozac or Zanax. Psychiatrists would insist that the garbage is in the heads of the residents, not on the streets.

The genuine problem is at the city dump (the Kidneys). The kidneys (city dump) are so backed up with waste yet unprocessed, trucks cannot get in the gates. 17 blocks of backed up trucks, not able to off their loads is a nightmare. Until dumping takes place, Toeville remains a mess.

Under ideal conditions, the toes can put out their collected uric acid garbage and know it will be picked up several times a day. Toeville's city dump problem, which has now become a joint, muscle and sleep problem, is now a body wide severe pain problem.

Uric acid irritates the delicate cartilage of all joints. It must be quickly removed. But, due to conditioning and big business selling the next new magic bullet, you are left without answers. Pain is killing you, but you are told there is nothing really wrong except the pain. Logically in this scenario you must use painkillers.

Unless you learn how to use nature to heal the body, it will get worse and worse. You are not a bad person, just misled, lied to and drugged.

The FDA, AMA and Big Pharmaceuticals need you to be medicated and spending every dime you can muster to alleviate your woes. They want direct access to your insurance and life savings. Is there a natural solution?

Something as simple as grapes or tomatoes reset your kidneys. The most severe problems may be reversed with use of green grapes. Tinnitus, including vertigo and arthritis can all see relief. Joints can regain their smooth pain free moment by just changing the diet.

Again, you are not a bad person, just one of the billions who have been misled, lied to and drugged.

47 Sugar: Love It or Flee From It?

There is very little that I can say about SUGAR. It is the biggest business on the planet and the most addicting substance man has ever created. You have never met anyone without some form of addiction to it.

Sugar is so dangerous that the mere removal of it from the diet can spell huge changes. Researchers believe that removal of sugar would eliminate 99.5 % of all health complaints.

Roger Bezanis

So debilitating is sugar and the sugar lifestyle that receptacles used for insulin needles are now common in busy public restrooms. Diet is the key to health and life. Business today is not in agreement with being healthy. Money is all that matters and money equals sugar, unless you chose the alternative.

Try to order a salad with nothing processed on it and the server will look at you like you have 6 eyes. Turn down bread with a meal and you are practically a leper. Read the quotes below and you decide if sugar has a place in your life.

"The average person loses more than 90% of their immune function within 15 minutes of indulging in this poisonous substance. This deficiency lasts for about 2 hours after the stress occurs." – Dr. Stoll

"The bottom line is that sugar upsets the body chemistry and suppresses the immune system. Once the immune system becomes suppressed, the door is opened to infectious and degenerative diseases. The stronger the immune system the easier it is for the body to fight infectious and degenerative diseases." – Nancy Appleton, Ph.D.

"Intensive research during the past twelve years on the relationship between diet and susceptibility to infection, not only in polio but also in common respiratory infections and tuberculosis, has convinced me that the human organism can protect itself against infection virtually completely by proper nutrition." – Dr. Sandler, 1952

"TB (Tuberculosis) increased dramatically in Japan, shortly after the Japanese acquired a cheap source of sugar on the island of Formosa (aka, Taiwan), in 1910. Britain experienced a dramatic increase in deaths from TB during the 1700s, especially among workers in sugar factories and refineries." – William Dufty (Sugar Blues, p. 77)

"If only a small fraction of what is already known about the effects of sugar were to be revealed in relation to any other material used as a food additive, that material would promptly be banned."
– John Yudkin MD, Ph.D., F.R.C.P., F.R.S.C., F.I. Biol., Prof. of Nutrition at London University.

The average American consumes an astounding 3 pounds of sugar each week. The average teenager is eating up to 5 pounds a week. If you don't think that advertising aimed at children is working, just consider the rising incidence of obesity, rabid rate of diabetes and childhood disease. Between 90 to 95 percent of these problems are due to the ridiculous amount of refined sugar we as parents allow them to eat.

None of this should be surprising, considering that highly refined sugars in the forms of sucrose (table sugar), dextrose (corn sugar), honey and high-fructose corn syrup, are in practically everything.

Making matters worse, foods such as bread, cereal, crackers, and rice convert to sugar in a few minutes of ingestion. Mayonnaise, peanut butter, ketchup, spaghetti sauce, and a plethora of microwave meals are loaded in white sugar. All of this attacks the kidneys and pancreas, which instantly kicks insulin production into overdrive. Insulin promotes the body to store fat. Eating manmade sweets can cause rapid weight gain. Recently it was reported that abdominal fat was directly linked to cancer, heart problems, kidney failure and even rapid tumor growth.

In the last 20 years, we have increased sugar consumption in the U.S. from 26 pounds to nearly 160 per person per year! Prior to the turn of last century (1887-1890), the average consumption was only 5 lbs. per person per year! Cardiovascular disease, cancer and morbid obesity were virtually unknown in the early 1900's. Look at crowd photos taken in 1900 compared to 2000 and witness the amazing fattening of Americans.

Being healthy is a choice; as long as we believe we are the victims, we continue to be victims. When you decide to be healthy, you have taken the first step to achieving that goal. Perfect health is a goal to be worked toward. It may never be reached, but the journey is well worth the trip. The alternative equals a life of constant aches, pains, and oddball diseases, compounding weight issues, excuses, denial and premature aging.

Do you want your health to improve or worsen? If you answered "improve" to this question, then the work I have put into this book is beginning to stick. The first step to making changes is changing your thinking process. Read this book as many times as you need to in order to know it.

In early 2007, the New England journal of medicine reported, "Sugar suppresses the immune system by up to 95% for as much as 8 hours after ingestion."

Compare that with the popular notion that sugar feeds cancer and parasites. Consider that sugar does not feed anything, but makes the body bankrupt in defending itself. All forms of sugar prevent the body from utilizing vitamin C. Some camps believe that Glucose (a simple sugar) coats tumors, making them impervious to damage. Regardless, sugar suppresses the immune system, leaving it moot. Sun, Sloth and Kinkajou bears are all known as Honey Bears. These three bear species consume large amounts of honey as part of their diets, which gives them their name. Honey bears are the only animals in nature that suffer with tooth decay.

In other words, even nature is not immune to the horrendous affects of the raw sugar coming from honey. Some research shows that honey derived sugar is even more damaging to tooth enamel than white table sugar. Do not make the jump to believe that raw fruit sugar is damaging, as it is not. Yet, fruit sugars found in pasteurized juices can be harmful.

White / brown / honey / molasses sugar is credited with creating the following problems:

Mineral imbalance	Obesity
Hyperactivity	Grey hair
Anxiety	Wrinkles
Depression	Colon problems of all types
Anger	Joint problems
PMS	Insomnia
Learning difficulties	Respiratory trouble
High blood pressure	Spontaneous abortions
Liver cirrhosis	Fertility trouble
Hypoglycemia	Prostate trouble
Heart trouble of all types	Skin disorders
Ulcers	Circulatory issues

Medical Nobel laureate (1931) Otto Warburg, Ph.D., discovered that cancer cells have a fundamentally different energy metabolism compared to healthy cells. They live on vast amounts of glucose (simple sugar). Cancer is anaerobic (in absence of oxygen) and sugar and lactic acid create an environment that is oxygen free, which allows tumors to spread. The key is that the body has become acidic due to processed food that is starving the system.

Tumor cells cannot exist in an oxygen rich alkaline environment. They need sugar and acid to starve the area under attack of oxygen. The body becomes fatigued and this is an early sign that something is wrong. Chronic fatigue or no energy can exist years before tumors are actually seen.

Keeping ones weight under control and within 5-10 pounds of their ideal is important to keeping the body from becoming acidic and toxic. Tumors are starved in the correct environment.

Sugar and Holidays

We are in a vast sugar cesspool and have no idea we are. How bad is it? Is it really true? Can it really be that bad?
Yes.

Consider what you are up against. The following are all built around sugar:

Halloween	Baby showers
Desert	New years Day / New Years Eve
Birthdays (family, friends, co-workers)	Super Bowl
Christmas / Christmas Eve	Boxing Day
Hanukkah	Save the Eagles Day
Kwanzaa	Amelia Earhart Day
Thanksgiving	Ben Franklin Day
Easter	Martin Luther King Day
Celebrations (general)	Chinese New Year
Weddings / Divorces	President's Day
Engagements	Purim
Father's day	Girl Scout Week (cookies)
Mother's day	Passover
Births / Funerals	Labor Day
Bar Mitzvahs / Bat Mitzvahs	Veteran's Day
Anniversaries	Boss Day
Valentine's Day	Administrative Professionals Week
St. Patrick's Day	Rosh Hashanah
Cinco de Mayo	Yom Kipper
Retirement	Dates and dating
Promotions	Happy Hour
Bridal showers	More...

All of the above celebrations practically beg for sugar. Is it really a surprise that the United States is the fattest country on Earth? Is it a shock that kidney problems, i.e. diabetes, hypoglycemia, gout, fibromyalgia, etc., are spiraling out of control?

We have a reason to eat sugar every day. We have to use discipline not to.

48 Food vs. Poison / Drugs

Question: What is the difference between food and poison?

Answer: Freshness and cooking or distilling.
Now I will tell you the rest of the story. Later in this book I will explain the importance / need for raw food. I am now going to explain this in such a way that it will probably change your life.

The coca plant is very popular in South America and is used even today in religious rights.

Mate De Coca, sometimes called Coca Tea is made by slowly brewing coca leaves over a low flame. When made correctly it has the stimulant effect of strong coffee. It has been and remains a popular South American drink.

The tea can be made stronger (via longer brewing at higher temperature) for healing applications. In the heights of the Andes its leaves are not only consumed via liquid ingestion, the leaves are also chewed to release their benefits. So common is the tea derived from the Coca leaf (and its benefits) that guides working on the Trail of The Inca (on the way to Macchu Picchu) recommend it for mild altitude sickness.

In parts of South America, it is considered a wonder concoction. It is revered as almost magical in its attributes. Interestingly, with such a fantastic reputation, how can a derivative of this amazing leaf be considered the lynch pin of world drug addiction? How can one compound so useful be at the apex or pinnacle of the war on drugs?

The Coca Leaf, if processed long enough, becomes cocaine!! Cocaine may very well be the most feared drug on the planet. Coca leaves, if distilled long enough, become so dangerous they become a pure poison. If you were elected World Drug Czar, you would want to eliminate cocaine from production and use. But if you did, tens of millions of people worldwide would be out of work. This would be a worldwide catastrophe. Illegal drugs, drug addiction, drug enforcement and drug treatment is a trillion dollar a year business.

But back to our story about Coca leaves. If you were to travel to the Andes and participate in a ceremony that employed the chewing of Coca leaves, it wouldn't be long until you felt the effects of a medium stimulant. Locals exposed to the leaves more often would feel an effect similar to that of strong coffee or black tea. Now imagine that you, in your eagerness to fit into this new culture, went a little overboard and chewed a pound of Coca leaves. What would happen? Would you die, get sick? What would become of you and your high Andes leaf experience?

At worst you would get an upset stomach, vomit or get diarrhea as your body rejected this over use of the leaves. They are placed between the cheek and gums (in front) just like chewing tobacco. This may also be the origin of chewing tobacco, as tobacco was not native to Europe.

At the end of your Coca Leaf experience, you would be in a state of slight hyper stimulation or highly energized but not dead.

Balance that against the amount of cocaine you would need to create a fatal experience.

Perhaps a gram of cocaine will kill. Why? Because that gram of cocaine is cooked residue of perhaps 3000 leaves. Is it more understandable why drugs are fatal in small amounts?

All drugs follow this same path from something natural to something dangerous all due to the intense distillation process. A gram of cocaine powder can kill, verses pounds of the leaves that will not.

This process of distillation is repeated to a lesser extent on a daily basis in kitchens and restaurants all over the planet. Heat kills most organic life. The longer anything is cooked, the less it resembles food and the more it resembles a drug. This explains the medicinal affects of mom's chicken soup when it is slow cooked all day.

To get a feel of just how bad cooking in a microwave oven can be, feel free to look up the following test. Its results were placed on the Internet. The test was conducted with houseplants and can be easily replicated. Testing was conducted with identical houseplants over a one-month period.

The test: Two identical houseplants were given equal amounts of water at the same time on a daily basis.

One plant received water that was boiled on the stove and cooled and the other received water that was micro waved and then cooled.

After one month of the exact same care, the plant that received the micro waved water was dead. Does this mean the boiling of food or water is better? This test would have to be repeated and studied with tap, purified, spring, microwave and boiled water to be fully relevant. It nonetheless proves that microwaving is harmful.

It is generally accepted that microwaving alters the molecular structure of anything it is targeted at. Consequently, it should not be a surprise that micro waving anything should be avoided.

49 Deadly Carbohydrates and Your Body

For a datum to really be understood and be useful, it must be repeated. Reinforcing your belief that the standard American diet equals death is a tragic thing to have to do. Electronic media continues to brainwash you, the reader, every day. Because of that, this little book needs to roar like a lion to even be noticed. Help me beat the drum. If you don't, we all die a little bit.

Roger Bezanis

We are now going to consider the staple of the American diet, BREAD!

Bread and all processed carbohydrates, but especially bread, immediately swell in the stomach. It then starts breaking down into sugar. Temporary euphoria takes over as you begin to feel wired and finally you crash. Metabolism comes to a roaring stop the moment that sugar and yeast collide with your system. That is why the body swells, instantly feeling larger.

Swelling is why men loosen their belts after a meal with bread. If you were to measure your waistline on a Monday morning and then eat bread several times during the day and for dinner, you would notice that your waistline has expanded by 1-3 inches by Tuesday morning.

When the body's metabolism is shut down or slowed, it cannot flush out waste. This causes the body to become acidic, which leaves the body open to disease and bacteria. Reduced circulation, lack of oxygen and limited energy makes living in a body difficult. Burning Mouth Syndrome and indigestion until all hours of the morning is not uncommon. Eliminate processed carbohydrates and live a leaner, healthier life. Eliminating bread is one of the more easy vices to give up. When you do, you will be shocked by the results.

Indigestion and the Acid Pump

Time for another pack of lies served up to you by your wonderful AMA and advertisers, "You have acid indigestion and it is caused by too much acid production in your stomach."

This statement is an ABSOLUTE LIE!

If you acted on this statement, you would forever have indigestion as the statement is backwards. Lipitor commercials for high cholesterol are no different. High cholesterol is a product of an overwhelmed or poorly functioning liver. Yet in Lipitor commercials, they warn you not to take it if you have liver problems. Hundreds of thousands take it every day and get worse. Still Lipitor is being sold and will continue to be.

It is the equivalent of adding gasoline to a fire in an attempt to put it out. I am just doing back flips on that one.

Do you realize that over the counter antacid sales exceed 20 million dollars a week? Do you realize that too much acid in the stomach is not the problem but the opposite of what is really going on? Here are the facts. Your stomach produces a small amount of hydrochloric acid to help soften food so that it can be digested. When the food is like slurry (a watery mixture of insoluble matter, mud, etc.), it passes on to the small intestines. Food that is poorly chewed eventually enters the small intestines as well.

When we eat breads, pasta, pizza, crackers, cakes, cookies, popcorn, sweets, etc., we overwhelm the acid producers and our stomach is shut off. All of these foods convert to sugar and in doing so leave the stomach a compost bin. The result is the body signals you by giving you an acid indigestion symptom. This is just the stomach asking to be made acidic again.

The solution is not to desensitize the stomach or try to block acid production, but to turn it back on. Here are a couple of things you can do to facilitate this. Eat an orange or tangerine (the juice alone will not help); a lemon or other citrus can work as well. The enzymes in the pulp of the fruit work to switch back on the pumps and acid indigestion is instantly reduced.

Try this; you will be amazed at how well this works.

What Are You Putting in Your Mouth?

We all like to eat. It is one of those simple pleasures that have spun out of control. We can eat 24 hours a day and have anything we want. We have more choices than ever before. Yet we are eating less real food. We are surrounded by food yet we are starving. We diet constantly, but we are the fattest nation on earth.

Oh, and eating is fun too. Science has improved our lives to the extent that we can mix our breakfast in a glass and eat protein bars all day long. Welcome to the future. Welcome to the Star Trek world of nutrition. Progress via science has really improved our lives. How did we ever get along without instant orange flavored drink, chicken nuggets, gummy bears, hot chocolate, self-heating soup cans and coffee? We all need microwave popcorn and frozen food. Don't we?

Clearly, we were in dietary hell before science came to our rescue and saved our lives, right?

Not even close. Look it up. You will see that the fattening of America continues. Some of our foods are closer to being plastic than food.

Do you realize that imitation crab is not actually a fish at all? It does not swim. It is closer to rubber than fish. Grab a bag and look at it. Read the ingredients: Sugar, sorbitol, meat or tapioca starch, egg whites, and vegetable or soybean oil. Natural and artificial crab flavorings are added. Carmine, caramel, paprika, and annatto extract are often used to make the crab's red, orange, or pink coloring.

There you are, eating imitation crab and trying to lose weight and you can't figure out why the weight is not coming off. It is not coming off because this imitation crab is not just imitation crab it is imitation food. Eating imitation crab is like chewing on filet of tennis shoe sole. Mmm,

mmm, mmm, "gotta get me some of that."

Eating rubber fish, what could be better? How about chicken nuggets? That is clearly better! Why? How? Well, they're actually chicken! But it is special chicken, very special chicken, made up of all types of chicken. And it is all mechanically separated from the bone. In other words, ground up, then mixed with, you guessed it, artificial ingredients and then PRESSED into the cute little fun-to-eat-shapes.

Then what do we do? We smother all of these delicious chicken-like bites in barbeque, honey mustard, or ranch sauce, with the main ingredient, you guessed it again, SUGAR.

I really want this book to sell, so I am going to coat the pages with sugar. Not only will this book sell because you can read it, it will sell because you will eat it before you finish reading it. Ha! When the book is gone you will have to buy another one! And another one!

Then I can advertise on Nickelodeon and show happy kids eating my book. I could be bigger than Dr. Seuss! Unsuspecting kids will love me!

I will be #1 on the New York Times Best Seller list and no one will actually be reading my book! The public will eat me right to the top. Sugar is a wonderful thing!

Why have they not invented Sugar-Salt? That way it will soothe all parts of the palate at the same time! Go ahead, tear out a page of this book and eat it.

I assure you this book is made of sugar! Just lick the page and you will see.

I am just joking.

Consider this: a body consuming sugar will have numerous symptoms including tendonitis.

50 Tendonitis, Bursitis and Arthritis

No doubt you have guessed by now that tendonitis is just a name an AMA researcher invented one day in the hopes of selling drugs and surgery.

Whenever an expert is presented with confusion, they must by definition of "who they say they are", come up with an answer. The honest response of "I don't have any idea" somehow sounds too unprofessional. Such is the case with tendonitis, bursitis and arthritis ("**the itises**"). With what you know right now in reading this book, you can discern more than the expert. You recognize that **"the itises"** are a kidney symptom, liver symptom or combination of both.

This is not to say that pulled muscles, torn muscles, strains, ragged ligaments and frayed tendons don't happen. They do, but what facilitated the pull or strain was a dirty filthy street that forced the back up of our Uric Acid Trash Trucks. All of this is due to overwhelmed kidneys. The fact that healing takes so long is also due to kidney weakness. Damage in a body with healthy kidneys heals at a sensibly fast rate. Filthy systems often never heal completely.

Because of this waste, all healing processes are slowed and injuries don't heal satisfactorily. In the end, a slight sprain, which should hurt a day or two, becomes a chronic problem due to constant stimuli of uric acid or lactic acid lingering in the area.

There is zero difference in how the body approaches Arthritis. It – **"the itises"** – is just an irritated joint due to waste accumulation. Arthritis does not exist. Corroded joints exist but arthritis is just a name for "I have no idea." Perhaps they slap a pseudo prefix on the symptom and call it "inflammatory arthritis" which equals "it hurts and there is swelling."

The CDC (Center for Disease Control) reports on their website that:

 1998: Doctors told 33 million patients that they had some form of arthritis, osteoarthritis, rheumatoid arthritis, gout or lupus.

 2005: Doctors told 46 million patients that they had some form of arthritis, osteoarthritis, rheumatoid arthritis, gout or lupus.

 They project that in 2030, Doctors will tell 67 million patients that they have some form of arthritis, osteoarthritis, rheumatoid arthritis, gout or lupus.

What is going on here? We are eating / poisoning our kidneys into failure. Diabetes statistics (another kidney issue) show the same trends.

Overworked kidneys cannot catch up. Therefore you are in pain. If you have concluded that you should not feel sore or stiff very long, you are right.

This is the simplicity of the body that I am continually speaking of. The attitude in the world today and for centuries to come will be to mask the symptom. This book and you can have a major affect in changing the minds of those in power that promote such archaic thinking.

Big business and Wall Street advertisers are not interested in this book. They want to sell you pain relievers. Sore backs equal big bucks. Pulled muscles equal bonuses and big houses. You do not have to buy into what the Wall Street advertisers are saying. They are making big money (billions) and they of course do not want to give that up.

Billions of dollars are sunk into arthritis research, a diabetes cure, etc. Because we are looking for a culprit outside of ourselves, nothing will change. You can change. But until you change, big Pharmaceuticals will keep doing business as usual.

The therapy is as simple as changing what you put in your mouth.

The culprit is what you sweeten your tea, cereal and muffins with. Including your coffee (a known diuretic) and all of those colorings, dyes, drugs, chemicals and preservatives that enter in our faux food supply. Lack of water, protein overload, poor diet, deficient sleep and 24/7 life styles can all cause these chronic problems.

It will take time, but you can master these issues and change your life.

In essence, when your kidneys are functioning at top capacity, you will notice the following body traits:

1)   Better flexibility with little stiffness.
2)   Better strength.
3)   Better endurance in all exercise.
4)   Faster recovery time after workouts.
5)   Resistance to pulled muscles.
6)   Better sex drive.
7)   Better sexual performance.
8)   Better reproductive performance.
9)   Better heart function.
10) Better balance or equilibrium.
11) Corrected blood pressure; if it is high or low it will correct.
12) Better afternoon and early evening energy.
13) Better sleep.
14) Better lymphatic system function.
15) Better bladder function.
16) Little if any cramping or soreness of any type.
17) Freedom of diabetic symptoms.
18) Freedom from Gout symptoms
19) Freedom from arthritis-like symptoms

With use and understanding of this book, you place yourself firmly in the driver's seat in your life. You are in charge of your own health care. Use this book and teach those around you.

51 Drought and the Extinction of Man

Man is being pursued by monster of such proportion that in less than 15 years all of the major population centers of the planet could disappear. Half the Earth's population could be wiped out.

We are aware of the accepted troubles of Earth such as rain forest defoliation and the diminishing ozone layer. This problem is so infinite that it affects those problems and makes them worse. Even the Polar ice cap decay is made small by the magnitude of this issue.

What is it? Water. It is no longer a plentiful resource. In fact it is no longer a resource at all. Water is a collectable at best. In the 1979 Mel Gibson movie, Mad Max, a world was imagined without gasoline. The fact is that a world without drinking water is far closer at hand.

When the day comes that water is rationed worldwide, health will no longer be of paramount concern. Daily survival based on getting the bare minimum of water will be the only concern. "What," you say? Balderdash! Earth is covered in water. We have water everywhere and on top of it all it rains and replenishes the supply. This is a half truth. Ocean water cannot be desalinized quickly enough to keep up with demand. Desalinization is running approximately 50 years behind our needs IF OUR NEEDS DO NOT INCREASE beyond the standards of today.

Therefore water is a mirage as what is available is not drinkable and what comes out of our rainy season is too infinitesimal to keep up with our demand. California and to a large part the entire planet is experiencing a severe drought.

Mandatory water rationing is on the very near horizon.

Unless you live in a third world country, you are used to turning on your faucet and seeing water pour out. We are spoiled by this expected life giving result. Whenever we want water it is there. It is always there. Most of you reading this have a bottle of water within easy reach. The fact is that drinkable or potable water is a rare commodity and this endangers mankind. Water is critical to life. Every system of our body must have water to operate. Only oxygen is more important than water to sustaining life. Yet water is quietly disappearing and there is no way to replace it fast enough.

The following are headlines from around the world:

- WORLD WATER FORUM DISPERSES POLICIES, PEOPLE IN TURKEY FEAR THE WORST
- SOUTHERN ETHIOPIA'S STRUGGLE FOR WATER GRIM
- DRY RESERVOIR LEAVES TAMPA FLORIDA ONE DAY OF WATER

Roger Bezanis

- SAUDI ARABIA TO JOIN BAHRAIN IN DRIVE FOR DESALINATION
- SAN DIEGO CALIFORNIA FACED WITH MANDATORY WATER RATIONING
- ATLANTA WATER RESERVES RUNNING OUT QUICKLY
- HOOVER DAM WATER LEVELS BELOW CRISIS LEVEL

DROUGHT FACTS

884 MILLION PEOPLE LACK ACCESS TO SAFE WATER SUPPLIES, APPROXIMATELY ONE IN EIGHT PEOPLE.

AT ANY GIVEN TIME, HALF OF THE WORLD'S HOSPITAL BEDS ARE OCCUPIED BY PATIENTS SUFFERING FROM A WATER-RELATED DISEASE.

THE MOST RELIABLE AND WIDELY-ACCEPTED WATER ESTIMATE TO PRODUCE A POUND OF BEEF IS THE FIGURE OF 2,500 GALLONS/POUND.

NEWSWEEK PUT IT ANOTHER WAY: "THE WATER THAT GOES INTO A 1,000 POUND STEER WOULD FLOAT A DESTROYER."

LESS THAN 1% OF THE WORLD'S FRESH WATER (OR ABOUT 0.007% OF ALL WATER ON EARTH) IS READILY ACCESSIBLE FOR DIRECT HUMAN USE.

AN AMERICAN TAKING A FIVE-MINUTE SHOWER USES MORE WATER THAN THE TYPICAL PERSON LIVING IN A DEVELOPING COUNTRY USES IN A WHOLE DAY.

POOR PEOPLE OFTEN PAY 5-10 TIMES MORE PER LITER OF WATER THAN WEALTHY PEOPLE LIVING IN THE SAME CITY.

WITHOUT FOOD A PERSON CAN LIVE FOR WEEKS, BUT WITHOUT WATER YOU CAN EXPECT TO LIVE ONLY A FEW DAYS.

THE DAILY REQUIREMENT FOR SANITATION, BATHING, AND COOKING NEEDS, AS WELL AS FOR ASSURING SURVIVAL, IS ABOUT 13.2 GALLONS PER PERSON.

The fact is that we as a planet are in a deepening hole regarding water. Los Angeles California is one of the largest cities in the world. It is built on a desert. It may become a ghost town in less than 10 years if the water table is not corrected. The date of this writing is 20 March 2009; by 2019 Los Angeles could be a memory unless something is done now.

This means that 18 million people will be displaced. Imagine 18 million refugees fleeing a city with nowhere to go. This is a real life-threatening danger. When the last drop flows out of Los Angeles, the city could become a dust bowl in just a few months time.

Lack of water is not just a California problem. It affects the entire country and the entire world without question. Where populations are densest the problems are the largest. It is that simple. Los Angeles not only faces water shortages but electricity shortages based on water shortages. One facility is the back bone of three states. This is an untenable environment that is teetering on collapse.

Hoover Dam produces the following quantities of water:

28.5393% Metropolitan Water District of Southern California
23.3706% The state of Nevada
18.9527% The state of Arizona
15.4429% Goes to Los Angeles

The Metropolitan Water District of Southern California supplies water to Los Angeles, Orange, San Diego, Riverside, San Bernadino and Ventura counties.

Hoover Dam Generated Electricity is Dispensed at These Levels:

5.5377% Southern California Edison Company

Nevada and other California cities use approximately 6.5% of Hoover Dam's energy output not included above. As you can see, one facility has a huge impact on very large population bases. Without help and a backup plan, these cities, counties and states are in jeopardy.

Hoover dam water levels are running precariously low. With no water to turn the generators to create power, there is no electricity produced. This is a worldwide problem. The above numbers only focus on three states affected by one facility. Every city on the Earth is facing the same kinds of problems.The solution is conservation and long term desalinization. Desalinization (cleaning ocean water) is 50 years away from being viable. Conservation works today and makes it possible for man to survive.

Americans and to a great extent the world believe that once they purchase an item it is there's to waste if they so chose. That is true a statement; ownership does have its privileges.

In regards to water, when this commodity is wasted, it is shortening mans' possible life span on Earth.

Roger Bezanis

Steps you can take to save water:

- Install a shower-minding water device that shortens shower times
- Install the new water saving dish washer
- Put in a water saving washing machine that saves hundreds of gallons a month
- Install an instant water turn off on all faucets in the house
- Install an ultra low flow toilet
- Install instant water shut off sprinkler heads that activate to prevent geysers
- Only eat at restaurants that use a "waterless" dish rinsing machine
- Replace seldom used lawns with a waterless substitute
- Shower devices save between 5-10 gallons per shower
- Instant water turn off faucets save 90% on shaving, 90% on brushing teeth, 100% on dripping faucets and 60% on washing hands.
- Industrial "Waterless" dish washing machines saves 1000's of gallons of water per restaurant, per week.
- Auto sprinkler shutoff devices do not allow a broken sprinkler to run unchecked for hours until it can be capped. These devices immediately shut down as water starts to flow unrestricted. The water pressure itself seals the sprinkler shut, stopping water loss cold.

These technologies and devices exist and work famously. To not understand and utilize them is paramount to treason against mankind.

Please go online and look up the websites below. These companies are acknowledged by the EPA as water saving leaders. You will also notice that I have included the EPA's own website. I encourage you to read their site and become a partner in saving water.

If you want to install the best water saving products, these are the sources to check:

www.waterconservationtechnology.com
http://buywatersense.com
http://www.epa.gov/watersense/pp/index.htm

Saving water saves the planet. Without water man will disappear from the face of the Earth. That is not a threat, it is a fact. No resource is more critical less oxygen. Every day the inhabitants of Earth steadily increase in population. Yet our ability to increase production of drinkable water is at a standstill. Every day we fall further behind. Today we stand 50 years behind need. Every day that number is growing as our supply dwindles.

These are not hard solutions to implement. Racing to put these simple solutions to work changes the outcome of this horrible situation. The consequences of failure are grim, therefore failure is not an option.

In the race for water every moment counts. Under your very noses there is a crisis of such immense proportion that it could wipe out more than half the Earth's population. Much of Earth's surface would be left a barren wasteland.

The time to act is now before you are too thirsty to act at all.

Please be a friend to Earth.

Your Friend,
Roger Bezanis

52 Food Additives: the same old poison

Many people are aware that Monosodium Glutamate (MSG) is toxic to the body and that many manufacturers of processed foods restrict its use. We see signs in the windows of restaurants and are thrilled that they say "NO MSG."

In the next few pages you will discover the ugly truth about this ubiquitous little ingredient. Most people in "developed" countries consume it every day and do not realize it. First patented in 1909, Monosodium Glutamate was produced in Japan and China. By the 1930's, Japan was creating ten million pounds yearly to add to its food supply. In 1948 it entered the American food supply. Its current popularity in fast food and canned products demonstrates just how pervasive this addictive substance has become.

The FDA itself, in a report dated August 31, 1995, stated that:
"Studies have shown that the body uses Glutamate, an amino acid, as a nerve impulse transmitter in the brain and that there are Glutamate-responsive tissues in other parts of the body, as well. Abnormal function of Glutamate receptors has been linked with certain neurological diseases, such as Alzheimer's disease and Huntington's chorea. Injections of Glutamate in laboratory animals have resulted in damage to nerve cells in the brain."

MSG is still being used. It is now autographed under numerous other names to hide its presence. Some of the well known yet safe "sounding" names for MSG include:

Monopotassium Glutamate
Hydrolyzed Protein
Hydrolyzed Vegetable Protein (HVP)

Calcium Caseinate
Yeast Food
Gelatin
Yeast Extract
Glutamic Acid
Sodium Caseinate
Hydrolyzed Corn Gluten
Textured Protein
Autolyzed Yeast

MSG radically affects the kidneys and creates Hyperinsulinemia which means large amounts of insulin are floating free in the blood. Abundant insulin in the blood is often present in "Type 2 Diabetes," which is a severe kidney condition.

In 1992, the FDA asked the Federation of American Societies for Experimental Biology (FASEB) to review the available data on MSG and make a report about the findings. In the 350 page FASEB report, the Federation concluded that an "Unknown percentage of the population may react to MSG and develop MSG symptom complex," a condition characterized by one or more of the following symptoms:

- burning sensation in the back of the neck, forearms and chest
- numbness in the back of the neck, radiating to the arms and back
- tingling, warmth and weakness in the face, temples, upper back, neck and arms
- facial pressure or tightness
- chest pain
- headache
- nausea
- rapid heartbeat
- bronchia spasm (difficulty breathing) in MSG-intolerant people with asthma
- drowsiness
- weakness

If these researchers were trained in my techniques of instant symptom analysis they would have noticed the same symptoms in seconds of exposure.

Again from the FDA – "These people, in addition to being prone to MSG symptom complex, may suffer temporary worsening of asthmatic symptoms after consuming MSG. The MSG dosage that produced reactions in these people ranged from 0.5 grams to 2.5 grams. A reaction is most likely if the MSG is eaten in a large quantity or in a liquid, such as a clear soup." MSG is also an incredibly addictive substance and to a great degree explains why junk food, which is loaded with MSG, is so addicting.

The following is a list similar to the list found in my chapter on salt and sodium. Foods that are rich in added sodium or salt are always rich in MSG in one form or another.

Potato Chips	Hot dogs	Sausage
Bologna	Nachos	Crackers
Dried Soup Mix	Canned Soup	Canned Pastas
Canned Chili	Flavored Noodles	Vegetable Juice
Canned Meats	Most Salad Dressings	Frozen Cured Meats
Frozen Vegetables	Frozen dinners	Gravy
Seasoning Mix	Cheese puffs	All types of jerky
Soy Sauce	Ice Cream	Sour Cream
Bouillon Cubes	Pasta Helpers	Seasoned Rice

"Since research indicates that the MSG is so pervasive and toxic at every level it is even linked to ADHD." As per his book "The Slow Poisoning of America" by John Erb (page 85):

Globally there are 1.5 million tons of MSG produced annually. Some Americans eat as much as four pounds of MSG laced foods a day. If MSG is given to dogs, the results can be unconsciousness, convulsions and eventually death.

You might remember the "Cheeseburger Act." G. W. Bush and his corporate supporters worked to push through a bill called the "Personal Responsibility in Food Consumption Act." Also known as the "Cheeseburger Bill", this sweeping law banned anyone from suing food manufacturers, sellers and distributors. Yes, the "Cheeseburger Bill" passed and was signed into law. You now cannot sue Jack in the Box for making you fat.

Reported by the BBC Friday, 12 March, 2004 — The study found that poor diet and lack of exercise caused 400,000 deaths in the US in the year 2000 — 33% jump since 1990.

Clearly the fast food industry is out to make a buck and as long as we keep buying they will stay in the junk supply business. The fact that MSG is addicting is a nolo contendere for the purveyors of poison.

The fast food business has now gotten away with stonewalling the public. You have little recourse other than to go on your merry way and stop complaining to them. They now do not have to listen. IT IS THE LAW. Without you to worry about, it is now business as usual.

FLUORIDE POISON

Dental Fluorosis is a health condition caused by an overdose of fluoride. In its severe form it is characterized by black and brown stains, as well as cracking and pitting of the teeth.

Fluoride stimulates abnormal bone development.

Clinical trials published in the New England Journal of Medicine and Journal of Bone and Mineral Research report that:

"High dose fluoride treatment increases bone mass but that the newly formed bone is 'structurally unsound'. Thus, instead of reducing hip fracture, the studies found that high doses of fluoride increase hip fracture."

Taylor Study, University of Austin: "Fluoride concentration of 1 PPM (parts per million) increases tumor growth rate by 25%" (this is the concentration used in the USA).

Clinical Toxicology of Commercial Products 1984: "Fluoride is more poisonous than lead and just less poisonous than arsenic."

Procter & Gamble, quoted in "Fluoride the Ageing Factor": "A seven ounce tube of toothpaste, theoretically at least, contains enough fluoride to kill a small child."
Dr. Limeback 1992, Canadian Dental Association Proposed Fluoride Guidelines,

"Fluoride supplements should not be given to children under three years old"

"Fluoride accelerates your ageing process." "Fluoride mineralizes the tendons, muscles and ligaments, making them crackly and painful and inflexible. At the same time fluoride interferes with mineralization of bones and teeth, causing osteoporosis and mottling or dental fluorosis." The process whereby teeth are discolored and crumble from fluoridation is known as dental fluorosis.

The US Public Health service has known since the research of its own Dr. HT Dean in 1937 that as fluoride levels rose, so did the percentage of children with dental fluorosis. This data was compiled following subjects in 15 major American cities.

The FDA (US Food and Drug Administration) requires all toothpaste manufacturers to print a warning on the label that, if more than a pea-sized amount of toothpaste is swallowed, the local Poison Control Centre should be notified.

The American Dental Association and other defenders of fluoride have testified and continue to insist that dental fluoride is a "cosmetic condition" and is not a health issue!

Dr. Yiamouyiannis cites the 1990 study of 541,000 cases of osteoporosis that found a definite connection between hip fractures in women over 65 and fluoride levels. The study was written up in JAMA (Journal of American Medicine Association). Several other major studies are cited with massive amounts of research, again all reaching the same conclusion.

Fluoride causes osteoporosis by creating a calcium deficiency situation. Fluoride precipitates calcium out of solution, causing low blood calcium, as well as the build-up of calcium stones and crystals in the joints and organs.

Dozens of other studies, like the Riggs study in the 1990 New England Journal of Medicine, showed that fluoride treatment of osteoporosis in the elderly actually increases skeletal fragility, i.e., more fractures. It's the same mechanism at work: incorrect mineralization, as we saw above. Thin old bones lose calcium; young bones age too rapidly by over-mineralization.

The above is what the study found but in actual fact fluoride does not rob calcium. It robs and weakens the magnesium in the bone that then makes the bones brittle.

Austrian and Japanese researchers both found that, "A concentration of 1 PPM fluoride causes disruption of the body's ability to repair its own DNA. Without this most basic cell function, cancer is promoted, and tumor growth is accelerated."

The unmistakable fact is that for the years 1940-1950, when none of 20 cities studied were fluoridated, the average cancer deaths were virtually identical. But after 1950, there is a major increase in cancer deaths in every single one of the fluoridated cities, while the non-fluoridated cities remain clustered together at a much lower level of death.

DEATHS DUE TO FLUORIDE PER YEAR

From Robert Sterling who wrote "Fluoridation Fraud": "...30,000 to 50,000 deaths each year from various causes may now be attributable to fluoridation. This total includes 10,000 to 20,000 deaths attributable to fluoride-induced cancer every year."

The dental community concedes that fluoride is ineffective at preventing the most common type of dental decay—pit & fissures. Pit & fissure decay—which is the decay found in the crevices of the chewing surfaces - accounts for upwards of 85% of dental decay now experienced in the US.

New evidence suggests that fluoridation is either unnecessary or doesn't work. Cavities have declined at similarly impressive rates throughout the entire western industrialized world over the past half-century.

This decline has occurred irrespective of a country's fluoridation status. Western Europe, which is less fluoridated than the US, has experienced the SAME decline in cavities as the heavily fluoridated US, and today enjoys the SAME low level of tooth decay.

Five peer-reviewed studies published in early 2006 have found that:

"Dental decay DOES NOT increase when communities stop fluoridation."

"High levels of naturally occurring fluoride causes a crippling bone disease known as skeletal fluorosis." According to UNICEF, skeletal fluorosis is endemic "in at least 25 countries across the globe" with the problem particularly acute in India, China and other developing countries.

Skeletal fluorosis comes in varying degrees of severity depending on the level of exposure. The earliest symptoms are characterized by joint pain that is difficult, if not impossible, to distinguish from arthritis.

If your local water agency is allowing the use of fluoride, your only options are:

1) Only drink bottled water or use a powerful filter that will exclude fluoride (not a small table top filter). Reverse Osmosis water filters are considered the best.

2) Never use tap water for anything except washing dishes.

3) Get a good shower filter.

4) Change your toothpaste if it contains fluoride.

The only filter that will take all fluoride and aluminum out of drinking water is a reverse osmosis unit. They range in cost depending on the replacement cartridges. Some companies sell their reverse osmosis treated waters on the mass market at your local grocery and liquor stores. At this writing they are Aquafina and Déjà Blue, but there may be others.

The second most effective filter is the human body. Half the fluoride you consume will be broken down IF YOUR SYSTEM IS CLEAN AND NOT TOXIC.

Therefore it is recommended to do a good body and colon cleanse once a year. Keep a close eye on the liver and kidney function as they must be in good working order twenty four hours a day.

By no means am I encouraging the intake of fluoride for any reason. Fluoride is a toxin and must be avoided at all costs.

To remain healthy it is always advisable to clean the system routinely either by diet, herbal cleansing, exercise or any combination of the three.

Your Friend,
Roger Bezanis

53 Dangers of Salt and Sodium

Salt and sodium are more insidious than sugar, as we never expect them to be so undermining to our health. Practically all-manmade food is a mix of sugar and salt and sodium. The reason, as "food / taste engineers" will tell you, is taste. Sugar is acidy on the PH scale, whereas salt is alkaline on the PH scale. Any chef will tell you that pleasing the palette is about balancing salt and sugar, as they are the most powerful sensors on the tongue.

Interestingly, sugar is the hardest of the trio to give up, as it is the most addictive substance on the planet based on sheer numbers. You do not know anyone who is not addicted to sugar. Even if we have given sugar up, we will always be addicted to it. Diabetes numbers prove this as its incidents climb steadily higher every day. Being an exaggerated or extreme kidney condition, this should not be surprising to anyone. Contact with any one of the three will produce the list of problems below:

A) Water retention

B) Increased or high blood pressure

C) Accelerated heart rate

D) Low back pain, muscle pain and joint pain

If you do the above, you will naturally eliminate all processed carbohydrates from your life. Yes, you are going to have to eliminate the terrible JUNK FOOD MONSTER as well. What makes up junk food? Junk food is basically a slang term for food with limited nutritional value, also known as empty calories. If you look on the label of some "so called food," you will see a chemistry lab concatenation of ingredients including:

Sugar	Corn sweetener
Sucrose	Maltose
Dextrose	Lactose
Honey	Glucose
Fructose	Molasses
Corn syrup	Brown sugar
High fructose corn syrup	

Many of these ingredients are listed as the first 5 ingredients on the label. What is the common denominator in all of these? S-U-G-A-R!

Sugar is wildly addicting, and junk food makers, knowing this, feed it to you by the tablespoon full. FDA Food label law requires ingredients to be listed in descending order of amount used. The first item on the list is the most prevalent down to the least prevalent on the bottom of the list.

Pay attention to the amount of saturated fat, unsaturated fat, hydrogenated oils, peanut oil, soy oil, and olive oil and canola oil. These processed oils are some of the worst things you can put into your body.

A few more words about bread:

If you want to see an immediate change in your weight, give up breads of all types, crackers, rice, grains of all types, pastry, cookies, doughnuts, muffins, pizza, pasta and rolls. If you cannot quite grasp this, just ask yourself, "If I planted_____ (fill in the blank) in the ground, would it grow?" If the answer is no, then you should not eat it.

"This week's topic is bread, a supposedly harmless subject, and a supposedly innocuous food item that we partake as food almost religiously two to four times a day. Bread, a supposedly harmless food, that when consumption is stopped, detoxification begins. It is common for people to experience severe cravings for refined grain products and often binge on them. There are more words of acute understanding that undermine the necessity of bread. There are more words that deplore why bread is so anti-health and its many implications when eaten. When starches are consumed, people wake up the next day and go through unpleasant periods of feeling foggy, hung-over, or sedated - Grain Damage by Douglas N. Graham, D.C.

The information on bread is nothing new, it just has been conveniently ignored. Man has been making bread for thousands of years. Well documented in ancient Egypt, common workers were given bread and beer (derived from yeast) as the centerpiece of the Nile diet.

Prior to settling in Egypt, nomadic ancient man ate a diet richer in protein as planting and harvesting was not an option. Farming and tending the land is a natural development of putting down roots. Ensuring survival requires life to adapt to the changing environment or go extinct. Whereas animals are forced to adapt to an evolving planet, man alters the planet to his needs. No water? Start building a canal. Perhaps a large mountain is in your way obstructing your view? Dynamite a way through. No rain? Start cloud seeding.

Moving away from a powerful nomadic hunter-gatherer to a more tranquil cultivation and domesticated lifestyle spelled mutation for man. Egyptians settling on the Nile 5200 years ago developed written language, monoliths, shipping and religion; they cultivated crops, created bread and ate grains. Because of the sugar conversion from grains and breads, for the first time in the archeological record, man developed chronic physical problems.

Tooth decay became rampant, malignant cancers appeared while he was losing inches off his height. His lifespan was noticeably shorter, his skull brittle and his brain tumors grew. Was Neanderthal man really as superior a being as his tremendous stature and physical strength would indicate? How did a smaller, weaker, sugar-craving smarter human oust this pre-historic superman? We may never know, as the Neanderthal gentleman is no longer here to defend his choices.

Summation: Man mutated or evolved in response to his dietary choices and lifestyle developments.

Consider the following:

"The milling of wheat destroys 40% of the chromium, 86% of the cobalt, 68% of the copper, 78% of the zinc, and 48% of the molybdenum. By the time it is completely refined it has lost most of its phosphorus, iron and riboflavin, as well most fiber. Wheat flour has been plundered of most of its vitamin E, important oils and amino acids. White bread also turns to glucose as quick as white sugar (This is the staple diet of the majority)."
– Klenner, Southern Medicine & Surgery. April 1951.

"It (sugar) ought to be against the law - and white bread also."
- Dr Kelley DDS, Sunday afternoon, November 7, 1971.

In simple terms, milling insults the kernel of grain via the grinding process. Milling grinds these kernels to a fine powder that is then renamed flour. Why is milling so horrific to all grain? Because once a kernel of wheat is broken and the germ or enzyme exposed, it is now no longer alive and thus bio-unavailable to the human body.

The germ or enzyme is nature's way of un-stressing the digestion of the body. It serves a dual purpose of pushing forth future generations of wheat stalk by carrying the genetic code necessary to sprout. Planting a scoop of even the best flour under the finest conditions will produce a yield of absolutely nothing.

Flour is dead in all forms. Planting a whole and complete wheat kernel produces wheat. Planting flour results in zero = dead substance.

Therefore, what is cracked wheat bread or whole wheat bread? A sales pitch, strictly a sales pitch. Cracked wheat is dead on grinding and then cooked to be certain of its destruction. Not to mention whole wheat bread has not one bit of whole wheat in it. If you were actually eating whole wheat, you would be gnawing on a stalk of wheat.

All foods carry enzymes prior to processing (as stated before).

Take a raw piece of steak and cook it "well done." Leaving it on your kitchen table for 6 months would produce a hard piece of leather. Natural drying out guarantees this expected affect.

Raw steak, if placed on your kitchen table for 6 months produces dust as it slowly disintegrates. The active enzymes assure this result.

Why does this happen? In raw food, enzymes are as vigorously energetic as nature intended. They are actively degrading tissue for later fertilization and seeding of the planet. To be sure, enzymes guarantee future generations and healthy soil. What happens to apples when they fall off a tree, if left alone? They rot (this is enzyme action) as the result of a robust ecosystem in action. Ignoring natural law and building an environment to meet his whims has poisoned man.

Enter big business as supported by your government. Here are your friendly U.S. Government food pyramid recommendations from 2003,

Per day serving suggestions are to eat:

6-11 BREAD (dead), CEREAL (dead), RICE (dead), and PASTA (dead)

3-5 servings of vegetables (lots of vitamins)

2-4 servings of fruit (sweet and good for you, also lots of vitamins)

2-3 servings of milk (source of calcium)

2-3 servings of meat, fish (source of protein and iron)

After scanning the above five points, if you can't see a connection to who is making "contributions" and is receiving favors from our government, then you are not looking hard enough.

Someone apparently has a vested interest in you staying fat, as the commerce of this country is dependent on what you eat.

If you followed the above guidelines, you would blow up like a balloon.

Addicting breads/ground grains and flours are "food-like" substances and must be eliminated from your life for you to achieve any kind of success commencing any diet. Processed carbohydrates are also known as simple carbohydrates. Simple carbohydrates quickly turn to addicting sugar in the system and then store as fat.

Complex carbohydrates such as tomatoes, oranges, grapes, onions, broccoli, apples, etc., contain natural sugar that is digested yet does nothing to contribute to "sugar poisoning." They convert from sugar to usable components in the body. The reason is because the enzymes contained in the fruit allow the body to utilize the sugars as fuel.

Manmade sugar-based carbohydrates are empty shells of energy, behind which there is nothing but vacant calories. Processed carbohydrates are guaranteed to become fat in the body. Bread is so free of any nutritional value, the makers embolden it with vitamins and minerals as a matter of course. Even with this bolstering, bread is still noticeably barely north of ingested cardboard.

Survive Better, Cut out the following:

White Bread	Tabouleh	Cake
Whole Wheat Bread	Pasta	Protein Bars
Squaw Bread	All cereals	Food Bars
Pumpernickel Bread	Oatmeal	Potato Chips
Unleavened Bread	Shredded Wheat	Corn Chips
Rice (white and brown)	Crackers	Pork Rinds
Kasha	Cookies	Puffed Rice

If you cut out just the list above you will feel a difference.

The above 21 items are just the beginning. If you are starting to think with the content of this book, then you are aware that cutting out the processed carbohydrates is not enough to fully change the lines of your body. Cooking food kills or destroys enzymes.
Therefore, the more raw food you eat, the better you will feel.

What to eat, FRESH OR RAW

Tomatoes	Squash	Potatoes
Onions	Cilantro	Hot peppers
Cabbage	Cucumbers (not pickles)	Pumpkins
Lettuce	Sprouts	Turnip greens
Spinach	Garlic	Turnips
Broccoli	Beets	Green Bell Peppers
Cauliflower	Kale	(not yellow or red)
Asparagus	Green beans	Fish / sushi
Radishes	Eggplant	(not cooked or seared)
Celery	Mustard greens	Steak Tartare
Zucchini	Okra	(not cooked or seared)

More on the Pursuit of Perfection

We all like to eat. The time of the day when you eat matters as much as what you eat. Family dinners and restaurants are the result of the socialization of man. However, eating at night is a sure way to add weight to your frame. If you only ate fresh fruit and/or vegetables after 4:00 p.m., you would soon see the scale registering a smaller you.

Successfully modifying the above paragraph would include eating only one type of vegetable or fruit after 4:00 p.m. This approach takes the stress off the digestive tract. In other words, you can sit down and eat all grapes for instance, but nothing else (not including water).

You can have melons if that is all you are having. Do not eat bananas at night as they are too heavy and can add bulk. Do consume: Strawberries, Grapes, Melons, Apples, Oranges, Tangerines, Tangelos, Guavas, Lemons, Cherries, Gooseberries, Mangos, Papayas, Pineapples, Tamarind, Kiwi fruit, Loquats, Passion fruit, Persimmons, Pomegranate and Tamarillo.

Something to Consider Regarding Raw Food

In the last one hundred years, there have been many movements regarding eating. Fad diets come and go with very little actual clinical study behind them. That is completely untrue when it comes to the eating of raw food.

Between the years of 1932 and 1942, Dr. Francis Marion Pottenger, Jr. of Monrovia, California (author of "Pottenger's Cats") conducted experiments on cats to determine the potency of standardized biological extracts. Because there were no extant chemical procedures for standardizing biological solutions, manufacturers of such derivatives had to use animals to determine their effectiveness.

He studied the adrenal glands removed from the cats, as they would harbor the remnants of the extracts being assayed. The decade long cat study demonstrated something odd and very alarming. The rate of mortality for cats receiving adrenalectomies (adrenal gland removal and dissection) was staggering. Clearly there was a relationship to diet and mortality.

To ensure the best possible health of his test cats, Pottenger fed them a diet of market grade raw milk: cod liver oil and cooked meat scraps from the sanitarium. These scraps included the liver, tripe, sweetbreads, brains, heart and muscle. This diet was considered to be rich in all the important nutritive substances by the experts of the day, and the surgical technique used for the adrenalectomies was the most exacting known. Yet, these cats were undergoing severe biological changes.

Why were these cats such poor patients? Why were they dying from procedures that should not have been fatal? In seeking an explanation, he began noticing that his cat specimens were showing signs of deficiency. All showed a decrease in their reproductive capacity and many of the kittens born in the laboratory had skeletal deformities and organ malfunctions.

As he added more and more cats to his experiments, eventually his supply of cooked meat scraps exceeded demand and he was forced to start using raw meat from a local meat packing company in Monrovia. These raw meat scraps were fed to a segregated group of cats each day.

The raw meat fed to the cats was composed of the viscera (1: an internal organ of the body; especially: one (as the heart, liver, or intestine) located in the great cavity of the trunk proper. 2 plural: HEART), muscle and bone.

Within a few months, Dr. Pottenger started to notice that the raw meat group appeared in better health than the animals being fed cooked meat scraps. Their kittens appeared more vigorous, and most interestingly, their operative mortality decreased markedly.

In contrast, the health of the cats fed cooked meat kept declining. The comparison was startling, yet they were polar opposites. The cats were beginning to reverse. It prompted Pottenger to undertake a controlled experiment to observe exactly what was happening. He wanted to find answers to such questions as: Why did the cats eating raw meat survive their operations more readily than those eating cooked meat? Why did the kittens of the raw meat fed cats appear more vigorous?

Why did a diet based on cooked meat scraps apparently fail to provide the necessary nutritional elements for good health? He felt the findings of a controlled feeding experiment might illuminate new facts concerning optimal human nutrition.

After extensive study, Dr. Pottenger proved that when cats were fed a cooked food diet, the prodigy and their parents would have numerous health problems. As generations of cats were born, the problems kept increasing.

These defects include:

Gum disease	Liver problems
Heart disease	Tooth decay
Personality problems	Miscarriages
Insomnia	Deformity

Various chronic diseases of the organs were so rampant that Pottenger started a separate study to compare humans to similar stressors.

He noticed the same kind of startling differences while studying twins and siblings reared in different environments.

The same exact health disruptions that plagued his cats were being reproduced in the human study. The results repeated themselves again and again among the twins. Whenever and wherever the diet was changed, the maladies followed. The findings from his human / cat study are often quoted. Pottenger's human study was conducted between 1932 and 1956.

Nothing has been added or subtracted from his findings, and the observations are valid. A careful study of the Pottenger study will reveal irrefutable evidence of disease and deficiency caused through diet. Feel free to look up Pottenger's work on the net; you will be amazed and shocked when you read the full extent of his work.

The above was not the only work done on the subject of what society and cooked food does to a body. Dr. Weston A. Price (author, Nutrition and Physical Degeneration) was doing a similar study on humans in 1938 – 1939. As a dentist, his focus was strictly on the mouth and gums. He was trying to understand why advanced civilizations had more dental problems than 3rd world countries.

The siblings that retained their more nature based diets enjoyed good health; the more civilized diet recipients became worse with each generation.

A summarization of Price's findings, for those now living a civilized / rural life style, gives us much data. Just as in Pottenger's cat study, the offspring were tracked as well as the health and disposition of the transplant.

The transplanted or rural relocated sibling reflected:

1. Rampant tooth decay.
2. Tooth placement now incorrect requiring braces.
3. Short stature with brittle bones.
4. Gingivitis common.
5. Narrowing of thighbones.
6. Cancer and malignant tumors.
7. Narrowing of skulls.
8. Deformities of the limbs.
9. Deformities of the skull.
10. Anemia
11. Nervousness

It is interesting that much of our even more damaging processed food had not been invented yet. In 1938 and 1939 the diet included white bread and sugars or candy that was not available in the native home or villages of the transplants.

Therefore, it is not a stretch to conclude that the above problems as well as today's problems (disease) are the result of our diet. The thought that man can safely adapt or adjust to our present (junk food diet) lifestyle is optimistic and idealistic.

Sugar Love It or Flee From It.

54 Salt/Sodium Difference

Note: Humans are the only animals on the planet that add salt to their food beyond what occurs naturally in their diet.

Note: If not for salt's food preservation properties, the America's may never have been discovered, as food storage would never have lasted the entire voyage.

A Brief History of Salt

Should you have visited a museum and gazed at an Egyptian mummy, you have looked at history preserved by use of salt. Remnants of the vast Nigerian and Mali salt mines are still found on the African continent. Salt has held a much-exalted place in man's history.

Salt is obtained either from shallow mines or distilled from soil.

Marco Polo (Italian Traveler and Explorer, 1254 - 1324, Venice, Italy) used salt as currency during some of his travels. For a time salt was as valuable as gold and even traded ounce for ounce. Polo was clearly fascinated by the profitable salt business as he watched it conducted all over China. He followed early Chinese junks as they traveled up and down the Yangtze River (it stretches from the interior of China to the coast). Merchants would conduct their salt business from ship to shore, as people would gather in great numbers to get this valuable element.

Early China was built on salt.

Marco Polo is also believed responsible for introducing the west to the great Kublai Khan. Through Khan (the then ruler of China) we first see the Peng-Tao (or Tzao)-Kan-Mu (the first known pharmacology work), circa 2700 B.C.

One portion of the text documented nearly 50 varieties of salt previously unknown to the ancient world. The Chinese had been extracting salt (almost 5000 years ago) and processing it for consumption via methods similar to those practiced by industry today. Salt can be found almost everywhere from West Africa to China, from the American North and South to Germany. In Medieval times, he who controlled salt production or stores controlled the politics and thus had the power. Our language is still sprinkled with the power of salt.

Salt was a currency and Roman soldiers were paid in the valuable white granules.

Salary: Salary (Roman payment), this word is derived from Latin salarium argentums or salt money, which eventually became the word salary. When salt became easier to mine and was therefore more common, its value declined and it ended up on our dinner tables.

Still sprinkling our language:
- Not worth / worth his weight in salt
- He is the salt of the earth
- Salting away
- With a grain of salt
- Back to the salt mines
- Below the salt (meaning common or ordinary)

Salt is sodium chloride. About 40 percent of salt is sodium and 60 percent is chlorine. Sodium is a life vital element found in fruit, vegetables, meats and legumes (nuts).

Salt is well documented in its ability to preserve everything from mummies to beef from decaying.

By the early 1800s salt was the number one preservative in the Americas. Food preservation was among the biggest problems of the day. The use of salt ensured an adequate supply of meats and grains for the upcoming winter and early spring.

Other than for industrial needs, modern man's need for salt has greatly diminished. Refrigeration has eliminated the need for preserving food to survive the harshness of the seasons. Therefore, all the salt we need for a healthy body is derived from our diet, if we eat a truly balanced diet. Since WWII salt has caused more problems than it has solved as a supplement.

Why Should We Eliminate Salt

Although a small amount of sodium (about 500mg) is essential to normal body functions, it is estimated that the average person consumes 4000 to 5000 mg a day. It is widely understood even by medical science that large amounts of dietary sodium result in high blood pressure (also called hypertension) and may lead to heart attacks, strokes and kidney failure. Man is no longer salt deficient, which is why health care professionals are advising us to eat far less added salt.

Healthy foods do not come in cans. Canned food is loaded with salt / sodium. Look at canned food sometime and you will be aghast at the sodium content. These so called foods are all worthless.

Do not eat anything pickled. Avoid foods such as sauerkraut, olives, relishes, dills and gherkins. They are all packed in vinegar and/or brine (heavily salted water), making them exceptionally high in sodium.

Cheeses contain salt for preserving as well as for flavor. Smoked or canned meat and fish products such as tuna, ham, bacon, cold cuts, corned beef and sausage are well seasoned with salt. Deli roast beef and turkey breast are often cooked with salt.

Beware Of Seasoning

Sodium is a part of many other ingredients added to prepare foods that often have no salty taste. Some are used in amounts that add a significant quantity of sodium to the final product.

Monosodium glutamate (MSG), a flavor enhancer
Baking soda (sodium bicarbonate), used to make quick breads and cakes rise
Sodium nitrate, a curing agent for meat
Sodium saccharin, an artificial sweetener
Sodium propionate, a mold inhibitor found in baked foods
Sodium citrate, an acidity controller found in soft drinks, fruit drinks, jams and jellies
Sodium, when consumed will, by its presence, throw off the functions of your body.

Think of sodium as a random renegade program that is fed into your computer (the computer is your body). This element feeds your computer wayward commands such as to store, delete, purge, format, copy, remove, etc., regardless of what the body needs to do. Sodium does not think, it is just reactive.

Other renegade chemicals that corrupt your body's hard drive are sugar, caffeine and all drugs. Life is hard enough without making it harder by poisoning yourself.

Roger Bezanis

What about Over-The-Counter Medications?

Medications can be another unexpected source of sodium in the diet. Over the counter products such as antacids, laxatives, bicarbonate of soda, pain relievers and other preparations often contain large amounts of sodium.

What Do Food Labels Tell About Sodium Content? If a nutrition label is not available, you can check the ingredient statement for the presence of salt or other sodium compounds. Ingredients are listed in descending order by weight, but since the specific weights aren't listed, it only gives you a rough idea of the amount of sodium.

Your best bet would be to never purchase anything that lists more than 120 mgs sodium per ample serving.

—-Consider the following; your FDA is lying right to your face—-

> **The Food and Drug Administration has also established the following guidelines for sodium claims:**
>
> **Sodium Free:** food contains less than 5mg sodium per serving. (No kidding. 5mg. really?)
>
> **Very Low Sodium:** food contains 35 mg sodium or less per serving. (Very low sodium...?)
>
> **Low Sodium:** food contains 140 mg sodium or less per serving. (So, this is low sodium!)
>
> **Light in Sodium:** food has 50% less sodium than original item. (What does that mean?)
>
> **Reduced Sodium:** food contains 25% less sodium than the original item. (Does this mean..?)
>
> **Unsalted, No Salt Added or Without Added:** Salt is used only if no salt is added to a food that is normally processed with salt, which means it could still be loaded with sodium. These strategies show just how dangerous government guidelines actually are.

The above points are the equivalent of our government issuing a proclamation:

> "We recognize that Russian roulette could be dangerous."
>
> "We recommend that it should be played with care."
>
> "Ideally with a 12 chambered pistol rather than the usual 6 chambers."

Why do you think that these salt / sodium guidelines exist? The answers are money and addiction. Foods containing added salt and sodium are addicting and this equals money in the pockets of those using it. If you also suspected that some of that money would end up being paid as kickbacks to the FDA or other agencies, remember I never said that. That was your idea.

Forgive me, but a LITTLE poison is still poison.

If this book has taught you nothing, except never eat anything containing sodium, salt or sugar, then I have done my job. Making these changes would dramatically alter the quality of your life. You would be on the road to the fountain of health and youth. You would actually start to appear younger. This happens every day. Do you deserve that?

You are surrounded by sodium, unless you give it up. This is a losing battle unless you decide not to fight it by not engaging in it in the first place.

Remember, it is best to never eat sodium.

The following foods are ridiculously high in sodium.

Anchovies	Gravy
Bacon	Ham
Baking Soda	Hot Dogs
Bouillon Cubes	Olives
Canned Soups	Pickles
Canned Tuna	Salad Dressings*
Canned Vegetables	Salsa
Cheese	Sausage
Cold Cuts	Sea Salt
Condiments	Soy Sauce
Cooking Sauces	Spaghetti Sauce
Cottage Cheese	Tomato Juice
Croutons	Vegetable Juice
Diet Soda	Ketchup
Fried Chicken	Mustard

* If the worst thing you ate was a little salad dressing that had some sodium in it, so be it. At the same time, if you are sensitive to it, drop it out as well. If you eliminate them from your life, except what naturally occurs in food, you will be lean and healthier.

I encourage you to do this. If you work hard at it, you will notice the difference.

How to Start to Ease into Being Healthy

Starting on this journey may not be easy as it is not what you are comfortable with. But unless you start, your body will eventually get very uncomfortable with waste your body cannot process. The first thing to do is, go to the grocery store and pretend you are shopping for food you would be eating based on this book. Walk down the aisles and notice what you would be eating and not eating.

Then, start over again, this time focusing just on what you would be eating. Walk around the market again. Take these same steps until you feel comfortable with the idea of what you are going to be purchasing.

Pick up the actual items you will be eating, hold them, look at them and get used to them.

Again, when you are comfortable with all of this you can go shopping. This may seem simple but it will prepare you for what is coming by allowing you to wrap your mind around the subject matter.

What Actually Happens When You Gain Weight

The human body is a carbon-burning, oxygen-breathing machine that expends energy based on its activity level. Putting on weight requires one or more of the following:

- Added muscle mass
- Slowed metabolism
- Decreased activity level
- Increased food intake
- Water retention
- Pregnancy

All six points above force the body to adjust its activities to accommodate the changes. The wildcard elements that cause the body to put on weight are:

Sodium: Which causes the kidneys to go "off line" and retain water, not utilizing it.

Salt: Which causes the kidneys to go "off line" and retain water, not utilizing it.

Sugar: Which causes the kidneys to go "off line" and retain water, not utilizing it. Sugar scrambles all of the commands that the body is trying to execute. Initially sugar causes a release of urine as the body goes into cathartic shock. It then commands the body to retain water.

Too much protein: Causes kidney overwhelm/poisoning. They go off line and the body starts retaining water as it tries to dilute the excess protein. Protein also interrupts sexual function in both sexes.

Drugs: Do all of the above while poisoning the body.

Alcohol: Scrambles all of the systems of the body and is a poison.

Waste that should be broken down isn't and the body can't utilize the fluid present to break down new waste. Interference with the kidneys always leads to disruption of the liver, heart, lungs, muscles, joints, pancreas, sex drive, etc.

On a digestive level, production of hydrochloric acid in the stomach comes to a halt as fluid is being diverted for other purposes. Therefore the food in your stomach is not being digested and is now a compost bin releasing foul gases.

Consequently, you develop varying degrees of indigestion, experience flatulence and begin belching as the food in your stomach rots and turns into putrid mulch. In the morning you have gained 1 - 7 pounds.

What caused this?

The body's inability to flush itself of toxic waste is the source of weight gain.

That is what goes on in your body.

55 Killer Caffeine

There is nothing like starting your morning with a good hot steaming cup of coffee.

I have never even tasted coffee and I know the above statement is true. How did a little insignificant bean from economically depressed countries take over the planet? Marketing! Repetition is the key and saturation is the result. Good marketing sticks to you like a long sleeve shirt in Florida at a mid August baseball game. There just is no way to peel it off.

Consider this: In the 1960s kids wanted to grow up to be an Oscar Meyer Wiener: "Oh, I wish I was an Oscar Meyer Wiener, that is what I truly want to be-ee-ee, 'cause if I was an Oscar Meyer Wiener, everyone would be in love with me."

What happened to Sara Lee? You might remember, "No-body doesn't like Sara Leeeee." When it comes to addictions, coffee has woven itself into the fabric of our very being.

Consider coffee houses	Coffee breaks
Coffee cake	Toffee candy

In the end nothing compares to coffee. Because coffee said there was nothing that compares to it. Coffee is practically a religion. If some clever pastor, rabbi, father, minister, monk, or other religious leader linked up with Starbucks...hmmmmm. Imagine the attendance!

Prior to 1985, coffee was an adult drink. Now, thanks to years of aggressive marketing, yearly coffee sales exceed water.

Roger Bezanis

It is second only to sugar as the most addicting substance on the planet. Shocking, you say? How many people do you know that are addicted to caffeine? Know anyone addicted to sugar? How about to heroin? Can you count those who are entrenched with cocaine? Sugar wins hands down.

Sugar is an ingredient in practically everything, even coffee and cigarettes.

If auto parts makers could perfect a way to coat parts with it, *everyone* would be a mechanic. Repairs would be ragged, but done in half the time. Men would meet in the auto parts houses not to talk as "gear heads" do, no; they would be sucking on break shoes and spark plugs. What about new innovations in cars, who cares!! Where are the fuel injectors?

Coffee and hot beverages are a real treat no doubt. But no one seems to care what caffeine is doing to the body. Caffeine is a common chemical found in natural sources, such as tealeaves, coffee beans, cocoa beans, cola nuts and carob beans. In the human body caffeine acts as an intense stimulant with such power, many people think they can't start their day without a little.

Caffeine causes your breath to quicken, heart to pump faster and blood pressure to rise (all of this is due to an intense attack on the kidneys). The kidneys under heavy duress start to release fluid (a diuretic response).

This completely upsets the balance of the human body as the caffeine has "reprogrammed the body."

This robs the system of fluid it needs to run on. But you feel great! Soon you stand in the restroom evacuating your bladder while starting to feel tired. Oh so very, very tired. As the kidneys spasm, blood pressure rapidly rises.

Suddenly you are jumpy, your low back hurts, you are nervous with shaky hands, which you think means that you need more caffeine. This is akin to shooting yourself in the foot and concluding that if you shoot yourself twice you will feel better.

Caffeine Comparison
Drink/Food - Amount of Drink/Food - Amount of Caffeine in mgs.

Mountain Dew, 12 ounces, 55.0mg

Coca-Cola, 12 ounces, 34.0mg

Diet Coke, 12 ounces, and 45.0mg

Pepsi, 12 ounces, 38.0mg

7-Up, 12 ounces, 0 mg

Brewed coffee (drip method), 5 ounces, 115mg

Iced tea, 12 ounces, 70mg

Dark chocolate, 1 ounce, 20mg

Milk chocolate, 1 ounce, 6mg

Cocoa beverage, 5 ounces, 4mg

Chocolate milk beverage, 8 ounces, 5mg

Cold relief medication, 1 tablet, 30mg

Source: U.S. food and Drug Administration and National Soft Drink Association.

According to the National Soft Drink Association, the following is the caffeine content in mg per 12 oz can of soda:

Product, Caffeine Content

Shasta Cola, 44.4mg	Pepsi Cola, 37.2mg
Jolt, 71.2mg	Tab, 46.8mg
Mr. Pibb, 40.8mg	Diet Pepsi, 35.4mg
Sugar-Free Mr. Pibb, 8.8mg	Coca-Cola, 45.6mg
Mountain Dew, 55.0 mg	RC Cola, 36.0mg
Dr. Pepper, 39.6mg	Diet Cola, 45.6mg
Mello Yellow, 52.8mg	Canada Dry Cola, 30.0mg

By means of comparison, a 7 oz. cup of coffee has the following caffeine (mg) amounts, according to Bunker and McWilliams in J. Am. Diet. 74:28-32, 1979:

Product - Caffeine Content mgs.

Drip, 115-175mg	Decaf, instant, 2-3mg
Espresso, 100mg - 1 serving (1.5-2oz)	Tea, iced (12 oz), 70mg
Brewed, 80-135mg	Tea, brewed, imported, 60mg
Instant, 65-100mg	Tea, brewed, U.S., 40mg
Decaf, brewed, 3-4mg	Tea, instant, 30mg

Energy drinks for kids are now out of control and are being consumed by even preschoolers. "Young people are taking caffeine to stay awake, or perhaps to get high, and many of them are ending up in the emergency department", said Dr. Danielle McCarthy of Northwestern University.

Dr. McCarthy conducted an extensive study in 2006 for the Chicago poison control center. Her findings were not surprising.

"Caffeine is a drug and should be treated with caution, as any drug is." - Dr. Danielle McCarthy

Anheuser-Busch and Miller Brewing Company now produce several "energy beers." This is a mix of beer and caffeine. A favorite is Red Bull and vodka. Bartenders often mix these two and call it a "Friday Flattener" or a "Dirty Pompadour." Concoctions like this have been popular for more than ten years.

In 2006, more than 500 new energy drinks launched worldwide. No doubt coffee fans are probably too old to understand why. We are building chemically dependent addicted kids almost as fast as they can be conceived.

The following list is taken from the "Caffeine Database." The caffeine content of the newest energy drinks aimed at kids is astounding. The following numbers are based on a per serving measure. Some of these beverages have more than one serving per can.

180, 90mg

Airforce Nutrisoda Energizer, 50mg

Ale 8 1, 37mg

Ammo, 171mg

Ammo, 75mg

Amp, 75mg

Amp Overdrive, 141mg

Arizona Extreme Energy Shot, 100mg

Arizona Green Tea Energy, 200mg

Battery, 106mg

Bawls, 66.7mg

Bazza High Energy Tea, 150mg

Beaver Buzz, 110mg

Blow Energy Drink Mix, 240mg

Bomba Energy, 75mg

Boo-Koo Energy, 360mg

Brawndo, 200mg

Burn, 118mg

Burn (UK), 45mg

Burn2, 199mg

Buzz Water, 200mg

Celsius, 200mg

Chic, 150mg

Cocaine Energy Drink, 280mg

Crunk, 100mg

Dare Devil, 240mg

Diablo, 95mg

Dopamine Energy Drink 120mg

Fixx, 500mg

Joker, 150mg

Jones Energy, 100mg

Kaboom Infinite Energy, 95mg

MDX, 82.25mg

Monster, 160mg

Morning Spark, 170mg

Mother, 106mg

No Name Energy Drink, 280mg

NOS, 250mg

Nuclear Water Antidote, 180mg

Pimp Juice, 81mg

Power Edge, 80mg

Power Horse, 80mg

Power Shot, 100mg

Rage, 200mg

Red Jak, 164mg

Red Line RTD, 250mg

Relentless, 160mg

Rip It Energy Fuel, 100mg

Rock Star, 160mg

Rock Star Juiced, 160mg

Rock Star Roasted, 225mg

Rock Star Zero Carb, 240mg

Rumba Energy Juice, 170mg

Sobe No Fear, 174mg.

Sobe No Fear Gold, 174mg

Socko, 160mg

Socko Slim, 160mg

Spark, 120mg

Fritz Kola, 83.3mg

Fuel Cell, 180mg

Full Throttle, 144mg

H2O Blast, 100mg

High Ball Energy, 75mg

Hogan Energy, 160mg

Howling Monkey, 160mg

Hy Drive, 121mg

Hype, 80mg

Spike Shooter, 300mg

Superfly, 150mg

Upshot, 200mg

V, 109mg

Vamp, 240mg

Viso Energy Vigor 300mg

Von Dutch, 160mg

Who's Your Daddy, 200mg

Wired X344, 344mg

It should not be surprising that at bedtime you and your kids can't sleep. The caffeine you had earlier that day is still upsetting your liver and kidneys! It also accumulates in your system. Not sleeping? Your sleeping pills contain - you guessed - it caffeine.

Does this make any sense?

But you say coffee helps me go #2 (bowel movement).

FACT: Ingesting ANY hot liquid instantly registers "sick" to the body. Why? The body is programmed to fight invaders by raising its temperature. The result is the body will rid waste from the heated area. In the case of the colon, you have an evacuation (bowel movement).

Temperature elevation = immune system response to bacteria, virus or irritant.

Every morning, as a result of boiling your intestinal tract, your body thinks it is sick. "**Every morning it thinks it is sick.**" Is there any question why you are looking old prematurely? Do you wonder why your body hurts?

The byproduct of breaking caffeine is uric acid. When caffeine is present we not only have a superheated body, we have a chemically heated body. Uric acid, a harsh irritant, raises body temperature by .5 - 1.5 degrees. This uric acid also stimulates the body to release. In other words, we have just thrown the body into spasm due to excess stimuli (uric acid and a hot beverage). Remember "Toeville"?

Throwing the body into panic mode is never, never, never a good idea. Caffeine causes the body to reject the normal biological processes that it should be running. Whatever the body was trying to do is shut down for hours.

The natural response to reading this chapter is to switch to decaffeinated coffee.

Roger Bezanis

Unfortunately decaffeinated coffee can be worse than caffeinated coffee. The decaffeination process leaves 6-20% of the caffeine behind. Yes, decaf coffee still has an appreciable amount of caffeine present in the final product. Therefore you are not free from caffeine, you are merely ingesting less. Caffeine is so potent a toxin that even a 1% residue is very damaging to the body.

The decaffeination process is often worse than caffeine due to the extraction process. The solvents that can be used to extract caffeine are formaldehyde (embalming solution), methylene chloride (known to cause cancer) and other solvents. There is no safe coffee of any type. Small quantities of poison are still destructive to the body. Caffeine free is safe, reduced caffeine or decaffeinated is not. Do yourself a favor and do not consume this destructive chemical or chemically laced morning cocktail.

If you are not clear about how dangerous caffeine really is, the next few paragraphs will make this very apparent. This information is available at doctoryourself.com.

The articles cited at doctoryouself.com incorrectly attribute emotional function to brain function. Therefore I will not print them in their entirety here. I have chosen to remove the brain references and focus on the "outcomes" from exposure to caffeine.

So-called allergies to caffeine are being widely diagnosed. Caffeine allergy is a laughable term and can be compared to an allergic reaction to bullet wounds. There is no such thing as an allergy to poison unless we are brainwashed to believe that poison is essential to life.

The work on caffeine / allergy / toxicity is correct when directing the attack at the liver. The liver must be allowed to wash the body free of waste. Caffeine completely disables the liver and is attributed to causing the mania listed below. When the body is "locked up" and retaining water it is at a toxic standstill and will behave in the following manner.

- Psychotic states
- Nervous breakdowns
- Irrational behavior
- Poor attention span
- Poor comprehension
- Mood changes
- Loss of organizational skills
- Delusions
- Hallucinations
- Paranoia
- Panic attacks
- Anxiety
- Toxic dementia
- Memory impairment
- Social anxiety
- Strained personal relations
- Inability to process information
- Brain damage (actually all organs are damaged by caffeine use)
- Vision impairment
- Loss of verbal skills

Caffeine related disorders were noted as early as 1936.

The general facts indicate that caffeine is the biggest contributor to mental health disorders on the planet today. The "beans" addictive qualities, prevalence, legal status, and rampant regular use, guarantee that these numbers will continue to escalate to epidemic levels. When society fully grasps the dangers of caffeine, it may be too late.

You now have the truth. Caffeine purveyors hate me. Therefore, if I suddenly disappear from the face of the earth, remember to look for me in or under the cornerstone of your corner coffee shop.

56 Hot / Cold Factor

When the body gets hot or cold for whatever reason, be it environmental or chemical, it does two things:

- **It tries to cool itself / it tries to heat itself**
- **It alters its function in response to the stimuli**

This is why we vomit and get diarrhea when we are sick. This is all an attempt to right the system. Just as sneezing is an attempt to clear the nose. Diarrhea is the colons attempt to sneeze.

Ancient medicine taught us that to break up constipation, a hot compress should be applied directly to the abdomen. This works the same way as consuming boiling liquid. The heat transfers to the bowel and this stimulates elimination. Again, the heat fools the body into a cathartic spasm as part of an immune response and the body evacuates.

Ergo, the body acts as if it were sick.

Consider this, when you eat hot food (as most people do), the body perceives the heat and wrongly perceives it as fever. It then starts to fight a nonexistent infection. Since survival is paramount, the body pulls resources from digestion and begins trying to fix something that isn't broken.

Now imagine that the body is constantly getting hot food. Having imagined that, imagine what happens to your body when digestion is not important and infection fighting is. If you think that the result would be that you would put on fat, you are right.

What about spicy food?

What happens when you ingest hot spicy food? Does it heat the body too?

Exactly right.

No doubt you have seen someone eating hot spicy food and sweating. Their brow is wet and beading with more sweat. To the body, hot is hot regardless of its source. Spicy food is like eating boiling food that does not cool. This is why after a meal of spicy food, the next evacuation or two will burn as the acids are still very potent even on the way out of the body.

When the body gets hot does it want to cool itself? Correct again. The fire-eater reaches for cold water to dilute the heat. Again the body does not differentiate between hot from spice or hot from heating. Hot is hot.

The chemical reaction causes an immune system response as the body tries to cool. Colon formulas are often loaded with hot peppers to cause the colon to heat and then evacuate. When you see African Bird Peppers in the ingredient list of a colon formula, heat is the purpose. The result is a hot rapid evacuation.

The temperature of the body elevates with any potent spice. The tongue is also on fire signaling that the liver is heating as a direct result. To prove this, take your temperature prior to eating spicy food. You will notice that prior to the meal your temperature is around 98.6. After your meal begins, you will feel hotter as your temperature has raised a few tenths of a degree or more.

The body attempts to reject anything hot either by vomiting, or eventually via a loose stool or diarrhea.

What about cold food?

One of the main reasons people tend to be heavier in very cold environments is a response to keeping warm. Fat is an insulator just like fiber insulation is in your attic and walls. Researchers have submitted work proving that the epicanthal "eyelid fold" (found in Asia) is a direct result of thousands of years of frigid climate conditions. In a cold climate the body must keep all vital components as warm as possible. This is the purpose of these folds that make Asians look like Asians.

As the peoples of the earth keep moving to warmer climates, these folds may eventually disappear.

What happens to the person who intentionally freezes or deeply chills some part of their body from the inside out? Eating bone-chilling food (like ice cream) slows the metabolism as the body is pooling its resources to stay warm. Eating ice cream or chewing on ice confuses the body and to some degree fat is the result.

Another interesting response that most of us have experienced is the cold drink / ice cream headache. This is simply the body locking-up and turning on the afterburners to fight off the intense sudden attack of cold on the system. Your headache is due to shock. The body goes into overdrive to heat itself. All systems are put on hold as you are temporarily freezing to death.

In a frigid environment the body needs fat for survival, as food is often scarce in such a locality. To support your body's needs you are forced to eat more and more to stay warm. Arctic conditions require the body to store fat for food and warmth. What kind of environment do you live in? Can you stay warm without fat? This is called hypothyroidism and is a western medical name for "The kidneys need help."

If not, improve your kidney and liver function. You will notice the difference.

What about Hypothermia?

Hypothermia is a slow or sudden drop in body temperature from 98.6 to as low as 86.6 where organ shutdown occurs. Remember the ice cream headache from above? Headache is one of the first symptoms of body temperature dropping.

The body contains 5 liters of blood. Should the body become extremely cold, it is vital to warm the body via the kidneys as 100% of our blood is circulated through them every 1-3 minutes. Therefore, warming the lower back (site of the kidneys) is paramount in cases of hypothermia.

If you are freezing, you need heat, not vitamins. Heat is more important than digestion under cold conditions. Cold is trouble to the body. To conserve energy you will get tired as digestion and the nutrient factory is switched off in an attempt to get the body temperature to rise.

Stage one: Goose bumps and slight shaking

Stage two: Shivering increases and muscle coordination becomes very erratic.

Stage three: Speaking is difficult and thinking is extremely clouded.

Stage four: Speech nearly impossible, body blue and puffy, walking nearly impossible. Organ shutdown eminent, yet brain death may take some time as freezing slows this process.

Summation: If we use common sense regarding what we put in our mouth, and therefore stay away from spicy, hot or freezing cold items, we will eat a far different diet. Most people will read this chapter and decide, nope, that is not for me. It was interesting but not for me. Yet some of you will make changes.

Your body will do its best to deal with whatever cards you give it, but you can stack the deck in your favor by just using universal wisdom about your life and diet.

If you are sure your body is smarter than you, your conclusion is thousands of years old. It is also exactly correct.

57 Importance of H_2O (Water)

Water is one of the basic building blocks of life. Without a steady supply of it all life would eventually perish. There are many theories on water. Such as, you should drink half of your body weight in water every day. Sometime in the past someone said, "The AVERAGE person exhales between 48 to 64 ounces of water a day (about 1 to 1 ¹/₃ liters) just breathing." These statements are almost wholly inaccurate.

Each individual is different as are his or her needs.

Have you ever exhaled on a mirror and noticed the temporary fog you created? The moisture you saw was the direct result of the millions of tiny droplets of water that are carried out of our lungs in every breath. Earlier chapters in this book make reference to the fact that the **body is a machine**.

This truth is undeniable as the human body exhibits every trait of being a carbon burning machine, including the production and release of gases. Some gasses are harmful (methane for example) and some harmless (water vapor). The way the body cools itself is via respiration, which is defined as:

   1: the placing of air or dissolved gases in intimate contact with the circulating medium of a multi cellular organism (as by breathing) b: a single complete act of breathing.

   2: the physical and chemical processes by which an organism supplies its cells and tissues with the oxygen needed for metabolism and relieves them of the carbon dioxide formed in energy-producing reactions.

Result? Every breath we take dehydrates us a little more. That is why you wake in the morning with a pasty mouth (you have been air drying all night long). Sleeping, as far as dehydration goes, is kind of like running a marathon every night. Perhaps you sleep with a jug or glass of water next to the bed to prevent this. In the end we are drying out nonetheless.

The amount of water we will exhale in a day is dependent on a number of factors:

1) Climate (the dryer or hotter, the more water lost).

2) Physical activity (the more active, the more water lost).

3) Diet (processed foods in the diet, the more water needed to digest them).

4) Use of Caffeine or any diuretics (diuretics cause your body to expel water thru urine).

5) Stress (stress causes the liver to work harder. The liver runs on water like a washing machine to cleanse and purify your system).

6) Drugs and other Chemicals ingested (this is such a wild card, that the body is wholly defenseless against these influences)

7) Condition of your kidneys

8) Condition of your liver

There is a patently false "old wives tale" known by many that, for every cup of coffee, you need 3 cups of water or 4 cups of water, or maybe it's 5 cups of water. These computations are flawed and have little practical application. Thoroughly examine the above 8 points and decide for yourself if the "so many cup rule" has any validity at all.

The best cup of coffee / water rule is "NEVER DRINK COFFEE." Well, that was simple.

There are even more factors that influence how much or how little water a person needs. Is someone toxic, i.e. are they carrying an undigested load of material in the body that needs to be flushed out? For 100 percent of us the answer is yes.

How much water do we need?

Let's say that you do not eat processed foods and have no caffeine or diuretics in your life. Let's also postulate that you are NOT THE LEAST BIT TOXIC to anything and are otherwise healthy.

Then you can follow your thirst.

Yes, you can follow your thirst. As I have stated again and again throughout this book, the body is constantly talking to you. The question is, are you listening and/or do you know how to listen?

If you get an impulse to drink water, drink water not soda, coffee, tea, or some beverage that would increase the load on your system.

Do not feel bad, as this is primordial rocket science. You are learning the basics of your body. The body no one ever told you anything about. There are many experts that indicate we must drink between 80 to 100 ounces of water a day just to get by. That is not true. Yet it is not false either.

Follow your thirst. It will tell you when to drink water and how much. But, if you successfully use the "drinking your body weight in water every day" and it works, keep it up. However, be willing to change as your body does. Perhaps you have heard "Drink half your body weight in water every day", same rule. It works only if it works. Stay in fluid contact with your body (no pun intended) and you will know what you need.

Perhaps you just drink a solid 120 ounces a day and you have been tested again and again for the amount of water you should drink. You know the rule. Rules are only good if they work. In this book, WORK = HEALTH.

Is there a time when you do not want to drink water?

Believe it or not, there is an answer to this question and for good reason. Your body must manufacture Hydrochloric acid to help digest your food. Without it, the food just composts in your stomach and eventually your intestines.

It all starts with the glands of the mouth, where saliva is produced. Saliva contains the enzyme ptyalin. Ptyalin, water and mucus combined with the act of chewing, helps your body to start digesting the food in your mouth.

You have heard "death starts in your colon." Well, "digestion starts in your mouth."

Next in line are the stomach and its glands, plus the intestines. In the stomach we find hydrochloric acid that helps to soften the food you just swallowed to make it more permeable for digestion. It is because of the mucosal lining of the stomach that the stomach is not destroyed by our Hydrochloric acid.

Once in the small intestines the other enzymes created in the body go to work.

Here are some of the enzymes involved in digestion:

Amylase: To digest carbohydrates

Bromelain: To digest proteins

Cellulase: To digest fiber

Chymopapain: To digest protein

Diastase: To digest carbohydrates

Glucoamylase: To digest carbohydrates

Hemicellulase: To digest carbohydrates

Hyaluronidase: To digest, proteins, adhesions & fibrin

Invertase: To digest carbohydrates

Lactase: To digest lactose and fats

Lipases: To digest fats

Maltase: To digest carbohydrates

Pancreatin: To digest proteins, fats & carbohydrates

Papain: To digest proteins, fats & carbohydrates

Pectinase: To digest carbohydrates

Pepsin: To digest proteins

Phytase: To digest carbohydrates

Protease: To digest protein.

Rennin: To digest proteins

Now imagine there was something you could do at every meal that would slow down or interfere with your digestion. Most people would never dream of doing such a thing. But that is just what we do if we consume water with a meal. If we do ingest water after a meal it should be more than 15 minutes after a meal. If you are parched during the meal, the meal is heavy in salt, sodium, sugar or spice. These elements are to be eliminated or greatly reduced in the diet.

This includes any beverage. Therefore do not consume fluids with your meals, as your digestion will slow to a snail's pace. What should be digested within an hour could take 4 or 5 hours or longer. Watering down or diluting the precious stomach acid that would otherwise start digesting your meal makes your metabolism seem sluggish when in fact the body is working the best it can under very trying conditions.

When we drink water, tea, soda, coffee or juice with a meal we are inadvertently telling the body to gain weight. After your food leaves the stomach, the gall bladder introduces bile or bile salts or bilirubin (terminology for bile) into the intestines to further dissolve fat, act as a stool softener and stimulate the peristalsis (squeezing motion of the digestive tract) of the intestines and the colon.

Food and a watery concoction (all mixed up) slow digestion. Can any of this be good? No. By over irrigating ourselves, especially at mealtime, we are doing a great disservice to our health. To reach a happy medium, sip water, as you need to throughout the day.

Your body will tell you when it is thirsty. Those who told you that when you feel thirsty it is too late, were trying to sell you water. Remember, if your needs change let your water intake change too. Should you be working out, you will of course need more water. These silly tables indicating you need so much water based on your body mass are just a bunch of flotsam and jetsam and completely worthless.

Water is the oil of the body. Without it we put on weight, grow old faster, have poor skin, poor energy, poor hair, etc.

Don't ignore water but don't drown in it either.

58 Disease Labels and Who Owns Them

Imagine that you did not have a name. Now imagine no one on the planet had names. Personal identification would be extremely difficult. The purpose of advertising is to separate, validate and inculcate (impress via repetition).

Your name achieves all three of those objectives when it is mentioned to someone you know. That is the purpose of advertising and of course labels. Labels convey a message and a reputation. Nothing without a name or a label is worth very much. Have you ever paid very much for anything that you could not identify or explain? The answer is of course no.

In the world of Allopathic medicine EVERY perceived malady must have its own special name or designation. Human frailties without names are not problems and NOT worth worrying about.

In the world of misguided and mistaken medicine, the word disease has lost its meaning and now means drugs and surgery. Earlier in this book I wrote that the true meaning of disease means DIS – EASE.

So-called diseases such as cancer and aids will never be cured until research stops looking for the magic bullet virus / cell / gene / fill in the blank. There is no such thing as a sickness gene.

There are chemicals that build up in the system / human body that eventually shut down the immune system. Who put those chemicals there? You did by choice or by lack of choice such as not moving your family away when the chemical plant was built a block away.

This is a hard pill to swallow. You are above the average man and can swallow it because you understand it. You reading this book now know it is true.

The word disease is a gold mine. Say the word and the eyes get wide and people go white with fear. Do not be controlled by fear. Consider the fear created and money made by the following list:

AIDS
Cancer
Diabetes
Legionnaire disease
Parkinson's disease
Hepatitis A-B and C
Erosive Acid Reflux disease

IBS (Irritable Bowel Syndrome)
Crones Disease
Alcoholism (now commonly called a disease?)
PAD (Peripheral Artery Disease, it has no symptoms? Wow!)
Restless Leg Syndrome (fidgety legs, hmmmmm?)

Again diseases make money. Clearly in the world of medicine, the name is everything. The above LABELS get your attention. There is little difference in the name West Nile Virus and Stuffed Crust Pizza. Both get your attention. In my opinion, disease is one of the most EVIL words in the English language. That is quite a statement. Why would I say such a profound or provocative thing?

As stated much earlier, disease means you are no longer responsible for your condition. Why? Your life has been stolen away by an invisible monster that attacked you as you slept in your bed. It is literally the plot line to the film "Invasion of the Body Snatchers." Disease means that something out of your control or influence **GOT YOU** and you now can do nothing about it.

Disease = VICTIM. Your American Medical Association is frothing at the mouth over the word disease. Disease and your agreement that there are such things, is how they support themselves and, in turn, the Food and Drug Administration.

The AMA names all disease and recommends the surgery to correct them. In turn, the FDA creates or hosts competition to create the drugs to treat the disease. Your American Medical Association owns the word disease. No natural health healer, practitioner (Chiropractor, etc.) or natural health company can legally name or even breathe the word disease (much less treat it).

A natural health healer would never name a disease as he or she thinks in simple terms. He thinks in terms of basic organ function and corrects that. The word disease by its very nature is meant to be confusing and mysterious. The mere mention of the word disease leaves the listener in distress trying to understand what it is. No disease or label for a disease can be treated, but organs can.

Weak kidneys: Can be assisted, But Diabetes (a kidney condition, cannot). Diabetes can be helped! The remedy requires awareness, responsibility and a little work. Call kidney exsurpo (exact source of the pain) swollen irritated kidneys.

Slow or poor immune system function: Can be helped and or improved, But AIDS cannot. AIDS (Acquired Immune Deficiency Syndrome) is gradual immune system slow down. When you know the component parts of the immune system (as laid out in this book) you can heal. All of this is really exsurpo liver, kidney overwhelm.

Slow or poor liver function: Can be improved, But Hepatitis, high liver enzymes and or cirrhosis of the liver cannot. Again, these issues are exsurpo liver overwhelm.

To be sick one MUST PARTICIPATE in their demise. Proper treatment does not cause new symptoms. Natural therapies produce healthy bodies which is the reverse of what drugs and surgery are capable of producing.

The body will not become ill unless you personally abet it or help it via ignorance which is a form of enabling. If you fall out of a tree which you climbed of your own free will, the broken arm you now have was by your choice. The best lawyer would not convince a jury that it was the fault of the tree. Who scaled the tree with the weak branch? Was it you? We are responsible for our own condition in life. No one ever said being healthy was fun or easy. Now you have got it.

All organs and systems of the body can be helped if you know who did it, and then name the exsurpo, which leads to the changes you will make.

All liver problems can heal if given the chance. Getting sick is not a signal to call the mortuary; it is a signal to DO SOMETHING ELSE. Because what you have been doing has not worked.

HIV is a harmless virus, which sits quietly inactive in the human body. It causes no known problems. But, since it can be found in a large number of people with weakened immune system function it has been assigned the label "Precursor of AIDS." This is all hogwash.

The reason the above three problems are out of reach for a cure is because the names, which say nothing about the source of the problem, keep them hidden. Since the problem (or disease) is not a thing, but a lifestyle (full of chemicals, preservatives, colorings, sodium, sugar, etc.), the cure is never even suspected.

To summarize:
All so-called diseases, such as AIDS (an immune system weakness) require you to confront the problem without panic and then fight to improve the weakened function. Sitting in fear and waiting for the latest drug to come out is slow suicide. Name the exsurpo (exact source of the pain) and take action.

Actively working to improve your system with diet, herbs and exercise is the right answer. You have never been "gotten" by a disease (label). You had to work hard to earn the condition. When you lift weights, the expected outcome is larger muscles and increased strength.

When you eat junk food, use chemicals, etc., you can expect the body to eventually become sick.

Not a popular point of view, but recognizing that you are actually the source of your problems never is. You are responsible for your condition. You can do something about it. If you chose to climb a poison tree and then fall out with a sickness of some sort, just remember you chose to climb the tree. It is also your choice to FIX YOUR condition.

The biggest and the least of us have the same chance to heal. Life style changes such as those mentioned in the chapter "The Hidden Keys to Weight Loss" and dietary changes such as those mentioned in the chapter "A Diet for a New Century" can change lives. We never just get sick. Anytime we use a disease label we reinforce the idea that these exist rather than simply physical disharmony. Understanding and using the term "physical disharmony" opens the door to healing. The term disease leads to confusion and the reliance on medical doctors selling drugs and surgery.

Using drugs guarantees a murky outcome and an unhealthy future. Poor health and sickness are the results of medical drug use. Just as if you lifted weights you would expect larger muscles and increased strength.

Choose to run your own life and heal yourself. Anything less is paramount to giving up your body and freedom to someone who will ensure that you never get well again.

59 Microbiology vs. the Sales Pitch

"Tell a lie loud enough, and long enough, and the masses will believe it" – Adolph Hitler

Question: What is the difference between?

Cancer	Herpes
Gonorrhea	Polio
Syphilis	Meningitis
AIDS	Tuberculosis
Diabetes	HIV
Chlamydia	

Answer: Gonorrhea, Syphilis, Chlamydia, Herpes, HIV, Polio, Meningitis and Tuberculosis can all be *isolated and seen under a microscope*.
Answer: Cancer, AIDS and Diabetes cannot be isolated and studied with a microscope.

Question: What else do the items on the list above have in common?

Answer: Every item on the record above that can be isolated under a microscope has been controlled. These substances include Gonorrhea, Syphilis, Chlamydia, Herpes, HIV, Polio, Meningitis and Tuberculosis. These entities are no longer mysteries and therefore do not receive hundreds of millions in grant money donated for research.

Answer: Every item on the list above that CANNOT be isolated and seen under a microscope are massive sinkholes for millions of dollars in wasted grant money. The items that are lucrative to research include Diabetes, Cancer and AIDS.

Conclusion: Cancer, Diabetes and AIDS will never be isolated under a microscope, as they do not exist as germs or parasites. They are conditions, brought on by an overwhelmed and toxic immune system. They are enigmas that capture our imagination.

—-Cancer, Diabetes and AIDS are conditions brought on by an overwhelmed and toxic immune system —-

Those seeking lifetime job security could do little better than to pursue shadows, witches, warlocks, AIDS, ghosts, fairies, evil spirits, Cancer, werewolves or Diabetes. These nebulous shadowy entities rivet our attention. These are the nefarious "monsters in the closet" of our youth.

Remember what Greek philosopher Plato said, "Everything that deceives may be said to enchant." We are enchanted with danger, mystery and superhuman evils.

Humans love imagining monsters hiding under the bed. We are enthralled with Stephen King, Jason, Freddy Kruger, Dracula and Chucky the killer doll.

Sequestering imagination from the equation, police work requires good evidence, not rumor, not hearsay. "Modern Medicine" is desperately trying to put the smoking gun into the hands of a killer that does not exist.

Rabid medicos are on a modern day "Witch Hunt" with the requisite ad hoc crazed mobs screaming with blood lust!

Wanted posters are posted everywhere. The hounds are frantically hunting for a trail to follow. Yet every trail keeps leading back to their masters. Unrelenting, the news warns us of terror lurking in every shadow. They tell us there is a monster out to kill us as we sleep! Every moment his relentless stalking brings him one step closer to sinking his teeth into our jugular vein to satiating his terrible thirst.

Few suspect it is actually slow death via poisoning by our own hand. You cannot arrest your murderer, if the murderer is you. Suicide is not glamorous. But invisible monsters are. Until you realize that you invented and fed the invisible fiend, it will never stop

—DISEASE BACTERIUM / PARASITES unseen by a microscope do not exist—

Yet drugs are produced for so-called diseases that cannot be isolated? How can we compose a therapy such as AZT, Radiation or Chemotherapy without knowledge of what we are trying to kill? These drugs and "treatments" are accepted deadly poisons. They work on the premise of differential toxicity.

The concept in "differential toxicity" is that the cure is deadlier than the so-called disease. Ergo, the doctors *hope* that the cure does not kill you. But if it does, your death is blamed on the so-called disease, never the treatment.
Does this make any sense? No!

How anyone can be administered these horrendous poisons and then recover is a testament to our monumental infinite power to heal.

South African deaths attributed to AIDS are factually malnutrition, which facilitates the collapse of the immune system. Not surprising to find malnutrition in the backwoods of a third world country. *Every* South African so-called AIDS case that received proper nourishment **recovered**.

The United States Government does not allocate funds to countries with deaths occurring due to malnourishment. AIDS diagnoses receive sympathy and American cash. Therefore, it behooves third world countries to report AIDS deaths in volume.

Whenever there is a national disaster anywhere in the world, the news media immediately jumps in and electrifies us with death. They pad the body count by attributing all deaths that occur during the calamity to the event, regardless of the actual cause. Fear sells newspapers. Deaths assigned to AIDS sell condoms and furthers the public terror of an invisible enemy.

Because of that, whenever AIDS research asks for money, it gets it.

Is there a conspiracy? Do men in black sneak around abducting citizens, then poisoning / infecting them with dirty injections or viruses? No.

These so-called diseases are actually conditions and all brought on and made worse by:

Roger Bezanis

Sugar	Alcohol
Salt	Hormones (supplemented or added to the
Sodium	food supply)
Drugs (over the counter)	Pesticides
Drugs (illegal)	And a junk food diet

*We are poisoning **ourselves every day***. AIDS, Diabetes and Cancer are getting a mega boost by "Big Fast Food."

What about the dangerous virus, HIV?
Everyone knows that HIV is the precursor to AIDS!

False, completely false! There are thousands of people who are diagnosed with the HIV virus, yet those same people do not develop AIDS. HIV is a dormant actor in the human body. It does not spread, it does not mutate. AIDS is a zero of influence in the human body.

What about how AIDS is spread?
Again, *everyone knows* that sharing needles, anal sex, vaginal sex and blood transfusions spreads AIDS.

Blood Connection

Sharing needles: Those who share needles have compromised immune systems as they are using drugs. Shooting heroin is deadly and destroys the immune system.

Anal Sex: This group (homosexuals) **in the past** used Amyl Nitrate as a recreational drug as well as many others. Previous drug use in this group is clear and not up for debate. All recreational drug use is well known to attack the heart, liver and kidneys. Therefore, anal sex has little or nothing to do with contamination and passage of this so-called disease. Use of cocaine, heroin, barbiturates and alcohol all tear down the system of anyone, regardless of sexual preference.

Vaginal Sex: It is believed that women can pass AIDS via vaginal sex to their boyfriends and husbands, not by kissing or any other method, strictly via intercourse. It is further believed that men can pass AIDS to their girl friends and wives via the same method.

Given that AIDS is **supposed to be passed** via direct blood to blood contact, are we to believe that there really are men and women having sex while simultaneously bleeding from wounds on their genitalia? The answer is emphatically no.

Regarding women, the vaginal cavity and uterus is very tough and some of the strongest, most durable membrane (skin) in the human body. So durable is this area of the body, it actively hosts new life, while withstanding baby kicks, twins, triplets, etc. Clearly the theories on AIDS are full of battleship size holes.

The conclusion is clear. We are being sold condoms, drugs, surgery and fear. Fear makes money. We have not a clue that we are the **sole cause** of our health conditions, good or bad.

Coincidence vs. Good Fortune

What form of contraception was almost out of business until so-called AIDS made it mandatory? That would be the condom. Do you think the boys at Trojan might have a hand in keeping the public fixated on an incurable non-existent disease? Do you think that maybe there is a secret division over there pushing AIDS stories into the news?

Fear not only sells newspapers, it sells condoms.

If we continue to ignore the affects of our diet and chemical lifestyles, we will all be victims. In the gay community, it is far more infrequent to hear about deaths caused by so-called AIDS. Why? The gay community, as a group, righted itself and made a conscious effort to be healthier. Drug use has dwindled while consumption of health food and regular ingestion of supplements has skyrocketed.

If we feed ourselves correctly, use supplements and detox our bodies, we can heal anything and stop chasing witches and warlocks.

We are standing at the precipice with a .44 Magnum clenched between our teeth. Do not pull the trigger. Put the weapon down and get busy improving your health.

Do not be fooled by the fear mongers telling you that little green men are hijacking your health. You control your health.

AMA/APA/FDA Drug Company Think

- You are a commodity of infinite value
- Your health is worthless
- Your sickness is a priceless gold mine
- Your insurance is a treasure chest to be dug up and plundered
- Your free will and ability to think is to be controlled

Roger Bezanis

Drug companies sell drugs via fear, while insurance companies sell fear and surgery. These two nefarious entities (drugs and insurance) want you to believe that every issue of life has a **drug answer** or a **surgery solution**. Once you have accepted this kind of sales pitch, you have given your power away.

Only you can guarantee your future health.

60 The Flu: the SUPER GERM

Flu, by all accounts, is one of the most controversial maladies that man has ever known. It is now widely accepted that the "flu" is the result of a 40 million dollar a year media campaign. We are asked to believe that germs follow a season. Like clockwork, they arrive twice a year in October and March. Between these times they mutate for no apparent reason.

It is the contention of many researchers that the "flu phenomena" is a conglomeration of scare tactics, real pneumonia and stress factors that aid the body in breaking down.

According to the CDC (Center for Disease Control):
The flu constantly changes; it can either mutate and "Antigenic Drift" or "Antigenic Shift" as much as twice a year. Antigenic shift indicates the flu abruptly changes without notice. Antigenic drift indicates it gradually changes.

To understand more about this medical enigma, read what is posted on the (Swiss pharmaceutical giant) Roche-Tamiflu website (below):

Introduced in 1999, Tamiflu is one of the only medicines proven in clinical trials to reduce the duration and severity of avian flu (bird flu) if taken within 48 hours of infection. It can also be used as a vaccine. Currently, the U.S. will have enough doses for 2 percent of the population by 2006. Many European countries have ordered enough to treat 20 percent to 40 percent of their populations. Currently, President Bush is meeting with vaccine manufacturers.

Read that last line again.

Currently, President Bush is meeting with vaccine manufacturers.
Aside from the clear political overtones of the above statement, the CDC indicates that Tamiflu would be obsolete in *"one season."* Yet Tamiflu sells billions in product every year.

Why would the US government get involved with business in the private sector? Why would a sitting president interest himself in the worldwide sales of vaccines? Could it be that vaccine sales support and line the pockets of government officials? Could our government be involved with helping to place lucrative manufacturing contracts into the hands of a favorite few friends and supporters? Finally, is the US government profiteering from flu?

Conspiracy-minded individuals would champion the truth of the above paragraph. If you think it is true, you are not alone. But sane individuals like me know that this sort of behavior would **NEVER** HAPPEN IN WASHINGTON.

George Bush is not getting kickbacks and lining the pockets of friends or supporters with profiteered cash. That would be illegal. No Democrat or Republican president, congressman, governor or mayor would ever do such a thing. Accept tainted money? Bite your tongue. Next you will be insisting that we are in the Middle East solely for oil. That is ridiculous; fighting a covert war for oil? Who would believe such a thing?

FDA Patent Connection
There is tremendous confusion surrounding who and what the FDA is. The Food and Drug Administration is part of "The US Department of Health and Human Services." To be clear, the FDA is a government agency.

All drugs that are sold in the United States, regardless of country of origin must receive an FDA approval patent. This patent insures 7 years of zero competitor competition (no generic knock offs) and allows the paying "customer" an exclusive market. Market protection is vital so that the paying company can recoup its investment.

The FDA 7 year patent costs 800 million dollars and must be paid prior to release of the new drug. In the United States today, even a marginally profitable drug can make over **one billion dollars a year** in sales. Patents are only granted to formulas derived via rigid laboratory process. The approved formula must remain unchanged for the entire 7-year period otherwise the patent is invalid.

The following is a paragraph from FDA NEWS
(http://WWW.FDA.gov/BBS/topics/NEWS/2006/NEW01423.HTML)

This season's approved formulation for the U.S. vaccine is identical to that recommended by both the World Health Organization and FDA's Advisory Committee. The formulation includes one strain that was used in last year's vaccine and two new strains. Seasonal flu vaccines do not protect against avian flu, which is caused by a different viral strain (bird flu).

Notice that last line again: ***Seasonal flu vaccines do not protect against avian flu, which is*** *caused by a different viral strain (bird flu).*

Did you notice while reading earlier, that Roche-Tamiflu is the ONLY drug approved for AVIAN flu (bird flu) and was supported by the Bush administration?

CDC WARNING - Avian Flu - Bird Flu -

The most common type of flu is avian influenza virus. Viruses found chiefly *in birds*, but rarely infectious to humans. The risks are generally low to most people, because the viruses do not usually survive human contact.

Tamiflu is only made for the avian flu and is a patented non-changing formula.
Bird flu is practically unheard of in humans. Why then is Tamiflu #1 produced, and #2 sold the world over?

The 1999 flu season (October-January) marked the arrival of the avian bird flu. Remarkably this event just "happened" to coincide with the October 27th, 1999 release of Tamiflu specifically for, YOU GUESSED IT - **avian bird flu.**

Was the avian flu warning for 1999 leaked to Roche in 1997? Was the avian flu on the FDA/AMA calendar in 1997 for announcement in July 1999? Do the FDA/AMA produce a schedule of upcoming flu's? Many do believe that this schedule does exist and was given to Roche.

Otherwise what kind of business acumen would it require to purchase an 800 million dollar patent for possibly only one year of sales? Tamiflu, based on CDC data, clearly indicates that Tamiflus' bird flu formula is practically useless.

Tamiflu should have been completely obsolete by January 1st, 2000 (four months after it was first marketed). Was the US Government helping Roche? Could we as consumers be brainwashed, uninformed, in fear and blind not to know this?

Again, Roche released its Tamiflu in October 1999, the same month that avian flu arrived.

Regarding the so-called ever-changing face of the flu, how could independent labs create vaccines completely in the dark without a blueprint or a little help? If avian flu is so rare and it shifts or drifts EVERY YEAR, THEN WHAT TAMIFLU IS SELLING IS A WORTHLESS FRAUD.

Keep Selling

The opportunity to make over a billion dollars a year in sales is what keeps Tamiflu on the market.

The business of making flu shots is the fine art of predicting the future or being handed a memo from the AMA / FDA hinting at what to manufacture next. Step two would be producing a non-offensive vaccine that does not poison the end user while making huge profits.

FDA PROTECTION

While under protection of the FDA, complaints are listened to, considered and for all intent and purposes ignored. The FDA "investigates" complaints until the 7-year patent protection phase has passed.

GLOVES OFF AS THE PATIENT EXPIRES

This explains why suddenly (November 27th, 2007) news started leaking out concerning rising deaths (300) while recently using Tamiflu in Japan.

Pay close attention to the dates in the next paragraph, i.e. (October 27th 1999 – November 13th 2006 = 7 years)

On November 13, 2006, the FDA alerted doctors and parents to watch for signs of bizarre behavior in children treated with Tamiflu. This warning was based upon federal health officials noticing an increasing number of such cases from overseas. Tamiflu (generic: oseltamivir phosphate) is prescribed to treat the flu is manufactured by Roche Laboratories, Inc. and was approved for use by the FDA on October 27, 1999.

However, analysts at Morgan Stanley Equity Research have said that Tamiflu is recognized as causing psychological disturbance, and apparent suicidal behavior.

The FDA said the 12 deaths **it** was reviewing included one suicide, four cases of sudden death and four cases of cardiac arrest. There also were single cases of pneumonia, asphyxiation and acute pancreatitis.

The 7-year patent has expired on Tamiflu. Therefore, pay attention as the heat on Tamiflu increases as the FDA's former customer" starts defending its interests. The FDA will now direct all inquires and law suits directly to Roche.

All signs and trails lead back to the Bush administration regarding the success and use of Tamiflu as it was brought to the world and the United States with his ample help. The world is also aware that George W. Bush is no longer president of the US. On January 20th 2009 Barak Obama was sworn into service as the new president of the United States. The result is of course new policies and new alliances. Do not be surprised if new flu drugs become very popular in the next four years. If this is the case the trail may lead right back to Mr. Obama.

Considering what you have just read conspiracy theorists will love what follows. *The Los Angeles Times* reported the following story on February 4th 2009:

Tamiflu no longer works for dominant flu strain

U.S. health officials say almost 100% of the type A H1N1 strain showed resistance to the leading antiviral drug. So far, the influenza season has been mild.
By Mary Engel
February 4, 2009

A milder than usual U.S. flu season is masking a growing concern about widespread resistance to the antiviral drug Tamiflu and what that means for the nation's preparedness in case of a dangerous pandemic flu.

Tamiflu, the most commonly used influenza antiviral and the mainstay of the federal government's emergency drug stockpile, no longer works for the dominant flu strain circulating in much of the country, government officials said Tuesday.

Of samples tested since October, almost 100% of the strain — known as type A H1N1 — showed resistance to Tamiflu.
(LATER IN THE STORY)
Tamiflu and Relenza have been stockpiled by the federal government for treating the public in case of the emergence of a dangerous pandemic flu. Four times as many Tamiflu doses have been stockpiled as Relenza doses.

Some microbiologists have argued that Tamiflu is more likely to develop resistance than Relenza. Therefore, they say, Relenza should make up at least 50% of the stockpiled antivirals....

Beware, take head and have a good sarcastic laugh if in the late 2009 or early 2010 a new Flu drug sweeps the planet and is the world's choice for battling the marketing machine called "The Flu."

The following was found on the MEDSCAPE page found on the internet.

FDA Approvals: Relenza and Eraxis

Release Date: April 6, 2006;
April 6, 2006 — The US Food and Drug Administration (FDA) has approved a new indication for Zanamivir (another name for Relenza) oral inhalation, allowing its use for the prophylaxis of influenza in patients aged 5 years and older; and Anidulafungin infusion for the treatment of candidemia and other forms of Candida infections (intra-abdominal abscess and peritonitis) and esophageal candidiasis.

Candidemia: Bloodstream infection with Candida, a yeast-like fungus. Persons at high risk for candidemia include low-birth-weight babies, surgical patients, and those whose immune systems are deficient.

Anidulafugin is a drug produced by pharmaceutical giant Pfizer. Therefore keep your eye on Pfizer there drug Anidulafugin receives American Presidential support.

Zanamivir for Inhalation (Relenza) to Prevent Influenza in Adults and Children

On March 29, the FDA approved a new indication for orally inhalable zanamivir (Relenza with Diskhaler, made by GlaxoSmithKline, Inc), allowing its use for the prophylaxis of influenza in patients aged 5 years and older.

Reflect on the lessons of this chapter. Tamiflu was approved in 1999 for seven year of patent protection from the FDA. Its protection term ran out in 2007. In preparation two drugs were approved for use on the flu Relenza and Anidulafugin between February and April of 2006.

The omnipotent power of the American Presidency is clear when we examine the fact that Tamiflu was rendered inert by its expiring FDA patent yet it hung around for 16 days after Barak Obama was sworn into office and George W. was back in Texas. This was all finally put to bed when the LA Times reported (above) on the demise of Tamiflu on Feb 4th 2009.

The flu is an amazing mix of history, media hype and lack of personal responsibility for our own wellbeing.

GOVERNMENT CONSPIRACY?

Is the US government behind the flu? Some think that our government is secretly helping to manufacture flu virus and then spreading it around the planet. Is our government behind this? Does the FDA/AMA or some other government agencies have a hand in poisoning the people of earth?

As exciting and Earth shattering as such a conspiracy of this magnitude would be, it is simply not the case. The FDA/AMA and our government do not need such a plan. The necessary factors that make bi-yearly sickness possible are already in place without any covert government help.

FLU GROUND ZERO

To understand the flu you must appreciate its roots. Flu is an astounding story full of mystery and intrigue. How a so called and "imaginary" SUPER GERM would take over the world is fascinating reading.

Influenza, or the Flu, was first noted March 20th, 1918 in the latter part of World War I.

Morning sick call at Camp Funston in Fort Riley, Kansas, was uneventful until soldier Albert Mitchell reported under the weather. By day's end, almost 100 young men had reported sick. Our newly trained "doughboys" were about to ship off for England and an uncertain fate.

IMPORTANT NOTE: Prior to their infirmary, soldiers at Fort Riley were VACCINATED with a **cocktail of bacteria** to protect them against the dangers of Europe. Injections were administered two days before the men became ill, exactly one week before they shipped out. Not surprisingly, vaccinations were never suspected as a venomous contributor to our so-called 1918 flu epidemic.

STRESS CONNECTION

Stress has been accepted as the leading cause of all sickness for the last 40 plus years. Why would these soldiers about to leave for war get sick? Imagine that you were about to go into a conflict that could cost you your life. Would you get sick? Would this be stressful to you? This postulation would mean that stress could make someone unwell regardless of his or her present health.

In 1918, stress was not a consideration in sickness. Today the world of health is a much different and forward thinking place. From MedicineNet.com
David Krantz PhD.
Chairman of the Department of Medical Sciences at the University Bethesda, Maryland

"The link between stress and heart-related problems has been widely studied, and researchers say that mental stress increases the body's demand for oxygen by raising blood pressure and heart rate. For people who already suffer from heart disease, this additional burden can increase the risk of heart attack, stroke, and even death. Stress can also act as a trigger for heart attack or stroke in people with undiagnosed heart disease."

Suzanne Segerstrom, PhD,
Assistant Professor at the University of Kentucky

"What happens is that certain components of the immune system become less effective at fighting off illness, especially those caused by viruses, when exposed to stress over days or weeks. Attitude plays a critical role in tempering that reaction."

"The main principle is that the effect on the immune system is not a factor of what's happening in the environment, but it's an effect of your perception of it. To the degree that you feel threatened or overwhelmed, the immune system will be affected more."

Dr. Segerstrom is saying that the actual threat is not as important as the perceived threat or YOUR reaction to either one. This explains how a whole family can get sick for no reason yet one or two family members are left untouched. The threat of loss or danger due to the "believed threat" of "catching" another's germs is more important than the germ.

To handle stress better, read about the LIVER in chapters 9,10, 11, 12 and 13.

Half of the Americans deaths in WW I are blamed on the flu
WW I lasted from 1914-1918. War claimed 20 – 40 million lives. Yet most flu deaths circa 1.5 million occurred at the end of the war 1918 -1919. Why would the there be so many deaths associated with flu occurring at the end of the conflict? Is there another smoking gun other than flu? Was something else contributing to these sudden deaths?

POISON GAS THREAT OVERLOOKED

American soldiers arriving in Europe were blamed for spreading flu. Little noted (at the time) was the escalating use of caustic poison gases. Even without poison gases, the stresses of war cannot be denied. The 1000-yard stare of soldiers who have been on the front lines too long is one example. Unmanaged stress makes any man sick.

Soldiers on both sides were terrified of the life stealing gas attacks.

World War I Witch Hunt
In search for an explanation for skyrocketing deaths from pulmonary catharsis, the flu was "invented" as an explanation. No one at the time understood the long term affects of chemical warfare on, the human body. Nor did they comprehend the contaminating affects these poisons would wreak on Earth's ecosystem and our food supplies.

The Germans invented Mustard gas and introduced it on the Eastern Front in 1915. It quickly gained prominence and was in regular use by both sides by late 1917. The three types of gasses used were Mustard Gas, Chlorine gas and Phosgene. Both sides viciously employed poison gas attacks. These attacks were unwieldy and relied on the direction of blowing wind. Meaning if the wind shifted your own gas could kill you. But according to statistics, half the Americans who died in WW I died from the flu, not consistent long-term exposure to poison.

The day-to-day threat of daily gas attacks was far worse than the attack.
Another validation of the so-called flu as the wrong source of death was that men age 20-40 were hardest hit. The ages with the strongest immune systems were hardest hit?

Hardly noticed in clouds of war, was the stark fact that even a non-fatal gas attack weakened the immune system. Soldiers and civilians downwind of the attacks were now open to TB, fevers, pneumonia and other respiratory disorders.

Roger Bezanis

Gas Attack Results:

Nausea and vomiting	Blurred vision
High Fever	Heart failure
Diarrhea	Low blood pressure
Coughing	Pulmonary edema (water in the lungs within
Burning sensation in the eyes	2 to 6 hours)
Watery eyes	Coughing up white-pinkish sputum

Notice that the above list matches the accepted model for flu and pneumonia symptoms.

CDC Pneumonia Symptoms

High fever	Nausea
Cough (with white or pinkish sputum)	Vomiting
Shortness of breath	Headache
Rapid breathing	Tiredness
Chest pains	Muscle aches

Why are these symptoms and chemicals relevant? Because these biohazards, released into the atmosphere lingered for months in our water, livestock, farmland (like DDT) and therefore our food supply.

Caustic agents (or gases) store in fatty human tissue and, like LSD, may be released at a later date causing toxicity or death. Just as hormones are changing humans in the 21-century, poison gasses were clearly mutating man in 1918–1919.

Man never wants to blame himself. But our actions clearly caused the so-called flu.

"Flu deaths" were heaviest in the countries where fighting was the most concentrated (the exception is the United States). American cities with high humidity featured the most so-called "flu" deaths. Were these gases traveling in the atmosphere and settling thousands of miles away? We now know that this is exactly what happened.

It has been postulated and then proven that an environment with moist, thick air creates an excellent incubator for reconstituting gasses such as mustard, chlorine and phosgene.

Interestingly, the death rate for 15 to 34-year-olds of influenza and **pneumonia** were 20 times higher in 1918 than in previous years.

Various physicians noted in their writings that patients with seemingly ordinary influenza (then considered "cold like" symptoms) would rapidly "develop the most viscous type of pneumonia that has ever been seen" and "it is simply a struggle for air until they suffocate" Another physician wrote that the influenza patients "died struggling to clear their airways of a blood-tinged froth that sometimes gushed from their nose and mouth."

Again notice chemical symptoms are consistent with so-called flu symptoms and mimics **pneumonia**. Was this early 1918 flu really flu, or a combination of gas attacks and pneumonia brought on the stress of war?

Needless to say, war is an aggressive act. The victor always spells out the terms of surrender. These terms become a further punishment and are often extremely harsh. World War I was no exception as surrender terms would be stern with no quarter given.

The Treaty of Versailles imposed tremendous such hardship on Germany, that she hedged in signing it. The British naval blockade of Germany was not lifted until the treaty was signed **at the end of 1919**. One result was that many German children starved to death. Reparation payments were very steep; the German government was literally broke. The Treaty of Versailles was so harsh; it was blamed as the major reason that Germany started WW II.

ON THE MOVE Refugees and Victims of War
Homeland exodus was rampant during 1918 – 1919. Homeless Chinese, Irish, Japanese, Scotsmen, Australians, Indians, Poles, etc. fled and headed to America.

Stress on the Move
Cramped boats, humidity and a lack of sanitation make for a stressful trip regardless of the final destination. Fearful of these "invaders" the United States "welcomed" these travelers by quarantining them, often without proper medical care. Consequently, many immigrants died before they even left their vessels.

From 1918 through 1945 immigrants looking for streets paved in gold were crowded into little villages in big cities. This is where the term "Little Italy", "China Town" etc., derived from.

Immigrants were blamed with causing the stock market crash, escalating crime, the blurring of American values and the weakening of the American social structure. Mass hysteria over the "unknown" is a flaw that can unhinge any civilization. How does this lead to today's mass hysteria over the flu?

Roger Bezanis

1957-The Hunt for the Smoking Gun.

In 1957 NBC news broke the terrifying story that the Spanish Flu had returned from the dead. It was back from its long 1918 - 1919 hibernation. If you carefully cull through the facts, you too will see there is always an event leading to flu claims. There is always a catastrophic event that leads to stress, which facilitates immune system weakness. What could have happened in 1957 to stress the American public?

Understanding What Led to the 1957 "Boogey Man Flu"

In 1953 the precursor of the IRS (the then Bureau of Internal Revenue) was under attack. Evidence of gross irregularities had surfaced and was front-page news and scandalous. Overwhelmed, the agency teetered on the brink of demise. Sweeping reorganization took place as the TAX MEN hired more agents, were given wide and comprehensive authority and thus became more antagonistic.

The agency renamed itself the **Internal Revenue Service** (IRS).

IRS in Action

TREASURY DIRECTIVE 15-42, of 1956, allowed the IRS via an audit to "collect" up to $500.000.00 in property, business, farms, stocks, paychecks and automobiles while seizing bank accounts and bonds, should the public be found cheating on their taxes.

The IRS Finally had Teeth!

The American public was of course terrified of the new money-eating monster, the IRS. Remember the threat of danger causes the immune system to shut down.

A Very Dangerous Environment Leads to Sickness

Abundant sickness was duly noted by an attentive news media. Suddenly, because the news media said so (and they are never wrong), the "Spanish flu" had risen from the grave to bite the American public again. The Spanish Influenza from 1918 was not dead; it was only hibernating. The Flu phenomenon was front-page news. The public was riveted to their newspapers, TV sets and radios.

The Hunting for "IT"

In a "plot twist" deserving of an Academy Award for "Best Screen Play", a multinational contingency of scientists was dispensed to Spitsbergen, Norway. Their assignment was to exhume mummified bodies buried deep in the permafrost. Victims of the 1918 Spanish flu were to be harvested for their tissue. It was hoped that frozen genetic material could be "revived" and used to defeat a flu monster that could wipe man from the face of the Earth. Stephen King would be proud.

Remember, if the news media says it, it must be true. Consider the power of the pen.

"Print is the sharpest and the strongest weapon of our party" - Joseph Stalin

1957 Flu in England
England was reported to have received the Asian flu, while America had the Spanish flu. How odd.

Additional Odd Data on the 1957 British Flu
6,000 Brits lost their lives due to so-called "flu"
0 Brits lost their lives to pneumonia
0 Deaths from the Cumbria, Nuclear reactor graphite core fire (reactor "melt down")

More 1957 British Nuclear Meltdown
Radioactive waste covered the county side, tainting milk supplies, killing cows and chickens, yet no human deaths were reported or *attributed* to *radiation*.

Death count oddities
Wherever death associated with influenza (a.k.a. flu) is calculated (68,000 in 1957) the flu death totals are always padded with pneumonia deaths. What is the purpose of linking these two seemingly different maladies?

"The death of one man is a tragedy. The death of millions is a statistic" - Joseph Stalin

To Be Truly Deadly and Threatening, Flu Must Come From Great Distance
Russian flu 1978
Hong Kong flu 1997 (chicken flu)
Spanish flu 1918 and 1957
Asian flu 1957

SWINE FLU 1976 (ORIGINATED AT FORT DIX, KANSAS)
The afternoon of February 5th, 1976, 19-year-old army Private David Lewis of Ashley Falls, Ma, entered the army hospital complaining of fatigue. Within 24 hours he was dead. It was

"claimed" that Swine flu killed him. Keep in mind his death somehow became considered an epidemic. Nationwide, private Lewis was the **ONLY DEATH** from swine flu in 1976. Yet **hundreds were reported killed** and seriously injured by **flu inoculations provided by the US government.**

Question: Since more deaths have been caused by adverse vaccine reactions than any other source since 1900, why are we still vaccinating?

Answer: Good question. There are numerous books on the subject, including: *"The Great Bird Flu Hoax: the Truth They Don't Want You to Know about the Next Big Pandemic"* by Joseph Mercola and *"A Shot in the Dark"* by H. Coulter.

Note: The news media supports sponsors who purchase ad time. Like it or not, advertisers influence what we think and do. The public is warned about "The next big THREAT or pandemic." The news, at sponsor request, warns the public that **IF** they are not prepared, they we will suffer grave consequences.

When there is an earthquake the news media does stories on earthquake preparedness. The result is, we PURCHASE bottled water, can goods, flashlights and batteries in large amounts and store them. Grocery stores love the added revenue provided by panic shopping. It is really no different than being warned that Halloween is coming. The difference is that little hungry candy seeking monsters do arrive at your door. Noise of a *possible* flu pandemic is a sales pitch created to instill the most fear possible for the greatest possible capital gain.

We react to what the media says as influenced by its advertisers. When the word "If" is heard, we react as if "If" meant the world had collapsed. "If" is synonymous with fear.

Remember all sickness requires at least one of the stimuli below:

#1 Stress (as stress will weaken the strongest of immune systems)
#2 Sugars
#3 Salts
#4 Sodium

#5 Drugs (over the counter)
#6 Drugs (illegal)
#7 Drugs (prescription)
#8 Alcohols

Our bodies are loaded with enough bacteria that if our immune system shut down right now, we would be dead in a matter of hours. The "SUPER GERM" theory is ridiculous.

We become ill with the seasons due to stresses brought about by changes to our home life, diet, etc. The idea that any branch of government would or could be ready in advance with their "healing" goodies is optimistic and unrealistic.

The flu is a product of an amazing sales campaign, which has taken almost 100 years to fully implement. The flu concept and its remedies do not follow the natural laws of nature or common sense.

The flu has never been identified under a microscope. If you cannot see it and isolate it, it cannot be tested against antidotes. Pneumonia can be seen but flu remains invisible. Flu is a ghost explanation that makes billions every year.

Lies that are commingled with truth are hard to detect. That is why the flu story is so hard to let go. The flu legend is based in history. The flu threat is based on a legend that 1) it exists, and 2) that it mutates twice a year.

Roche - Tamiflu brilliantly capitalized on this empty yet potent legend and is selling strong seven years after it should have been off the market. The flu is one of the best marketing campaigns witnessed less AIDS and cancer.

"Terror marketing" creates petrified automatons that will do whatever they are told. Witness the instant affect of broadcasting the word flu. Suddenly we become hypnotized spending machines grabbing up vaccines in excess of 25 billion dollars a year.

We are allowing our NEWS MEDIA to dictate how we live our lines. We are the victims of a government funded ad machine. Profit based fear spewing marketing is not only affective; it is unstoppable unless we are constantly vigilant against it.

About the flu:

- Marketing—-It is promoted via TV, radio, print media and Internet.
- Marketing—-It arrives in March and stays until April.
- Marketing—-It returns in October and leaves in January.
- Marketing—-Every year it mutates and therefore needs a new vaccine.
- Marketing—-It is always predicted before it arrives.
- Marketing—-Forward thinking scientists somewhere in the world devised a vaccine that will eliminate flu before it exists and ruins our lives.
- Marketing—-The flu vaccine is mass-produced and distributed just in time to ward off the "bug"

Roger Bezanis

October - January

October starts the holiday season, which equals family, shopping frustrations, financial worries, overeating, partying and alcohol. Consider the stress of this bombardment. Is it any wonder why people are sick during the holidays? Halloween = sugar poisoning, Thanksgiving for many, equals family and food stress, Christmas / Hanukah / Kwanzaa, etc., equals financial woes, family woes and general holiday overwhelm. Follow that up with New Years Eve.

March - April

Tax season, which is full of stress over money. We are buried in new tax laws, deadlines, payments, complicated forms and worry. Note April is tax month worldwide.

Worldwide, flu seasons just happen to coincide with the most mentally, physically and financially stressful times of the year.

This is the totality of what flu season is. The CDC keeps stumbling over itself contradicting its own information. Flu vaccines are a joke and potentially dangerous. Stress is the only consistent factor in the so-called flu. If stress is understood and handled, "flu" becomes a non-factor.

Stress is guaranteed to devastate immune function and is underneath all sickness. Notice those around you who never get sick. How is that possible? They will tend to be those who have less stress, handle stress better or take excellent care of themselves or all the above.

Flu is a mindset, not a microbe or virus. Get your stress under control and be healthy. Make your own decisions about your health.

Get active and make sure those around you know what the flu score is. We are up against a multi-billion dollar a year INDUSTRY.

We as a group can fight flu and make the truth known. Only then can the flu myth be eradicated.

If we all work together, it might only take 20 years or so to make "flu season" a memory. Until then our lives are at stake. We have to win this battle. Imagine a future where mention of the flu does not instill fear. Imagine that the word flu makes people laugh at how stupid we were "way back then."

Tell everyone you know what the truth is.

61 What is Fibromyalgia?

Fibromyalgia is another name for a hodgepodge of organ symptoms that have appeared under one umbrella and then called Fibromyalgia.

MedicineNet.com defines it this way:
"Fibromyalgia is a chronic condition causing pain, stiffness and tenderness of the muscles, tendons, and joints. Fibromyalgia is also characterized by restless sleep, awakening feeling tired, fatigue, anxiety, depression and disturbances in bowel function. Fibromyalgia was formerly known as Fibrositis. While Fibromyalgia is one of the most common diseases affecting the muscles, its cause is currently unknown. The painful tissues involved are not accompanied by tissue inflammation. Therefore, despite potentially disabling body pain, patients with Fibromyalgia do not develop body damage or deformity. Fibromyalgia also does not cause damage to internal body organs."

That is a mouthful!

What you have just read is amazingly wrong. Here are the facts. There are two distinctly different forms of Fibromyalgia (both of which are of course not diseases).

• Skin based, where the skin burns, tingles or is numb. This version may be accompanied by restless sleep, awakening feeling tired, fatigue, anxiety, depression, blurry vision, headaches and muscle pain in the right shoulder region.

• Muscle and joint based, where the joints are sore, stiff and tight. The muscles may feel the exact same way. This type of irritation can include left shoulder pain, ankle pain, low back pain and general muscle soreness and stiffness.

These two types of problems, that are now commonly called Fibromyalgia, are actually liver & kidney problems. Yes, you read that right. Fibromyalgia is nothing more than exsurpo liver and kidney overload.

If this so called disease was anything more than a kidney and liver overload, I wouldn't have been able to successfully treat myself twice! Thousands have discovered these simple facts about this oddly named kidney/liver overload problem.

Read over the kidney symptoms & then read over the liver symptoms in the chapter "How to Do Face Reading." As you read it, did you notice that all of the Fibromyalgia symptoms were kidney or liver symptoms?

I have personally experienced both variations of Fibromyalgia; trust me, they are not fun. What I did then was treat myself for liver issues and/or kidney issues and within a week the symptoms were gone.

Mind you, I went hog-wild crazy taking herbs for liver (during one incidence) and kidney herbs another time. I really indulged myself so that if it was possible to beat, I could. I rapidly eliminated these problems both times. Anyone trying to tell you that your symptoms are anything more than kidney and liver symptoms is trying to sell you something.

Don't buy it. You are being lied to. Go out and treat yourself. Please take some time and research herbs for the liver and/or kidney and use them; you will notice a huge difference in a short time if you act vigorously enough.

You can do this; it is very effortless to feel better. Get used to using the word exsurpo to train yourself in finding the real source of all of your problems.

62 Heart Disease and Ear Piercing

The body will try to adapt to any situation. If the left leg is hurt the right leg will bear more weight. When the kidneys are in trouble it is the liver that steps up and takes some of the load and vice versa.

Approximately 5000 years ago the Chinese developed the practice of Acupuncture. The practice has performed miracles for thousands of years. Acupuncture is the practice of using very fine high-grade surgical steel needles to gently pierce and stimulate an energy meridian of the body to bring about a healing.

These pre-sterilized and disposable needles are used "only once." Since your body is a dynamic environment of interrelating and interconnecting networks, it is appropriate to address them as needed. Some people will find great benefit from the subtle and broad changes through this practice. Western science has focused its attention on the obvious networks such as the nervous, circulatory, endocrine and lymphatic systems.

On the other hand, when Acupuncture points are stimulated, they cause an increase in the production of endorphins and simultaneously activate the immune and endocrine systems. Acupuncture can relieve pain and has been used for all maladies. Millions of patients have enjoyed the benefits of Acupuncture and Traditional Chinese Medicine. They report the elimination or reduction of pain, and increase in function, and a greater sense of vitality and well-being. As you have read earlier in this book the ear is the domain of the kidneys and the heart. If you have studied traditional Acupuncture you know that there are far more points on the face than those mentioned earlier.

Isn't it nice when different modalities converge and agree? In late 2004, I started wondering if an Acupuncture point could be destroyed or continually stimulated if punctured via piercing. I took this question to several different Oriental Medicine Doctors (OMD's) and they all agreed that not only is that possible it is factual.

On the face reading chart you have learned that the ears are represented on the upper lip, nose and ear lobes. I then asked, since that is true, does that mean that women with pierced ears are more susceptible to heart disease than men? That was also confirmed. I was buried in e-mails when I returned home. I then wondered if piercing is the culprit. If that were the case, then wouldn't it also be true that ear piercing among men would have been on the rise in the early 1980s and then leveling off and declining since. Ear piercing among men was on a steady climb since 1980 and topped out in 1986.

When I looked into this that was exactly what the numbers showed. The numbers in several studies support my conclusion regarding both men and women. See below.

The American Heart Association reported the following regarding women statistics:

• Cardiovascular Disease (CVD) remains the leading killer of women in the U.S. and the world. CVD kills nearly 500,000 U.S. women each year, claiming more lives than the next seven causes of death combined, including cancer.

Consequently, women's awareness of heart disease has been on the rise. The American Heart Association's first national survey in 1997 found that only 30 percent of women spontaneously listed heart disease as women's leading cause of death, a figure that increased to just 34 percent in the 2000 survey.

In 2003 that figure jumped to 46 percent, a significant leap.

From the BBC, regarding men, latest available figures show that in 2001 there were around 79,800 deaths from cancer and around 79,500 deaths from heart disease in the UK. This compares with 10 years ago, when there were 84,250 male deaths from cancer and 100,600 from heart disease.

It is estimated that by 2010, deaths from heart disease in UK men will have fallen to 30,000 while there will be 85,000 men dying from cancer. Perhaps there is another unknown reason for all of this heart disease. In the end, if you can reduce your risk it is far safer and healthier.

Roger Bezanis

Diagnostic Face Reading and Acupuncture both agree that constant meridian point stimulation is not healthy. If this were a healthy activity, Acupuncture would have given us this information 5000 years ago. Also, remember, my research indicates that each impaired ear lobe indicates a 30% increase in heart issue tendencies.

Eyebrow piercing is swelling in popularity. We know that the eyebrow represents the lower part of the bladder; does that mean that bladder issues will mount as eyebrow piercing gains in popularity?

Yes, that is exactly what it means.

Therefore, if you have piercings and continue to put them in, you do this at your own risk.

Eyebrow piercing has become extremely popular among young woman. Statistics illustrate that there is a direct connection between bladder infections and eyebrow piercings. In the past 10 years bladder infections among women have increase exponentially. These maladies are blamed on lack of cleanliness, Candida, unprotected sex and myriad of other reasons. Until we start paying attention to piercings we will not find the true smoking gun.

Fact: Data reveals that 8 million women a year visit their doctors for the treatment for a urinary tract / bladder infection. If you compare male and females statistics women suffer these infections four and a half times more often than men.

Fact: Eyebrow piercing is a female dominated phenomenon.

Remember, the bladder meridian (via face reading) intersects across both eyebrows. Does that mean that bladder issues will continue to rise if eyebrow piercings continue to escalate in popularity? Yes, as stated above, that is **precisely** what it means.

What about nose piercing? When we pierce our nostrils we are irritating the heart meridian and therefore creating heart arrhythmia. Regarding tongue piercing there are a number of conflicting ideas. Depending on the placement of the piercing it can interfere with the lungs, heart or digestive tract.

I was working with a young woman who attended one of my seminars. She had been constipated for five years. If she did not take large doses of an herbal colon formula she would be not have eliminations for two to three weeks. I noticed that she had a tongue piercing and explained how it could be interfering with her digestive tract. She indicated that within days of getting her piercing she became constipated five years ago.

I begged her to take it out. Three weeks later she finally complied and took it out. Her constipation was eradicated 48 hours later. She has not been constipated since.

Destroying any meridian with piercings guarantees to put tremendous strain on the body.

The evidence damming tongue piercings is present at every turn. Tongue rings clearly torment the stomach and digestive tract. How important to the body is the tongue? When a piercing is taken out the tongue heals itself in hours. As little as two hours after the tongue piercing is removed; the hole is healed. The speed that a body part heals is an indication of how important it is to the survival of overall organism.

I have studied dozens of tongue piercings and all of them have led to vomiting, constipation, ulcers and varying degrees of sickness.

The location of piercings does not matter. Wherever they are placed they are interfering with the flow of energy in the body. When we see tracks of piercings along the outside of the ear we can expect kidney issues. Nose piercings irritate the heart. Bottom lip piercings aggravate the reproductive system. Piercings below the nose and above the upper lip (simulating a beauty mark) confound the heart.

Belly button rings interfere with the kidneys and reproductive system. Consequently there is much empirical evidence linking these types of abdominal jewelry with pregnancy havoc and sexual malfunction for the wearer.

Many people have asked me if clip on ear rings are healthier than piercings. The fact is that I have not fully investigated them yet but we all know about the cousin to acupuncture, acupressure. Acupressure is well known to increase circulation and healing in a body needing repair. The hands are well known as amazing instruments of healing. This is not debatable as we know that massage and all of its "touch" variations including Reiki healing change the state of the body.

With these salient points at hand (no pun intended) it is not healthful to wear clip on earrings or do any piercings whatsoever.

Pierce and clip on at your own risk.

63 Pressure and the Body

Consider that every organ of your body hates pressure. That is a strange statement, is it not? Think about it. What does it take for a bullet to pierce your skin? High velocity = pressure! The body is fairly safe from anything that cannot in some way exert pressure or move rapidly. Do this simple test. With your right hand squeeze your left hand until it hurts. Why did it hurt? Pressure!

Pressure equals pain. Remember in the explanation of Quantum Physics? Energy and mass must be in equal amounts or one is pushing hard on the other. This is pain and this is pressure. Why does a Chiropractic adjustment work? The bone is putting pressure on nerves and surrounding organs. The energy flow is interrupted and we feel pain.

This sounds too simple to be true. But the body in all of its complexity is very simple. Screwing it up requires our participation in misunderstanding its simplicity and trying to make it complex. Consider this, what is blood pressure? Answer: The pressure needed to move blood from one point to another. When blood pressure is high, it indicates that the kidneys are being pushed "offline." Offline, meaning: not in charge of their own actions or processes. What weakens the kidneys? Pressure they don't create.

One way we pressure-damage our kidneys is by sleeping in the wrong position.

When we sleep flat on our back the pressure of the body is equalized from organ to organ. When you feel full from a meal it is due to the exact same pressure phenomena. This also explains why going to bed on a full stomach is difficult for your body as extra pressure is now being exerted on your vital organs.

Have you ever seen a man lay on a bed of nails? The reason he is not hurt is due to the fact that his weight is distributed evenly over the entire bed of nails not just one.

When we slumber lying down, the more surface area that we can distribute weight over, the more healthfully we will sleep.

When we sleep either on our right or left side, pressure is not equalized.

The pressure exerted by the body compressing or squashing down on the side that you are sleeping on (next to your sheets) is excruciating. This can be witnessed via increased blood pressure on the side that is down. Based on hundreds of tests, the side that is down will have blood pressure as much as 70% higher than the side that is up. If you sleep on your left side you are crushing your left kidney and corresponding organs.

To sleep on the other side creates problems for those organs. Better break out your anatomy book to see what you have been doing.

The increase in blood pressure can reach 200 / 155. The side that is not down will have normal blood pressure (120 / 80 or so).

Imagine squeezing your left thumb until it turned blue and went numb. That is what we are doing by Sleeping on one side or the other rather than flat on our back.

How long does it take for blood pressure to rise while sleeping or lying on your side? Answer: 30 – 60 seconds!

Even the New England Journal of Medicine recognizes that blood pressure should be taken while standing or laying flat. Sorry to scare you, but, the above is true. If you sleep on your side for any length of time you are doing damage to the organs on the down side. This news is a real problem for couples who love to spoon (sleeping on their side while touching front to back). Regardless of age, lifestyle, gender, race or size, the results are always the same.

When your eyes drift shut
Sleep not on your front, left or right
Sleep flat on your back
And deliver your body from its plight.

Sleeping flat on your back is healthy. You can sleep your way back to kidney health!

A special note on flying

Flying a minimum of 150,000 miles a year for almost 20 years, some might think that I know a few things about flying. Experiencing turbulence, hard landings, cramped seating and airborne sleep are all common and almost expected. Like many of us, I have lost luggage and detest long lines snaking through security. The privilege of flying comes with these accouterments.

Most people have no clue why they feel so poorly throughout their body when they fly. The following succinctly explains what is causing these phenomena. Unless you live in Denver, Colorado or Mexico City , you ill equipped to the high altitude of flight. These cities rise above a mile above sea level.

Airline cabins are pressurized to 8000 feet of elevation. Meaning that when you fly, you are experiencing pressure (remember the last section on kidneys and pressure?) 7 to 8 times greater than what you are used to. The results are a lack of energy, muscle pain, joint pain, heart arrhythmia, vertigo, frequent urination (or no urination at all) and decreased hearing. What do the airlines feed you? Salty nuts, salty crackers, sweet cookies and alcohol! All of this is very detrimental to the kidneys.

Yummy! All poisons at sea level! Ingesting them while flying is like receiving "kidney punches" (punches to the kidneys, also known as "rabbit punches," now illegal in pro boxing). Now you know why you feel so bad on arrival. When you fly, drink lots of water, and if you have to eat, bring fruit (ideally grapes), the body you save will be your own.

When flying, be sure that your liver and kidneys are functioning at optimum capacity. Alcohol may seem like a fun treat or a good way to relax while in the air. But is a false promise. The effects of alcohol are even more severe while flying. Alcohol is a poison. Do not involve yourself with this toxic substance while flying. If you do, you are more susceptible to liver and kidney damage while traveling. Your flight / vacation experience can become a disaster.

No one disputes that the FDA is based on bribes and corruption. If an honest FDA received an appeal to approve alcohol for human consumption today, it would be flatly denied. All alcoholic beverages would be labeled poisons.

64 The Truth About Alcohol

No one disputes the fact that the FDA business model has no interest in your welfare and is based on bribes and corruption. Not surprisingly, if the FDA was asked to approve alcohol on its merits today it would be labeled a solvent and flatly denied.

Alcohol not only has light solvent attributes, it acts as a preservative similar to formaldehyde. This is the derivative of the phrase "You are pickling your liver with that stuff." It is known to erode the stomach lining and paralyzes sensitive tissues on contact. Some believe that alcohol would be better if labeled "for industrial use only."

These strange and popular elixirs have acquired slang names such as booze, sauce, brewskis, hooch, hard stuff and juice. Regardless of the name, the damaging effects on the body do not mitigate. Freedom of choice and freedom in personal destruction are protected by our laws unless they draw too much attention or create too much of a mess. Laws pertaining to alcohol are not meant to prevent its use but to keep the noise created by it damage down to a dull roar.

Every year, more money is spent promoting the use of alcohol than any other product. Perhaps through its elaborate and creative marketing, the most basic, yet important facts about alcohol are entirely overlooked or ignored. Alcohol at all levels is a drug and a poison. Without question it is the most commonly used and widely abused psychoactive drug / poison in the world today.

Alcohol is blamed for 100,000 deaths each year.

5% of all deaths from diseases of the circulatory system are attributed to alcohol.

15% of all deaths from diseases of the respiratory system are attributed to alcohol.

30% of all deaths from accidents caused by fire and flames are attributed to alcohol.

30% of all accidental drowning are attributed to alcohol.

30% of all suicides are attributed to alcohol.

40% of all deaths due to accidental falls are attributed to alcohol.

45% of all deaths in automobile accidents are attributed to alcohol.

60% of all homicides are attributed to alcohol.

Drinking coffee or taking stimulants do not assist a drunk person in sobering up. The result is a wired drunk person. Only time can sober up a person, not black coffee, cold showers, exercise, or any other common "cures." Alcohol leaves the body of virtually everyone at a constant rate of about .015 percent of blood alcohol content (BAC) per hour.

Thus, a person with a BAC of .015 would be completely sober in an hour while a person with a BAC of ten times that (.15) would require 10 hours to become completely sober. This is true regardless of sex, age, weight and similar factors.

The best treatment for alcohol is not to drink. If it was not such a mega money maker, alcohol would have been banned long ago. In the old west it was almost a joke what alcohol was and was doing to the body.

In a dusty yet bustling mining town like Deadwood, a filthy and tired miner would ride into town. Stumbling off his horse he would saunter into the Gem Variety Theatre and Saloon where he would be met by Al Swearengen, who would direct him to the bar. There a burly bartender would ask the immortal words "What's your poison?" The frontier mixologist would then pour the poor sap a watered down drink cut with a solvent. Hours later if he could still stand, our Levi wearing gold digger would slither out to his pony.

Today we dress a little nicer and we likely drink exactly what we think we are being served, however, when we leave we seat belt ourselves into a 3000 pound gasoline burning-missile capable of taking out an entire crowd if we lose control.

Roger Bezanis

Alcohol impaired drivers kill a new victim every 30 minutes, nearly 50 people a day and almost 18,000 people a year. In the U.S., the annual indirect alcohol related death tolls soar above 82,000 people. Indirect causes of death include cirrhosis of the liver, falls, cancer and stroke. If we include complications of the kidney and heart (caused by alcohol) the numbers jump above 250,000 deaths per year!

Traffic fatalities are the single greatest cause of loss of life for persons 6-33 years of age. About 45% of these totals involve alcohol. Underage drinking costs the United States more than $58 billion dollars annually. If this money was used constructively it would purchase every public school student a new computer once a year.

Young people (under 20) claim that their frequency of alcohol (which is a drug) use exceeds marijuana and cocaine use combined. Not surprisingly alcohol kills 6 times more young people that all other illicit drugs. Every 30 days, 50% of high school seniors dink while 32% report being drunk at school at least once a month.

Problem drinkers average four times more days in the hospital than non drinkers. This FDA sanctioned drug kills six times more youth than all other illicit drugs combined.

The example you set at home is being programmed into your children. You are setting a standard that may be emulated by your children. Many try to justify drinking by standing behind bible verse or teachings. They will site that Jesus and others drank wine.

The fact is that wine from over 2000 years ago had an alcohol content of about 1% versus the 11.5 to 17% of today's wine. The fact is that safe drinking water was practically nonexistent in much of ancient times in Egypt and the Middle East. The Nile was a washing machine, bathtub, sewage facility, boating channel and finally a water supply depot. Water was not safe to drink as it was full of filth, therefore it makes sense why beer and wine was consumed so readily.

No one is disputing the authenticity of any religious texts, but the Earth has changed much since the time of the bible. Some of God's creations can no longer be safely eaten. Such as fish. Today's fish is laden with mercury, acetone, benzene, dry cleaning solvents and other chemicals. The damage to our seas is now so bad that we are being issued government warnings. Mercury levels are so high in our seas we are issued warning not to eat Tuna.

Alcohol had a purpose 2000 years ago as a safer avenue than water. Today our water can be rendered safe easily. Our needs have changed as our problems have changed. Today water is safe to drink and therefore the germ free safety of beer and wine is superfluous to the human condition.

Short Term / Immediate Effects:

Even at small amounts, alcohol significantly impairs the judgment and coordination required to drive a car or operate machinery safely.

Low to moderate consumption of alcohol (1 - 2 drinks week) can also increase the incidence of a variety of aggressive acts, including domestic violence and child abuse.

Moderate alcohol intake (2 - 4 drinks a week) includes dizziness and talkativeness. The immediate effects of a larger amount of alcohol include slurred speech, disturbed sleep, nausea, and vomiting.

"Hangovers" are another effect after large amounts of alcohol are consumed — symptoms including headache, nausea, thirst, dizziness, and fatigue.

Heavy alcohol consumption (5 or more drinks a week) can cause death or at the least addiction (alcoholism).

Sudden cessation of long term, extensive alcohol intake is likely to produce withdrawal symptoms, including severe anxiety, tremors, hallucinations, and convulsions. Alcohol causes permanent damage to vital organs, several different types of cancer, gastrointestinal irritations, such as nausea, diarrhea and ulcers.

Daily consumption of alcohol leads to malnutrition and nutritional deficiencies. A regular drinker literally begins to starve.

Other effects: sexual dysfunctions, high blood pressure and lowered immune system function.

Mothers who drink alcohol during pregnancy may give birth to infants with fetal alcohol syndrome. These infants may suffer from mental retardation and other irreversible physical abnormalities.

In addition, research indicates that children of alcoholic parents are at greater risk than other children of becoming alcoholics.

In the end what you put in your body is your choice. Like it or not you are a role model and your choices may become the choices of your children.

There are no non role models. Therefore let's all set a good example.

Roger Bezanis

65 Grapes and Your Kidneys

There are foods that are remarkably credible for healing the body..

One of them is a grape. The organs that love them are your kidneys. That is correct, they LOVE grapes. You can heal more problems of the kidneys by eating grapes than with most supplements.

I have been using grapes this way for everything under the sun in regards to kidney issues, including diabetes and high blood pressure with excellent results. For the past 8 years, grapes have proven themselves as effective as any herb or therapy. My testing indicates the following fruit and vegetables are amazing at correcting kidney issues of all types;

-Grapes in general = The best aid for the kidneys

-Light grapes = Mild kidney repair

-Dark grapes = Intense kidney issues

-Tomatoes = General kidney health and reproductive system tonic

-Cinnamon = Intense kidney issues and diabetic symptoms

-Mango = Powerful aid to the kidneys

-Water melon = Excellent for soothing irritation

-Fresh cranberries = If eaten fresh help break down stones

-Coconut water = Terrific aid in assisting the kidneys in filtering.

-Radishes = Open up circulation in the kidneys

-Cucumber = Increases energy in the kidneys

-Onion = Powerful blood cleanser

The power of grapes is beyond reproach. They far exceed the power to heal even when compared to the list above. If you focus on eating grapes do not be timid about process, just eat them fresh. Organic produce makes a huge difference. But do not let the lack of available organic produce stop you from eating grapes and other fresh produce. The key is to eat a least 3-5 servings of fresh produce every day.

If you cannot buy organic produce, use a pesticide "removal wash" to clean off any residue. What does matter is that they are eaten often (3-4-5 times a day). Anyone with sore joints, regardless of the reason, needs to indulge in these little green, red, black and purple wonders.

The only type of grape that does not work is any grape that is fermented (wine). Raisins show no benefit at all as they are not live. Go back and study what the kidneys need and you will see what kinds of issues the eating of grapes can solve.

As stated above, I suggest eating grapes 3 to 5 times a day or as often as you have symptoms. Remember that food is the oldest and safest drug on the planet. Mother Nature made no mistakes and intended for us to utilize it. When we ignore it, we pay in pain and discomfort. Even Vertigo (dizziness) has been aided with use of grapes as the kidneys regulate the ears and the inner ear regulates your balance.

Poor kidney function as well as liver function can interfere with our sleep. Keeping grapes at your bedside might be more important than water. When you wake up, eat a few grapes and you will be back to sleep in no time.

The next time you notice that you have low back pain, knee pain, ankle pain, wrist pain, finger pain or left shoulder pain, pick up three (3) grapes and hold them in your left hand. Now notice the pain again and see if the sensation in the joint is not reduced. I invite you to read the chapter on Quantum Physics and also the Energy Balancing Technique as these chapters explain the phenomena.

The healing power of grapes is beyond compare. Eat them often.

What Does Fresh Fruit Mean?

Fresh fruit or fresh vegetables are defined as recently picked and alive.

Fresh fruit seeds can be planted and will grow. The enzymes of fresh fruit break down and will cause fruit to rot if not eaten in a timely manner. This is nature cleaning and fertilizing itself, guaranteeing its future.

I am often asked about eating trail mix that has fruit added. The fruit in such a mix is no longer whole and no longer enzymatic or alive. This type of fruit is worthless to the body.

As mentioned before, raisins are not alive and if planted would not grow or produce new grapes. Fresh means fresh. Sealed bags of mango are not fresh. Fresh fruit needs air and goes bad in a few days of purchase if not eaten.

Fruit or veggies that are dried, pressed or in air-tight sealed bags are not fit for consumption. Is this making sense now? If you are going to eat fruit or vegetables, eat them fresh, not out of a can, sealed bag or box.

66 Sexual function

As stated earlier in this book, the kidneys regulate the entire reproductive process, including sexual performance, pleasure and fertility.

One of the many functions of the kidneys and the liver is to break down and then wash excess protein from the system. Both organs swell when too much protein is present. The question is how much protein is too much? When you eat a bite or two of some type of meat or nut protein and notice that you feel low back pain or pain in general, you have just discovered your limit.

If you remember the earlier chapters on kidneys, I wrote that protein poisoning of the kidneys could bring them and the body to a halt. Kidney overwhelm / poisoning is real and happens every day.

How did we become a nation of beef / meat / nut eaters? Like all advancements, it was advertising.

Prior to WWII, meat was more of a luxury. Since 1945, beef and chicken lobbyist have become very aggressive. The result is the public would soon be eating more of their goods. Looking at supporting kidney issues, the result of excess protein in the diet skyrocketed since 1947.

If you are old enough, you remember the 1960s and the 1968 "threatened" beef shortage. People were actually eating canned dog food. The big news from this time period was that "one table spoon full of peanut butter contained more protein than an 8 ounce steak."

Nuts (also known as legumes) are the most concentrated form of protein we can eat. Nuts are the protein equivalent of the atomic bomb. For instant protein, nuts are very potent.

How could this be a problem? How could there be a problem in the fact that there is more protein in a handful of nuts than there is in the equivalent amount of beef, chicken and fish. But there is!

The result was simple. People were living on nuts. They were suddenly eating 400-1000 times more protein than they needed. Beaten up and overwhelmed, weakened kidneys do not run well.

My testing has proven again and again that kidney health can be greatly improved by monitoring protein intake. Today everyone's kidneys are weak and protein is a huge irritant.

The public, not knowing this and hearing the advertising, eat more and more protein. The result is more back pain, frequent urination and all of the other kidney symptoms, plus the new hitherto unseen problem, sexual malfunction.

The kidneys regulate the entire reproductive system of both sexes.

They can't do the job of protecting and cleaning your blood if they are off line. Protein pushes them off line and into slower response time. Thanks to protein, your reproductive organs are taking a massive hit.

Remember this all started in the late 1960s. Then protein heavy weight loss diets became all the rage in the early 1980s. By 1987, Viagra had appeared as a result of "erectile dysfunction," which did not exist in large numbers prior to 1980.

Do you follow what happened?

    We poison our kidneys for 6 years

    We notice erectile dysfunction

    We start taking the NEW drug designed for the problem.

Interestingly, when women are fed a diet high in protein from nuts, they have the same problems men do.

    Lack of interest

    Lack of lubrication

    Lack of orgasm

Like it or not, we have eaten our kidneys right into a corner. In our western pursuit of protein, we eat nuts on top of the meat we eat and add nut butters to that.

Another interesting aspect of any addiction to poison is that we will crave it regardless of the outcome. The human body always craves what it is most toxic to.

Why would your body crave something that is poisoning it? In the case of the kidney, that is very simple. The body does need some protein, but when the kidneys are not operating at capacity, the body keeps asking for protein that cannot be digested. Imagine being thirsty yet only able to splash your face with water. Water would keep being asked for, as your thirst will not quench.

The question becomes: where does protein come from? I will cover this at more length in the section on raw food. All fruit and vegetables have a trace amount of protein in them. To heal the kidneys a protein fast is an excellent idea.

Fad protein rich diets will continue to cause a further rise of erectile dysfunction. Go on the net and you will see for yourself that the fad protein craze matches the rise in products for erectile dysfunction.

Avoid all nuts including:

Pistachios	Sunflower seeds
Almonds	Sesame seeds
Pine nuts	Brazil nuts
Pumpkin Seeds	Walnuts
Peanuts	Etc.
Cashews	

The type of nut does not matter: raw, roasted, fried or any other variation that you can imagine. Let your body be your guide. Eliminate nuts and you notice the difference.

Find herbs and herbal combinations from the list of herbs for kidney and liver and start testing. You will be pleased with your results. Relax; you will be fine. Just clean up your diet.

67 Magnesium

Most of us have heard something about magnesium. Perhaps it was in combination with calcium. Perhaps you have taken or remember Milk of Magnesia. You may have taken magnesium in many forms but it is what it does that is important.

When people hear the term Osteoporosis they think of bones breaking due to lack of calcium.

This is again all thanks to advertising. Could the "powers that be" want you needing hip surgery by giving you bad advice? Did you know that using calcium by itself does just that, make bones brittle?

Perhaps they think of an old man hobbling around on a cane and falling and breaking his hip. Either way, the pictures that come up are not attractive. How would you feel if your house burned down after you had spent most of the day fighting the fire?

You fought the blaze with every bit of courage and determination you had. You stood there staring down flames that nipped at your ankles but nothing you did worked. You even used a heavy-duty fire hose and yet at the end of the afternoon your house was reduced to ash. So what exactly happened?

As mentioned above, bones are like the ashes of your house and the calcium is like the gasoline you were pouring on the fire that you thought was water.

Yes, it turned out you were using a hose that was pumping only gasoline.

You were trying to put out a fire with gasoline! You were pouring explosive fuel on your fire and expecting to put it out.

This sounds ludicrous, does it not? Consuming gasoline instead of water? The terrible, sad and tragic thing about this made up story is that it happens every day. Calcium when consumed alone, destroys bone. People try to keep their bones from deteriorating but what they are using is causing more damage.

As a public, Americans are preached to on a daily basis. It is now accepted that TV has a hypnotic effect on humans. You are being brainwashed every night and do not notice. We are told to take calcium supplements to prevent bone loss.

If you don't take magnesium with calcium in a ratio of 1 to 1, the body will use its own magnesium to break down the calcium.

Yes, magnesium is the tool or the element / mineral that breaks down calcium.

Where do you think that magnesium is stored in the body?

Is it in the: A) Liver? B) Bones? C) Kidneys? D) Brain? E) Muscle?

Did you say B, the bones?

If you did, you are right. When magnesium is leached from the bones for any reason, the bones become brittle and are prone to breakage at any age. Magnesium is the answer to brittle bones. Again, your bones become weak and brittle when you take calcium because the body now must use its own magnesium to break down this rogue calcium. Therefore, supplementing calcium without equal amounts of magnesium is dangerous and at the least not healthy.

On the other hand, magnesium is vital at any age. After oxygen and water, magnesium is clearly the most important element to the body other than food. Magnesium is involved in close to 400 different body processes. When magnesium is eroded away, or leached from the body, the body starts weakening in the following areas:

Energy   Kidney function
Digestion   Adrenal function
Muscle function   Brain function
Bone formation   Immune function
Cell health   Bladder function
Heart function   Nervous system

The following substances rob the body of magnesium, some of which will not surprise you, as I have been preaching their evils throughout this book.

They are:

Sugar   Diuretics
Salt (added to food)   Sodium
Drugs   Fast foods
Tobacco   High calcium
Distilled water   Antacids
Caffeine   Alcohol

The elements listed here are just deadly to the body. Research indicates that 95 % of the American public is deficient in magnesium. To be sure your magnesium is being assimilated, use a form that dissolves in water. If you take magnesium tablets, you are now dependant on systems of the body that may be weak. To ensure absorption use a mix that dissolves in water.

I could list all of the problems that are improved when magnesium is used correctly. If I did, I would fill the next 3 pages. It would be hard to come up with a single body process that is not enhanced by use of magnesium.

Please look magnesium up on the web. Go to your favorite search engine and type in magnesium and read a few pages on it. Magnesium is remarkably well documented again and again. You will be shocked and wonder why I didn't include more of it here.

Be smart and use magnesium correctly and never, ever use calcium by itself.

68 Sports Injuries

Watching sporting events has been one of man's favorite pastimes since he invented competitive trials thousands of years ago. Injuries are par for the course as bodies smashing into bodies do break.

Yet there is something very interesting in the injuries we have today as opposed to 50 years ago. In one study it was reported that injuries in pro sport increased by 33% between 1991 and 1999.

Aberration: Professional baseball has more hamstring and knee injuries than football, soccer, hockey or basketball. At a much slower pace and as a non-contact sport, how can such data be true? Yet it is without reservation clearly the case.

Football features lethal career-ending injuries such as shattered bones, the never-ending concussion, patella tendon blowouts, medial collateral ligament (MCL) and the anterior cruciate ligament (ACL) ruptures.

Yet knee, leg and joint injuries are most common in the comparatively docile sport of baseball. No other sport creates the nagging injuries of baseball.

Basketball, by the numbers, is a safer sport than baseball yet far more violent. Football is off the scale with brutal collisions. Yes football players do play with incredible pain, but they stop when they cannot walk. Why then are football players somehow immune to baseball-like injuries? What is at work here?

Is it diet related? Is it lack of conditioning? In comparison to basketball, the frequency of baseball injuries is shocking. The game of hoops involves constant movement and pounding, yet muscle pulls/injuries do not occur nearly as frequently. Why then are there so many hamstring injuries in baseball?

The answer seems to be one of bad habits. Certain activities separate a large percentage of baseball players from players in other sports.

The terrible trio is chewing tobacco, sunflower seeds and Gatorade.

Before you bust a gut laughing yourself to death, consider this. All muscles need fluid in continual circulation to run properly. Pain equals the absence of circulation, oxygen and energy.

What does salt, sodium, sugar, excess protein and Nicotine all do? They shut down the kidneys. They also shut down the body's washing machine, the liver. When waste is not moved, it becomes solid and causes havoc. Suddenly knee cartilage shreds. Muscles tear or are pulled and damaged. Scenarios like this are common where fluid is not free to wash the system free of waste.

The cocktail of the above items is a promise of disaster.

Roger Bezanis

Gatorade's own website spells out their formula for doom: water, **sucrose syrup, glucose-fructose syrup,** citric acid, natural and artificial flavors, **salt, sodium citrate,** monopotassium phosphate, ester gum, **sucrose acetate isobutyrate,** red 40, blue 1). This yummy concoction is practically a 100% guarantee of KIDNEY and LIVER TROUBLE.

What sport features all of these irritants being ingested during the playing of that sport?

Baseball and baseball alone, is the sole owner of these insults to kidney and liver health.

Toxic kidneys cannot wash the system free of lactic acid and uric acid, the byproducts of physical activity. You already know that the kidneys monitor your joints, tendons and ligaments. Weak kidneys equal weak muscles equal appalling injuries.

A toxic liver cannot wash the waste accumulating via the kidneys and remains stagnant, preventing any inner-body cleansing at all.

Pro basketball, football, soccer or hockey players do nor use chewing tobacco, eat sunflower seeds and guzzle sports drinks during a game.

Yet Gatorade is part of other sports too. I am certain that if those "sports drinks" were replaced with water, we would reduce injuries across the boards.

Chewing tobacco is an aberration all to itself, found almost entirely in baseball. Considering the earlier segments of this chapter, it is no stretch at all to conclude that what goes in the mouth is more involved in physical performance than anyone ever dreamed of possible.

Remember, pain is the precursor to damage, and is caused by the interruption of oxygen, energy and circulation to any part of the body. Electrical impulses cannot move through a massy or junked up joint or muscle.

Nicotine, sugar, sodium, salt and excess protein are all factors weakening the kidneys and therefore weaken strength, endurance and recovery time.

Pain is the absence of circulation, oxygen and energy. Do not interrupt it or **you will feel the pain.**

69 Clear-Cut Answers

This chapter is devoted to a collection of data that has much use but is not dense enough to warrant its own chapter. Year after year I am asked the same questions again and again. Here is the data you will be asking for.

Stated much earlier, the body signals you as to what it wants and needs. Every pain or signal is a request for action. You job is to identify the exsurpo and aid your body correctly.

What you do with those signals will absolutely determine how well you live and enjoy your life.

Right Elbow Pain

Your right elbow and upper right forearm indicate the health of only one part of the body. These symptoms are indicators of one organ or an entire system interruption. It is also very reliable.

Right elbow pain, stiffness or right elbow joint crepitus (crunchy joints) indicate:

- Digestive disturbance
- Stomach issues
- Colon issues
- Intestinal issues
- Liver issues (this is the exsurpo = exact- source-of pain)

This can be further defined as acid reflux, indigestion, heartburn, acid indigestion, ulcers, parasites, stomach irritation and bloating.

The above problem(s) will lead to the symptoms:

Symptom: Right elbow soreness or pain. The right elbow is a reflex pain point for the digestive tract.

Symptom: You may occasionally feel pain directly in the stomach, intestines or colon.

Symptom: You may feel no symptoms in the stomach and only feel irritation in the elbow. When you correctly treat your digestive system, pain localized in the elbow decreases.

When you feel these symptoms, address them by treating your stomach with citrus or an herbal. Your stomach will immediately show change unless the disturbance is caused by H. Pylori. If it is H. Pylori, Goldenseal or Echinacea will make an immediate change.

The condition brought on by H. Pylori is similar to ingestion. You may have heartburn or even acid reflux. But unlike indigestion it does not react the same way and is therefore not treated by the same methods. H. Pylori bacterium is caused by a microbe overgrowth that has seized a foothold somewhere in the colon. It can be successfully combated with light to moderate herbal antibiotics such as those mentioned at the end of the last paragraph. Results in handling H. Pylori microbes are often seen in less than 24 hours.

Itchy Face or Dry Face

An itch or dry patch on the face corresponds to the organ associated with that region of the face.

As the face is dominated by the liver or the kidneys, these factors are also either liver or kidney issues.

The next time you have an itch, try drinking some water or take an herb or formula that you know (via your own testing) is fantastic for the function of the organ asking for help. You will be amazed at what happens. This is not a cute parlor trick or hocus-pocus. It is simply the direct response to a direct communication, directly from your body to you, and the correct response back to it. Remember finding the exsurpo is the key.

•• Every itch, from your neck down (not including your face) is your LIVER asking for help.
•• Every itch of your scalp is your BLADDER / KIDNEYS asking for help.

Treat the direct organ along with the liver or kidney for best results.

Supplement Use and Label Recommendations

Supplement bottles do not think. The clock does not think. Your body computes how to improve your health 24 hours a day.

Maybe you have found and herbal supplement that really works. Many produce excellent balancing in the body.

Question: The bottle says take _____ 3 times a day. Is there a better way to take my supplements?

Answer: Take your supplements based on your body's symptoms. Your body tells you what it wants when it wants it. You would never spend all day Monday scratching an itch that you were not going to have until Tuesday. You would of course scratch your itch when you had it.

Taking supplements is no different. When you take supplements for an ache or pain and the pain goes away, you have done something right.

Now wait for your ache or pain to come back and then take your supplements again. Yes this may mean that on some days you take them six times. But on other days you may not take them at all. Let your body tell you when to take your herbals.Finally, you will also learn what is making you feel so bad that causes you to need your supplements. How? Because pains and aches always follow the absorption of a stimulant that caused it. Such as, eating a Snickers bar (or whatever) that "turned on" the pain. Pain never occurs without a cause.

All Low Back Pain

This is solely and only a kidney irritation (may be modified by the transverse colon). Drink water, eat grapes and or take a supplement to turn back on your kidneys as they are slightly off. Remember, addressing the transverse colon with citrus or a gentle colon formula can modify low back pain.

Spasms/Pain Or Cramps Above The Right Hip

This is the location of the ileocecal valve. It is the valve that opens and closes, letting matter move from the intestines to the ascending colon. Sugars, parasites, breads, processed foods, alcohol, processed oils, caffeine and heavy protein can block it, causing irritations. When very severe pain is present (in this area) accompanying a very high fever, suspect that the appendix is at issue. When this occurs, seek medical attention immediately. If the appendix ruptures and goes untreated, death can result in 24 to 72 hours.

Right Shoulder Pain/Fuzzy Vision/Irritated eyes/Bad Mood

This is solely and only a liver issue (may be modified by the transverse colon). Drink water, eat citrus and or take a supplement to turn back on your liver as it is slightly off.

Ketones and Protein Intake

Ketones are waste particles derived from fat / protein and are irritants to your kidneys. When the body is fed more protein than it can use, it signals that it is overwhelmed. We may see floaters: clear shapes passing through our vision (undigested protein). Men may notice very foamy urine (as it hits the toilet water) first thing in the morning. The foam will break-up very slowly like soap foam. I believe most people consume seventy five percent more protein than we need on a weekly basis. Most Americans could cut back their protein intake to two times a week, as protein cannot be stored in the body. Ketones build up in excess and can poison and even kill cells of the body. Too much protein or more protein than the kidneys can synthesize can lead to calcium loss via the urine and lead to bone loss (sometimes called osteoporosis).

An over abundance of protein can also rob us of our vitamin B6, as it is required to break down protein.

Kidney Details

The kidneys hold 20-25 percent of the total volume of blood in your body. This is why car makers have moved seat warmers from our seats where they warmed the buttocks to the backrest where they now warm the kidneys and blood. If your body is overheated, the fastest way to cool the body is to cool the low back.

The kidneys strongly react to the "big five"
- Sugar
- Salt
- Sodium
- Caffeine
- Alcohol

The must filter:
- Uric acid this builds in the joints and creates arthritis)
- Lactic acid which is the result of exercise as it lingers in your muscles
- All waste water from the liver.

Most pain and stiffness in the body are the result of either weak kidneys or a weak and tired liver. If you focus your personal therapy on these two organs you can create miracles in the body. Only the colon is as overwhelmed as the liver and kidneys. Therefore be sure that your full body detox includes powerful liver herbs, kidney herbs and excellent herbs for the colon.

Vaccines

It is becoming clearer that vaccines are extremely dangerous and over the last 100+ years have cost millions their lives. Why would this be the case? Vaccinations use a microscopic amount of dead bacteria as a catalyst to get the body to react. A dead bacterium isn't harmless or it wouldn't cause the body to react.

Using poisons to treat the body is clearly not a good idea and uses the principal of differential toxicity (the hope that the poison is more poisonous to the bacteria than it is to you).

Allopathy commonly uses such an approach (such as with the FLU), but it should be avoided. If you shift your focus away from individual hairs that turn grey and instead address the organ regulating the hair, which is the kidneys, you can achieve great results.

Acne is not just a skin condition; it is an accurate reflection of how well the organs connected to that part of the face are running. The skin anywhere else on your body reflects only the liver, but on the face we have subdivisions.

When you identify the correct organ at the bottom of a symptom, you can even identify what caused the problem in the first place. Treat the body as a whole and remember that what you do to one part of the body affects all of it.

Trouble Eating Wheat or Gluten

Commonly called Celiac disease, Sprue or "Celiac Sprue," it is a permanent adverse reaction to gluten (a byproduct of wheat). Gluten is a composite of the proteins gliadin and glutenin. These exist, conjoined with starch, in the endosperms of some grass-related grains, notably wheat, rye and barley. Gliadin and glutenin comprise about 80% of the protein contained in wheat seed. You are already aware of the body's aversion to excess protein; here is another indicator of this condition.

What is so unusual about this "reaction" is that it is common among the entire population. Why are there those who do not notice it? Because some people are so toxic they cannot perceive the reaction, or do not connect their discomfort with this aversion.

No one should ever eat bread, crackers, cookies, cake, doughnuts or any yeast bearing substances of any type.

What Kind of Meat or Heavy Protein Can Be Ingested?

This is a tricky question to answer as some people like me need very little or even none. If you must have meat protein, try sushi (raw fish), steak tartare (thinly sliced raw steak) or even a raw egg in a smoothie. If you do eat raw nuts, a little goes a long way. Eating 5-10 nuts a day for many will suffice.

Why cooked protein is so dangerous is because cooked protein is foreign to the body. The enzymes that made it digestible are now gone or destroyed. Placing a piece of raw steak on a plate and leaving it there undisturbed for six months will produce dust, as the steak enzymes consumed the meat.

Cooked steak left alone for six months will produce a hard piece of leather, as the self-digesting enzymes are dead from cooking. Cooking results in indigestible substances that compost in the gut.

Should I Add Enzymes To My Diet?

The answer is flatly no. Enzymes, to be viable, must be found in their whole natural uncooked source. The reason enzymes are destroyed is due to cooking. Enzyme supplements must be cooked or processed to extract the enzyme residue and then encapsulate them. Enzyme supplements are just another sales pitch and sinkhole for money.

Whole foods are the answer to correcting your health as they are self digesting. The lack of effort / energy used by the body in the digestive process, means that, energy is now available to *heal the body*.

70 Parasites in Your Dinner!

Par·a·site: noun 1. Biology, an organism that grows, feeds, and is sheltered on or in a different organism while contributing nothing to the survival of its host.

Truth: All parasites live on and are enhanced by receiving sugar. The type of sugar to avoid is white table sugar or added sugar. Sugar that occurs naturally in fresh fruit or vegetables is not a problem.

No one likes the idea of being taken advantage of. Some of us may like watching the 3 Stooges but no one wants to be a stooge.

Stooge: noun; the partner in a comedy team who feeds lines to the other comedian; a straight man. One who allows oneself to be used for another's profit or advantage; a puppet:
Slang: A stool pigeon.

No one likes being the victim of someone or something that is taking advantage of their kindness, thoughtfulness or hospitality. Have you ever had a houseguest who decided to stay a while? Remember how that made you feel? Parasites are not guests at all. They are stealthy microscopic warriors out to survive and need your blood to do it.

Do you remember how frustrated you felt when you saw an individual taking advantage of someone you cared about? Remember how hard it was to keep your mouth shut and let them find out for themselves? Or perhaps you risked your friendship and took the role of protector by alerting your friend to the danger they were in. If you did, then you know how difficult it was to get your point across.

On the other hand, how could your friend have been so blind? What if the stooge was you? What if it was happening right now? Read on. If you are a radical like me, you say that 100% of the public has parasites. The conservative right says it is only 90%. As you can see, there is not much difference between the left and the right.

Parasites are blamed for every malady /disease and ache or pain known to man. Parasites are now believed to be a leading cause of many prostate issues. Some see this being an issue in as many as 60% of prostate related issues. They may very well cause most, if not all diseases. I am of the attitude that we all have parasites and in a strong body (one that is healthy) the parasites do not get a good foothold and your body can defend itself. My belief is not a common one but when did adversity ever stop me? It is clear to me that if our bodies are weakened through diet and lifestyle, we can fall victim to such attack.

In a weak enough state, even a cold can be fatal. Regardless of what side of the fence you are on, it is safe to say that parasites are the opposite of money. You don't want more now. You always want less. You don't want more at a later date. You want none. And when faced with the option of not having them, you don't want them ever.

Parasites have caused the greatest loss of life in history. The black plague, Yersinia Pestis, a species of rod shaped bacterium, ravaged Europe from 1347 to 1352. Unless treated immediately it is nearly always fatal.

It first appeared in recorded history in Athens in 430 B.C. and appeared again in 532 A.D. in Europe. But in 1347, the epidemic started in Asia and killed countless numbers before the oriental rat flea, a common pest among rats, hitched a ride to Italy during trade with the Far East.

Once a person was infected symptoms began showing up in 1–7 days. Death could come in 24 hours. Yersinia Pestis developed into 3 forms of plague, bubonic (death rate about 75%), pneumonic plague (death rate almost 100%), and septicemic plague (death rate not charted). All forms have been responsible for enormous mortality in many fearsome epidemics throughout Mankind's history.

Yesinia Pestis was identified and named during another outbreak in Asia in 1894 by Swiss-French bacteriologist Alexandre Yersin. Thanks to the ferocity of these breakouts, we are left with something else rather haunting.

A nursery rhyme you have known about and probably sang to yourself since childhood.

Ring around the Rosy

Ring around the rosy
Pocket full of posies
Ashes, ashes
All fall down

What the Rhyme really meant

Ring around the rosy
This was the mark of the plague on the skin (the rosy) a red or black circle.

Pocket full of posies
It was believed that posies could ward off the plague.

Ashes, ashes
There is much conjecture as to what Ashes, Ashes meant. Most agree it referred to the burning of the dead. Yet there is another variation, "a tissue, a tissue" (indicating a runny nose). There is also the variant "ahchoo ahchoo" for sneezing or Ashen, Ashen, referring to the grey pall of the dying.

All fall down
We all die.

With this translation this innocuous little nursery rhyme has a taken on a deep and tragic meaning. Parasites can come to us from hundred of locations. The parasite menace is so overwhelming that most cannot conceive of the danger.

Common Ways To Get Parasites

The ocean   Any raw meats
Rivers   Mosquito bites

Streams	Oral sex
Lake	Cockroaches
Ponds	Ants
Cats	Kissing / Mononucleosis
Your cat box	Flies
Dogs	All insects
Birds	Tap water
Other animals	Open air buffets
Salad Bars	3rd world travel
Sushi Bars	Hose water
Raw pork	Animal Pet Kisses
Raw fish	Pets Sleeping in your bed
Raw beef	Eating food after it has been on the floor or ground
Raw chicken	

Eating food that has fallen on the floor or ground is a very bad idea. Slow motion stop action photography demonstrates that when anything crashes onto the floor a plum dust is sent airborne immediately coating the item dropped.

Truth: All parasites live on and are enhanced by receiving sugar. The type of sugar to avoid is white table sugar or added sugar. Sugar that occurs naturally in fresh fruit or vegetables is not a problem.

Par·a·site: noun 1. Biology, an organism that grows, feeds, and is sheltered on or in a different organism while contributing nothing to the survival of its host.

After rereading the definition above ask yourself if your parasite problem is being ignoring or are you actively taking measures to prevent and eradicate them. Even STD's are parasite based. The fact is we are living with parasites right now. The reason you are not dead is because your immune system is keeping them in check.

There are four ways to handle the unavoidable little terrors called parasites:

1 Do a parasite detox as needed as often as once a year

2 Keep your immune system strong and let it do your fighting

3 A combination of the above

4 Do nothing and hope for the best

There are many good formulas available for parasites but the key is to do a detox long enough.

Roger Bezanis

Doing a parasite cleanse for a week is does not scratch the surface of the problem. If you are going to start a parasite cleanse be sure that you do it for at least 3 months.

The proper protocol for a parasite detox is:
-Taken 3-5 times a day

    6 days a week (always take one day off to rest)

    3 weeks ON

    1 week OFF

    3 weeks ON

    1 week OFF

    3 weeks ON

When you have followed the 3 month protocol above you are done unless you have picked up new parasites in the final days of the detox. If so you may need to do an extra week or two.

The reason you are doing a parasite cleanse for 3 months is because parasites are insidious. When attacked the little buggers burrow deep into the system for safety trying to survive. That is why you give a full week off between the first month and second month and second and third month.

The first month addresses all parasites that are present and not able to escape herbal animation. The second month picks up any micro vermin out hunting for food after their "week off" from devastation. The third month collects any stragglers and the final month destroys any final eggs that have hatched. There really is no better way to handle parasites other than not to get them in the first place.

Do not be fooled by the folly being offered by medical doctors (MD's) regarding parasite infestation.

The worlds of allopathic medicines aka "Big Pharma" also have their so called answer for parasites. It is called Vermox. They suggest that Vermox is effective in one week. This is absolute folly. Treating parasites for a week is akin to throwing water balloons at an armored car. The active ingredient in Vermox is called Mebendazole. It is for worms such as hookworm, whipworm, roundworm and threadworm. They suggest that you use this treatment twice a day for three days. Please do not use Vermox or its protocol as it strengthens the parasites making them resistant to treatment.

I have met many people who attempted Vermox treatment. They continued to have parasites for months and for some years after the cure.

The best herbs for the detoxification of parasites are:

Black Walnut

Wormwood

Clove

Garlic (also good for vampires, a type of
  parasite. Take that, Dracula)

Chinese Wolfbane

Pumpkin Seed

Prickly Ash Bark

China Bark

Grape Fruit Seed

Citrus has an irritating affect on parasites. That is one of the reasons why in traditional Sushi bars an orange is served at the end of the dining experience. Oranges and all citrus aid in digestion as well as make the digestive tract almost fully untenable for parasites. In such unfriendly environs evil insidious parasitic cultivation is severely hampered.

If you are suffering with parasites, please do something about it. It is easy to do. One final note; I was working with a woman who had no success with any form of parasite cleanse over a 15 year period. She too had used Vermox as mentioned above. Begging me to help her I agreed but not via formulas. This woman was failing not because the formulas she was using were all bad. Many companies make good parasite formulas. She was failing due to what she was doing behind closed doors. She was covertly making herself sick.

At first she insisted that her diet was sound and healthy. I knew otherwise as there are never exceptions just secrets that are explained as exceptions. She was taken aback by my poking and prodding but that did not stop me. Her diet was the key. I had to find the right locks to put that key in. Upon detailed inspection and much cajoling it was revealed that she was a full fledged sugaraholic.

Definition: -Aholic

-a- Combining form extracted from alcoholic, occurring as the final element in compound words, often facetious nonce (present time) words with the sense "a person who has an addiction or obsession with some object or activity: workaholic; chargeaholic etc.

This woman had been riffed with horrific health for 15 years and was bringing it all on by her own hand. The irony of this story is that we are all our own executioners. When it comes to food and "food like" fast foods, we are born addicted. In the next few years medical science will announce that sugar addiction occurs in the womb. The fact is it does now. We are just waiting for Duke or Harvard to make those findings public.

Regarding this woman, she was feeding her parasites like pigeons on a park bench. I begged her to give up her candy bars, cookies, breads, cereal, Coke, sugared coffee, sweet tea, chocolate, etc. I patiently explained that she would never get well otherwise. She called me three months later jumping for joy as she was a new woman. For the first time in a decade and a half she was alive again.

She had followed my instructions to a "T" and did not use any formulas. With hard work, her efforts to eradicate her parasites by changing her diet was a major success. Also vanquished was her arthritis, diabetes symptoms, heart palpitations, high blood pressure, bad moods, insomnia, fuzzy vision, constipation, poor skin and more.

The power to be healthy is in each of our hands. If we surround ourselves with healthy "real food" we cannot help but be healthy.

Hookworm

The hookworm is the diarrhea and cramp-causing intestinal parasite. Heavy infestation with hookworm can be serious. Hookworm infections occur mainly in tropical and subtropical climates and affect about 1 billion people—about one-fifth of the world's population. One of the most common species of hookworm, Ancylostoma Duodenale, is found in southern Europe, northern Africa, northern Asia, and parts of South America.

Hookworms have a complex life cycle that begins and ends in the small intestine. Hookworm eggs require warm, moist, shaded soil to hatch into larvae. These barely visible larvae penetrate the skin (often through bare feet), are carried to the lungs, go through the respiratory tract to the mouth, are swallowed, and eventually reach the small intestine.

This journey takes about a week. In the small intestine, the larvae develop into half-inch-long worms, attach themselves to the intestinal wall, and individually consume small amounts of blood. When there is an infestation, the small amount of blood consumed becomes quite large and can lead to anemia. The adult worms produce thousands of eggs. These eggs are passed in the feces (stool). If the eggs contaminate soil and conditions are right, they will hatch, molt, and develop into infective larvae again after 5 to 10 days.

Hookworm infection is contracted from contact with soil contaminated by hookworm, by walking barefoot or accidentally swallowing contaminated soil. Children, because they often play in dirt and go barefoot, are at high risk. Since transmission of hookworm infection requires development of the larvae in soil, hookworm cannot be spread person to person.

Chronic heavy hookworm infection can damage the growth and development of children. The loss of iron and protein retards growth and mental development, sometimes irreversibly. The first signs of hookworm infection are itching and a rash at the site where the larvae penetrate the skin. These signs may be followed by abdominal pain, diarrhea, anemia, loss of appetite and weight loss.

One further symptom, though not common in Hookworm infections, is anal itching. As their waste is produced, it can cause irritation of the anus. Hookworms can also cause difficulty breathing, enlargement of the heart, as well as an irregular heartbeat. When Hookworm infections go unchecked, the symptoms can be very severe and, in infants, may even lead to death.

Pinworm

Pin·worm: Any of various small worms that is parasitic on or in cattle, horses, rabbits, and other mammals. Pinworms (Enterobius Vermicularis) are a species that infests the human intestines and rectum. A common variation of the name pinworms is threadworm and is the same thing. The pinworm is about the length of a common staple and lives for the most part within the rectum of humans. While an infected person is asleep, female pinworms leave the intestines through the anus and deposit eggs on the skin around the anus.

The symptoms of a pinworm infection are caused by the female pinworm laying her eggs. Most symptoms of pinworm infection are mild, and many infected people have no symptoms or, at most, some itching around the anus, disturbed sleep, and irritability. Should pinworm infestation be heavy, your symptoms may be more severe and also include loss of appetite, restlessness, and insomnia. As infections get worse, so will your symptoms, such as insomnia, voracious non- stop itching, loss of concentration, mood swings, loss of productivity (as all you can think about is the itch that you can't scratch in public).

Within days of infection, Pinworms begin attacking the liver directly and indirectly via the byproducts (waste) left in the blood due to their presence. Liver issues can be very severe during Pinworm infestations. If this is not clear to you, review the symptoms of liver weakness in the chapter on the liver. Pinworms are the most common parasitic worms in the United States among school age children. Infection or contamination of preschoolers runs a close second with day care centers coming in at third. Adults are not immune to pinworms but are not as likely to have pinworm infestations, unless the worms were acquired from their infected children.

If you thought the movie Alien was scary, consider this: pinworm eggs can survive up to 2 weeks on clothing, bedding, or other objects. Infection is acquired when these eggs are accidentally swallowed. Also consider this, within a few hours of being deposited on the skin around the anus, pinworm eggs become infective (capable of infecting another person). At night, the adult worms can sometimes be seen directly in bedclothes or around the anal area. In hotels the comforters are cleaned only twice a year, unless severely soiled. Therefore it's a good idea to

Roger Bezanis

have the comforters removed by the housekeeping staff upon your arrival.

When pinworms are suspected as a problem, your doctor can order a microbiology test to verify his suspicions one way or the other. Be aware that these tests can take 3 - 5 weeks to receive after testing.

The tests involve acquiring a smear or sample of the debris around the anus using transparent tape or a pinworm paddle. The eggs adhere to the sticky tape or paddle and are identified by examination under a microscope. The test needs to be done in the morning prior to showering and prior to bowel movements as washing and wiping will remove the eggs. Fingernail samples also may produce eggs for examination. Pinworm infestation can be treated with herbal formulas or with over the counter products.

Treating pinworms correctly can take up to 3 months. Always consult your health care provider before treating a suspected case of pinworm.

Always consider treating the entire family if a member is infected. Beware that infected playmates, schoolmates and close contacts can bring about a re-infection.

Tapeworm

They live in the intestinal tract, attached with a rounded head equipped with hook-like structures that attach to the intestinal wall. Once secured to the wall, the worms begin feeding. The host unwittingly feeds the visitors, as the tapeworm has no digestive tract. The tapeworm is also called a flat worm and is shaped like a hollow strip. The worm is made up of proglottids (worm segments), starting below the neck. An adult worm can reach a length of 15 or 20 ft. As a segment dies off it separates and is removed in the bowel movement of the host.

A tapeworm is a true hermaphrodite, having both male and female reproductive organs. Self-fertilization does take place but it is more common that a second worm will be necessary. Human tapeworm infestations are most common in regions where there is fecal contamination of soil and water. Tapeworm incidence will be higher where light cooking or raw meat consumption is most common. The beef tapeworm is the most prevalent tapeworm in the United States. This happens when a host cow becomes infected while drinking or grazing.

The round-bodied embryos, equipped with sharp hooks, hatch and bore through the cow's intestinal wall into the bloodstream, where they are carried to the muscles. Here each embryo encloses itself in a cyst, or bladder; at this stage it is called a bladder worm. During the bladder worm stage, the embryo develops a miniature head. It remains encysted until the primary host eats the muscle. If the head has not been killed by sufficient cooking of the meat, it sheds its covering and attaches to the intestinal wall, of the human host, where it begins growing.

sIntestinal tapeworm infestation frequently occurs without symptoms; occasionally there is abdominal discomfort, diarrhea, constipation, or weight loss. The most serious tapeworm infestation in humans is caused by the ingestion of T. Solanum eggs through fecal contamination. The embryos migrate throughout the body, producing serious illness. Interestingly, the dog tapeworm embryo encysts in various internal organs of humans, most commonly in the liver.

The cysts produced by these embryos are called hydatid cysts, and the infestation of the liver is called hydatid disease.

Heartworm

Heartworms are found primarily in dogs but can be passed to humans via mosquitoes. They can be hard to eliminate and can be fatal. Heartworm symptoms usually can't be detected until advanced stages. Symptoms are similar to congestive heart failure and include coughing, difficulty breathing, lack of energy, etc.

Adult heartworms live in the heart and pulmonary arteries of infected dogs. And as mentioned above, rarely in humans, but they can be affected. They have been found in other areas of the body, but this is unusual. Heartworms survive up to 5 years and, during this time; the female produces millions of offspring. These offspring live in the bloodstream, mainly in the small blood vessels. 30 different species of mosquitoes can transmit heartworms. The female mosquito bites the infected dog and ingests the blood borne offspring during a blood meal. From there mosquitoes can pass the parasite young to unsuspecting hosts.

When fully developed, the infective larvae enter the bloodstream and move to the heart and adjacent vessels, where they grow to maturity in 2 to 3 months and start reproducing, thereby completing the full life cycle.

Roundworm

The roundworm is the most prolific internal pest known to man. There are more than 20,000 species documented at present. They are often passed from dogs to humans through accidental ingestion of eggs. They can be found throughout the world and even in Antarctica and oceanic trenches. There are more species of roundworms than species of man and animal combined. They possess a complete digestive system with a mouth that attaches to the intestines with sharp projectiles. They are thin, round voracious little feeders. The skin of the roundworm secretes fluid made of keratin that protects the body from drying out due to digestive juices. Roundworms have a simple nervous system, with a main nerve cord running along the ventral side. Simple or not, they are very debilitating to the host.

Protozoa

(Greek protos = first and zoon = animal) are single-celled creatures with nuclei that show some characteristics usually associated with animals, most notably humans. The most common protozoa variants are; Flagellates, Amoeboids, Sporozoans, Apicomplexa, Myxozoa, Microsporidia and Ciliates.

Most protozoans are too small to be seen with the naked eye, being around 0.01-0.05 mm. To detect protozoa you need a microscope. The common symptoms of protozoa are anemia, back and muscle pain and occasional diarrhea. The organ that is most often attacked by protozoa is the kidney.

Amoeba

Genus of protozoa that moves by means of temporary projections called pseudo pods, and is well known as a representative single cellular organism. They are found in sluggish waters all over the world, both fresh and salt, as well as in soils and as parasites. The Amoeba itself is found in freshwater, typically on decaying vegetation from streams, but is not especially common in nature.

However, because of the ease that they may be obtained, they can cause havoc with humans. The most well known species is A. Proteus. Each has a single nucleus. The name "amibe" was given to it by Berry St. Vincent, from the Greek amoibe, meaning change.

Giardia

A genus of Protozoa that is parasitic in the intestines of vertebrates including humans and most domestic animals. Giardia reproduces and lives in the intestines and may produce minor symptoms include diarrhea, abdominal cramps and nausea, flatulence and/or weight loss. It is passed via unwashed hands of an infected person, or by drinking groundwater polluted by the feces of infected animals such as dogs and beavers (hence the nickname "beaver fever"). Once it migrates to the small intestine it multiplies quickly.

Symptoms, when present, occur one to three days after infection. In some cases the infection becomes chronic. Giardia is common in tropical climates and can hold aggressively in developed countries. Interestingly, men and very young children in close contact with each other are most susceptible. Anywhere where hand washing is not common or not mastered, Giardia can be found. Microscopic stool analysis or testing for antibodies to the parasite is the best way to detect them. In most cases, if the body is healthy and strong, no treatment is necessary.

Toxoplasmosis

Toxoplasmosis is an infection caused by a single-celled parasite named Toxoplasma Gondii. It is found throughout the world and infects more than 60 million people in the United States. Infestation with the Toxoplasma parasite may carry very few symptoms because the immune system usually keeps the parasite from causing illness.

How can humans get Toxoplasmosis?
1) Touching your hands to your mouth after gardening, cleaning a cat's litter box, or anything that came into contact with cat feces.
2) Eating raw or partly cooked meat, especially pork, lamb, or deer.
3) Touching your hands to your mouth after contact with raw or undercooked meat.
4) Organ transplantation or transfusion, although this is rare.

If a woman is pregnant when she is infected with Toxoplasmosis, the infection can be transmitted from her to the baby with catastrophic consequences.

What are the usual symptoms of toxoplasmosis?
Flu like symptoms
Swollen lymph glands

Muscle aches and pains that can last several weeks. If anyone develops more severe symptoms it is because their immune system is weak or they are actively weakening it with use of sugar and drugs, including OTC (over the counter drugs). If you have any of the symptoms mentioned in this chapter and you suspect that you may have parasites, see your health care practitioner and be fully examined. It is important in any treatment for parasites that the therapy (whatever it is) is administered long enough, usually 3 months.

Vermox is often given by the medical profession for parasites and is a one-dose treatment. I have seen this approach fail again and again.

I will leave this up to you whether you think a one-dose treatment of anything can be successful. Always follow your doctor's protocols and recommendations. Should you decide to add something else to your treatment of your own design, or that is purchased somewhere else, always let your doctors know, as the two approaches may not work successfully.

Roger Bezanis

71 How Can You Change?

I grew up playing sports. I played football, baseball and was a shot putter. I was completely out of control in football and played the roving linebacker position of Monster Back. I was just as intense in baseball. If I could have tackled a pitcher I would have.

I was remarkably fast but it was not always this way.

In elementary school I was the fattest, slowest running kid in the school. I was not really that fat, I was in a school that was in good shape. Nevertheless, when on the grounds many of the other children playing called me "Fatty!" In the 6th grade we had a national physical fitness test. Part of that test was to run 3 laps around a 600-foot track (100 yards). I could not stop running. I was hypnotized looking at those dashed lines disappearing under my feet. I ran (fully clothed) 25 laps until I was made to stop.

For at least two hours I was drenched in sweat.

The next day I was playing sock ball (like baseball) and I hit a ball to the shortstop. The kid I hit it to was much faster than me, yet I beat him to first base (much to my surprise), then to second base, on to third and then home plate. All the while the boy was yelling "Fatty slow down, slow down fatty."

Something dramatic had happened!!

I was remarkably fast the rest of the day. I had gone from being the slowest runner in school to really fast overnight. The next day I sought out Roger Lane, the acknowledged fastest kid in the school.

When we raced, we were dead even. Wow! How remarkable. Can you expect this? Anything is possible.

At age 34, I decided to rebuild my softball career. I was out of shape and overweight, but that did not stop me. Two left knee surgeries when I was 24 did not stop me. What stopped me was my right leg. One afternoon I had just lined a clean single to right center and was racing to first base when my right upper leg (the rectus femoris muscle) decided that my day was done.
I was suddenly in great pain and nothing I did relieved it. I was yet again knocked out of action. I suddenly had a fist-sized knot in my upper leg. No massage or treatment (less surgery) would relieve the knot or the pain. I again hung up my bat and glove.

For the next 10 years I did not play again.

Three years ago (age 44); I took up softball again (after I had lost 63 pounds). There was no reason to believe that I could still play. I had blown out my knee twice playing softball when I was 24 years old. Now at 44 I was going to play softball again?

That is just what I did.

Yes, fast-forward ten years (44 years old). The fist size knot was still in my upper right leg but I decided to celebrate my 44th birthday at the batting cage. For three straight days and about three and a half hours, I swung away. My right leg was sore but I pushed through it. The sports bug had hit me again and I decided to take up organized softball yet again. I had just lost the 63 pounds I mentioned at the beginning of this story and I felt good.

Amazingly, the knot in my leg was almost completely gone!!! Did years of herbs, weight loss and three and a half hours of the batting cage change me again?

The following Monday I was walking in and out of my office and as I was walking up the steps, my leg hurt like it hadn't in ten years. When I sat down to massage my right upper leg something happened. The knot was now gone!! This is no exaggeration. The knot was gone.

I have been playing off and on ever since and I have recaptured my speed that I earned that day in elementary school.

Nothing should have fixed my leg, but something did. To be very fair, here is what the influential factors were:
   a) I had switched to a completely raw diet 3 months earlier.
   b) I had been taking herbs for kidney (sometimes 7 times a day) for three weeks. Remember, the kidneys regulate all muscles, tendons and ligaments.
   c) I was exercising intensely (batting cage).
   d) I had decided to not be stopped by my leg.

Any one of these factors or a combination of all of them could have played a role in this major change. In the end, something changed, and without figuring it out further, it would be accurate to write that I changed and my body changed with me. Remember, ten years without playing and at the age of 45 years old, I am again playing like a high school kid.

I have since been relaying this story to numbers of doctors. Most do not understand the relationship of intention over the physical world and have attributed this change to the use of the herbs and diet.

In retrospect it is clear to me that weak kidneys led to my leg and knee problems years earlier. It is also clear that circulation was the key to all of these problems. If there is no circulation or energy flow there is not life.

I have said it again and again, when there is reduced circulation oxygen or energy flow there is reduced life / energy / strength.

All of this leads to injury.

72 Power of Intention

What we believe becomes law. You may have heard it or just always believed it. Regardless of how you came by it, it is very true. Here is a story that illustrates this simple point, I have at least 20 of these stories, but this is one of my favorites.

In the early 1990's, I was on my way to Anaheim, California near Disneyland for a convention. While driving to the hotel I either ate something or was exposed to something that swelled my left eye. It was puffy, red and it hurt like hell. I looked like I was a refugee from a horror film or on the losing end of a fist fight. It felt terrible and looked worse. Since I had never missed a day of work in my life (now there is a story of intention right there) I was not about to be stopped by a neon red, throbbing, bulbous eye.

At the time, I had not developed any formulas for eyes so I was stumped. I tried things to get the red out and nothing worked. I looked like a reject from Animal House, not a lecturer or expert on anything. Something had to be done. So I used my cell phone and called anyone with a clue. Nothing seemed to work. I was destined to look like a red-eyed freak. I had to come up with a solution. I bought a pair of cool looking shades and attempted to look ultra cool (by hiding my eyes).

As I left my hotel room in my suit and cool sun glasses, feeling self conscious like a man with a third eye that throbbed, I had visions of people pointing and gawking at my eye. I realized I would get nothing done unless this eye thing went away and I mean soon. Walking onto the convention floor no one even noticed me. Everyone was looking cool; half of them had sunglasses on. It was going to work out!

But I still had this sinking feeling of not trusting people in sunglasses. Therefore, I didn't trust myself behind sunglasses either. If I didn't trust me, who would? In about 10 minutes of working something happened. My eye swelling and pain went completely away. I was cured and just in time. When the day was over, I walked back to my hotel room and, as I walked, my eye started throbbing again and it was starting to swell again. This was not good at all. It was also very odd.

What was going on here? My eye allowed me to work but not relax. The next morning the exact same thing happened:

Dark shades	Short walk
Short walk	Big swelling
A few minutes of work	Lots of pain
No swelling or redness	No rest
Day over	Repeat

This continued until the end of the weekend when I was driving home and all the pain and swelling went away. My only thought was that nothing was going to stop me from working. My intention to make things work was senior to the physical problem.

We might all have these stories. If you do, champion them. You are a powerful human being. The fact is we all are. Part of being able or powerful is deciding to be powerful and able. If you have no reality on this, that is okay. Perhaps one day you will. The fact is that nothing ever changes until someone has identified a problem and decided to change the condition. You are this powerful and can do things like this, but you have to decide to effect change in your own life and not be a victim.

You make a difference. Make it a point to get this book into the hands of people who need it and want to read it. Do not forget how important our kids are. They are the future of our planet; they need this information and instantly "get it."

Help me heal this planet. It is all of our responsibility.

The choice is yours how you will help.

73 Shopping for Supplements

How fun is it to shop? Some of us live for it. Some of us can't stand it. Others just don't care one way or the other. If you have ever had the experience of standing in the supplement aisle of your health food store and staring at the bewildering wall of bottles confronting you, you will love what comes next.

I have been preaching, "Your Body is Smarter then you are" I am going to reinforce this in this short chapter.

The intelligence in your body that you are not fully aware of is always active. This is a simple little trick that you can use again and again.

Stand in the aisle looking at the wall of supplements and see what bottle you are drawn to. Walk over to it and pick it up. Then, find the nearest herb book, usually in the aisle for easy access, and read what it says about that herb. Compare what is known about that herb to what you know about your symptoms.

Did this bottle of herbs match your symptoms? Do not be surprised how often what you are drawn to is just what you need. If every bottle is emanating some sort of energy, and your body is energy, being drawn to a bottle makes sense.

Do not be afraid of using this. No one will know what you are doing. You also can do several dry runs to test yourself.

Do not expect to only be drawn to herbs you know. You will be picking up all sorts of odd combinations and herbs. This is because your body knows more about itself than you will ever know. You are employing the body's innate intelligence. It is just your body trying to help you. You may initially find that you are not very good with this technique. If that is true, your ability to use it will increase, as your system gets healthier. Stick with it. If after a few months you still can't use this little trick, figure you are in the 3–5% range of those who cannot do this.

There is another group of people (that I am not a part of) who can detect energy of organic objects. They can pick something up and feel whether something is good or bad for them. I don't have a clue how to train someone how to do this, as I don't have the ability. If you do, my hat is off to you. If you want to test it for yourself, pick up a bottle of supplements or 5 or 6 and see if you feel anything.

Regardless of what approach you take, best of luck and be healthy. Choose to be healthy.

74 Those Who Want Help

Try as you may, some people, no matter what they say, do not want help. There are people who will buy this book and never open it. They will just add it to their collection. Some people will read some of this book and tell everyone how good or bad it was as if they were an authority. Still others will call me with after having found punctuation errors. They will gleefully spring to their phones or computers attempt to reach me so that they can criticize my work. What shabby, shabby work. One woman called me and glumly said "You aren't a very good writer are you?" I wondered if she had so much as written her name before. Yet she chose to be critical of my work.

This person who called could not receive help. It was clear that she only wanted to be right. When you analyze them these people as I have; you see a shell of a person ignoring the lessons that would save their life.

Beware when someone asks you for advice. These people tend to be sponges and just absorb more and more opinions that ruin their lives. Some people will ask you for advice or, if you are a practitioner, come in and ask for help. They will not have any intention of following anything you have said. The best way to handle anyone asking for advice is not to give it to him or her. People can't ignore advice fast enough. Just look at all the advice that you have given out. How many people are actually following what you have said to do? How many times have you said or thought, "I told you so." If someone comes to you with a question answered in this book, hand them the book and have them read the chapter concerning it. You will have done more good than you know in more ways than one.

Many husbands do not listen to their wives and vice versa. The same thing is true with friends. Distance equals intelligence for most people and they do not even know it. Many mothers know what it is like to beg your child to eat something and have them steadfastly refuse. They are later shocked to learn that the same child while at a friend's house "discovered" and now loves what she could not get the child to even taste. With that in mind use this book as your authority reference guide. It will convey what you could not. Use it like tool. Think of it like a shovel to move concepts into understandings which leads to action. You and your friends are welcome to hear me speak around the country. The web is a great reference library to find out what and where I am teaching.

The web is loaded with information and current pictures relating to my work. Please use these assets as much as you can as they are useless unless you are helping people heal by becoming better informed.

I am here to help but I cannot do anything until someone is ready to listen. Pain is a fantastic motivator when it comes to health. If someone is in enough pain, they will go to great lengths to get better. Pain diminishes pride, dislike and prejudice it is the factor that levels the playing field when someone has been resistant to taking help.

But even in the case above it would be vital that they read the chapters in this book that pertains to them. Why? This book is authoritative and is not you. You will be saying the exact same thing this book has said. You may be parroting entire sections. But because you are saying my words they may not have as much impact. When this happens and you are not reaching your patient, hand them my book.

The written word is king. Use it.

This book is your friend and as such, it will never abandon you. The impact of these pages are without out boundaries, don't forget that. This book is your tool as the words in it spell something. What do they spell? T-R-U-S-T. It is shocking to think that your husband or wife would listen to a stranger and not to you, but those are the facts. If you have been with this person long enough, you have seen it again and again.

I was once speaking to a CA (Chiropractic Assistant) and she told me how constipated she was. She would have eliminations once a week at best unless she used an herbal formula to help move her colon. Keep in mind that constipation is defined as having less than one-elimination per meal eaten. In questioning her about it, she indicated that she drank 2 to 3 pots of coffee a day and hated water and refused to drink it. But she also did not want to be constipated and also did not want to take her herbal laxative.

Her conversation with me was like someone talking to me while hitting themselves over the head with a cast iron frying pan. What they are saying is, "Gee whiz, my head hurts, can you make it stop?" bang, bang, bang, "This is a headache right?" bang, bang, bang, "I don't know why my head hurts!" bang, bang, bang, "But I sure wish it would stop", bang, bang, bang.

Get the picture? This was absolute insanity. How could someone complain about knife wounds while cutting their arm with a knife? But there she was. When I explained the relationship of diuretics and elimination, she seemed to understand. When I told her she would have to give up her coffee or forever be constipated, she told me "I would rather die first."

Hearing that kind of statement was like being kicked in the head. I was stunned. So I tried to reason with her, I said, "If you were on your death bed, and you hated corn on the cob, to you it was the most vile thing on the planet, and the doctor told you that if you just eat a stalk, you would live, but if you don't, you will be dead within 24 hours, what would you do"?

She said, "I would die." I said okay.
That was the end of that. You can't help everyone.

Concentrate on those that want help and save your grey hair.

Do not risk disaster by commingling with people who don't want you to succeed. Some people have it wired up that if you succeed, **they fail**. To them, all success of any type means failure to them. They want you to stay fat and unhappy, sick and tired, or frazzled and weak. Just imagine if you got healthy. Minimally, they would have no one to compare stories with. You do not have to help everyone.

You may meet someone who absorbs all your free time and energy in an attempt to get them feeling better, but they never get better.

I have met many people who love the attention from being sick. They are thrilled to know that you are up all night worried about them. Cut them loose. They are poison to your practice, Mr. or Ms. Practitioner. If you are focusing 60 percent of your ability and attention on only 3 of your patients, set them free.

They just want attention with no intent of ever getting better.

My Mother's Story

This next story makes it clear that only those who want help can be helped. Notice that until my mother wanted help she was just a sinkhole for attention.

My mother's name was Mozelle. She was a little feisty woman who taught me to work hard and be a good listener. Thanks to her I never missed a day of school or work and have a booming voice. Around my house my mother's "inside voice" was at times deafening. She spoke very loud ; some would call it yelling. Me, I got a loud voice out it.

Some of my first memories of her were lengthy sessions of her complaining how sick she was. My mother was as healthy as a horse by most people's standards. Nevertheless she was always complaining of this and that. Eventually I learned to ignore her. She really did not want help, just someone to listen to her.

She would call me, drop by, write me, flag me down on the street and block intersections just to gloat about how sick she was. Like Freddy Kruger (of Nightmare On Elm Street fame) she would even complain to me in my dreams. Then one day in 1986 she had a battery of tests done on her year old medicine ball sized abdomen. These tests confirmed that she had cancer. Cancer that, if she knew was there, would cause her to fold up like a tent. My mother so loved the idea of being sick.

Good for her, she could not stand/hated her doctor. She disliked him so much she refused to speak to him. Under the circumstances, the doctor asked me if I would pass on the bad news. They thought she might only have six months to live.

Roger Bezanis

She never spoke to him again.

I conveniently (for my mom), neglected to tell her what the doctor told me.

A day or two later she asked me if I could help make her feel better. Honored, I agreed and then proceeded to give her various vitamins, magnesium, grape juice, other herbs and fresh juices. This went on for 3 months. Her abdomen reduced to a normal size and she felt great. She lived another 20 years before she succumbed to Alzheimer's disease in 2002. I took great solace in the fact that cancer was not listed as her cause of death. There was not a trace of cancer found in her body. My mother was very sweet in her last year of life. I do miss her.

The point of all this is help those who really want to be helped.

Share this book with your friends or spouse because that is the least you can do. Better than that, become the best you can be and set an example of what is possible.

It is our choice to change our conditions in life. We can transform the world we live in if we all band together.

Choose to be healthy; it is well worth the work.

75 Extremism and Extremists

Extremism is an interesting subject for this book. Yet it has a direct correlation between your humble author (yes, I am an extremist) and you the reader. Extremism is not so unusual; it is actually revered and held as normal when lives are not at stake. Extreme devotion to the eating of chocolate would not be healthy. Yet extreme devotion to saving lives such as in a trauma emergency room would be a healthy and applauded lifestyle.

It is safe to say, we all have some extreme tendencies or habits from time to time. Here are a few:

Crossword puzzles	Knitting
Playstation or X-Box	Surfing the Internet
Cleaning	Magic
Shopping	Exercising
Organization	Eating
Collecting	Traveling

Habits that are part of a balanced life that include, proper finances, health, family, friends and work are considered normal and social. When habits require secrecy to be carried out, then it becomes correctly labeled harmful.

A good rule of thumb to determine if an activity is social or harmful is to ask this question:

"Would I feel embarrassed to carry this activity out while being seen on my roof"?

If the answer is yes, then you should examine the activity. Perhaps it is not the kind of activity that includes you in the race of men but excludes you from all men. Heavy statement, I know. But remember any man who profoundly isolates himself is slowly dying, be it obvious or not. Humans, craving only solitude and isolated, are on a spiraling road to blackness.

Mixing social activities and living alone is not a crime; it happens every day. Keep in mind that isolation is not the goal in this scenario. Man is looking for companionship.

Extreme extroversion and a need for the company of hundreds 24 hours a day is also a dilemma. Therefore a happy medium between these two opposites would be called normal and healthy.

On a professional level, being an extremist is by all means not an awful, terrible thing. Living in the midst of extremists has brought us much social and economic change. If it were not for Edison's extreme fascination with the light bulb and all things new you would be reading this book by candlelight.

Famous extremists in history (good and bad)

Alexander the Great	Michael Jordon
Hippocrates	Tiger Woods
Harriet Tubman	Louis Pasteur
Henry Ford	Jacques Cousteau
The Wright Brothers	General George S. Patton
Adolph Hitler (made the list for obvious yet not wholesome reasons)	Stephen Hawking
	Booker T. Washington
Albert Einstein	Benjamin Franklin
Christopher Columbus	Oprah Winfrey
Kobe Bryant	Roger Bezanis (I've always wanted to see my
Harry Houdini	name on a list with Oprah & Kobe Bryant)
Napoleon Bonaparte	

As you can see from the above list (which is very short and could go on for pages) extremism, at its best solves global/social issues. At its worst causes death and destruction. Therefore we can say that the intent of the extremist activity will establish its social or humanitarian value.

Roger Bezanis

Extremism is only considered ghastly when it obsessively endangers the life of the participant or that of others he or she is contacting (See Adolf Hitler).

Extremism that saves lives is always welcome. A thrill seeker who chooses the life of a fireman or the life of a Navy Seal or Special Operations tactician is a welcome extremist. If focused or channeled, extreme behavior can be very powerful and useful to society.

All of this talk about extremism is very interesting and has a direct relationship to the next section of this book on addictions and eating disorders. These problems all revolve around out-of- control extremism.

76 Eating Disorders and Addictions

An addiction is an overwhelming urge to repeat some activity or habit over and over again. An addiction may involve a certain time of day or a certain type of stress or environment. The longer any habit is practiced, the more it ingrains itself into the fabric of the individual. Due to this imprinting, and its repetitious nature, it can be hard (yet not impossible) to re-pattern the body to a new condition or state of better health.

There are five classes of substances (all manmade) that are extremely toxic to the body. The five toxic classes are:

Manmade sugary substances (acid)

Manmade salty substances (alkaline)

Manmade chemicals that create sedation

Manmade chemicals that create stimulation

Manmade chemicals that create hallucination

When consuming a toxic substance, the body will crave the exact same material 24 hours after its first ingestion. This has been proven 1000s of times on test. If you look in your own experience you will also find that your more negative cravings follow a schedule.

Yes, if you ingest xyz toxin today at 5:00 p.m., you will crave the exact same xyz substance tomorrow at 5:00 p.m. This speaks to the 24-hour clock that the body runs on.

Seeing that the body is attempting to create balance, toxic substances confuse the body and trick it into making the toxin part of its daily program. This is why an addiction is so hard to beat. The toxin may mimic hormones or amino acids and or vitamins that the body desperately needs.

Psychiatry does not understand these phenomena and believe that an addiction is a brain problem. It is strictly a toxic body problem manifested and or made worse via an overwhelmed liver. Bulimics do not binge on oranges or fresh fruit to latter vomit. No addiction is impossible to defeat as it is modified by the individuals personal will power, which is infinite. Again, all craving rules hold true for bulimia, which involves a habit and a toxin. There is no urge to vomit up food taken directly from nature such as oranges, apples, grapes, melons, etc. Only artificial foods / junk / manmade / man processed foods become toxic to the body.

The above paragraph gives the clue to beating the habit / addiction.

What you are about to read for some may be the most important part of this book. Over the next several pages I am going to investigate, answer and offer solutions to Bulimia / Rumination and Anorexia.

The solutions I give can be used for any addiction. Later you will read the chapter Control = Cause, in it you will discover how I handled my stuttering. Out of control habits only remain so because no one is controlling them. When the source realizes that he or she is the source of their affliction, healing can take place.

The practice of bulimia and bulimics are fascinating. They are the equivalent of the modern day vampire. They are the un-healthy immortals of the food / nutrition world.

77 What are Bulimia and Rumination?

Definition: Bulimia (*pronounced— BAH-LEE-ME-AH*) is the secret (hidden from others) practice of eating, usually to excess and then either vomiting or taking bowel purging substances to ensure evacuation the next day or sooner. Bulimics tend to believe "they are alone and the only one" which leads to isolation in order to continue their self-abuse.

The bulimic may have a treasure chest of supplements that they take on a daily basis. They may be "health nuts" and know the fat, sugar, salt content and calories in an amazing amount of foods.

They may be voracious pill poppers and use all manner of vitamins and or supplements. Often experts on metabolism and digestion and disorders of the gut, they are a virtual resource book of health related information.

Some bulimics take supplements to support their habit upwards of 10 times a day. All of us live by or with life's consequences and rules. Bulimics have found a way to bend those rules.

The rules of healthy eating are:

- Eat in excess = get fat
- Eat just enough = maintain weight
- Eat small amounts = weight loss
- Eat too little to sustain life = death

The formula / existence of a bulimic runs as follows:

- Eat a lot = Vomit or laxative = No weight gain = Hide the habit = Repeat
- Eat a lot = Vomit or laxative = No weight gain = Hide the habit = Repeat
- Eat a lot = Vomit or laxative = No weight gain = Hide the habit = Repeat

The literary world says that vampires are never satiated. They are dead and yet have to rely on the blood of other living beings. Likewise, the Bulimic is never really satisfied, as the urge to eat is never fully satiated. Both are stuck in a repetitive cycle of eat and hide, eat and hide.

- **Bulimics and anorexics are extremists/perfectionists.**
- **Bulimics and anorexics do not want to be the way that they are.**
- **Bulimics and anorexics are terrified of what will become of their bodies if they stop their practice.**
- **Bulimics and anorexics seek total (or close) control of themselves and their surroundings to feel safe and happy.**
- **Bulimics and anorexics feel it is almost (but not quite) out of their control to discontinue their habit.**
- **Bulimics do not actually expel all the contents of their stomachs as some food always gets through. This is proven as the body still produces stools. It is further demonstrated as the bulimic does not wither away to skin and bones, unless there is another factor missed such as parasites / cancer, extreme laxatives, etc.**
- **Bulimics believe they are too smart to ever be caught. Bulimics are the chameleons of the nutrition world, as they appear to be like all of us, but in fact are very different.**
- **Bulimics tend to gulp their food taking large bites in a frenzied struggle to hurry ingestion so that it can be removed before it does damage and digestion occurs.**
- **Bulimics and Anorexics need isolation to carry out their starving, binging and purging, as it is not a socially acceptable activity.**

What makes these conditions or states tenable are man's free will, worries, stresses, misunderstandings of nutrition, micro awareness of self, desire for perfection and wholesale choices in getting and ingesting sustenance.

Man (and to a slight extent the ape / monkey) is the only species on the planet that eats for pleasure. This is where free choice comes into play. A rattlesnake never turns down a mouse meal unless he has just fed and can take any more.

Conversely, when it comes to a meal, man wants the first and second course, two helpings of desert and then a snack before bedtime.

Some might argue that "but my cat (or dog) puts his nose up at food he doesn't like". That is learned behavior. In the wild, food is food for a hungry animal period.

Elephants do not seem to be concerned about how much weight they are gaining. Lions and tigers are not trying to look better than the alpha male or matriarch of the pack. Man is he desperately wants to fit in and be young forever.

Rumination/Bulimia

There is an additional level of bulimia seldom noted called rumination. **Definition:** Rumination is derived from the Latin word ruminare, which means to chew the cud. It is the voluntary or involuntary regurgitation and re-chewing of partially digested food that is either re-swallowed or spit out.

This type of regurgitation is effortless and is similar to belching. Rumination does not involve nausea or gagging.

I am an expert on this subject as I have had this ability since I was a small child.

Since so little is known about this ability / phenomena, that for the next several paragraphs, I am going to spell it out very clearly.

Rumination Factors:

- **Food is swallowed and then returned to the mouth for more chewing. It is considered a pleasurable activity to re-taste food no longer available for tasting.**
- **The larger the piece of food, the easier it is to ruminate.**
- **Food can be returned to the mouth prior to reaching the stomach. This indicates that esophageal control is also a factor.**

- Flexing the stomach muscles and pushing the content up to the mouth achieves rumination. The esophageal sphincter is a valve that is meant to remain closed after food passes into the stomach. In rumination the esophageal sphincter is flexed open and allows food to pass back up the esophagus and to the mouth. There is no pain or discomfort. It is simply the flexing of a muscle.

- Some rumination is performed before the food gets to the stomach as it is flexed back up the throat before it passes the esophageal sphincter.

- The esophagus and esophageal sphincter is so sensitive it is possible to correctly identify what kind of food particles are being returned to the mouth to be re-chewed.

- The food is not bitter or acidy until after about 35 minutes in the stomach left undisturbed as digestive acid takes over.

- Dairy products such as milk become acidy faster than other more dense foods. This means they increase the speed of the digestive process.

- Yeast bearing foods such as bread, crackers pastry, cereals, cake, cookies etc. foods also become acidy quickly in the stomach and are then more difficult to extract.

- When a ruminator is sick and the body needs to or is trying to vomit, the ruminator resists vomiting. When sick, the body is actively rejecting something. This reaction seizes control of the stomach and esophagus and to a great extent renders the free will of the ruminator a non-factor.

- Rumination may be achieved by flexing the diaphragm (that sits under the stomach) to push up from below the stomach, thus pushing the stomach content up the esophagus.

- It is believed that infants involuntary ruminate. There is no way to validate this postulation, because infants do not explain their actions. Clearly rumination is not involuntary later in life. It is clearly a voluntary action.

- Watery fluids are the most difficult to ruminated.

- Thick fluids can easily be ruminated.

- Once food is mixed with water it is much harder to ruminate.

- Food mixed with water has very little appeal to the ruminator as the water has diluted the taste of what they have eaten.

- Tomato based products quickly become acidy in the stomach.

- Mixing different food types slow digestion and makes rumination possible for 2-3 hours after digestion.

If monsters are scary, as we do not know much about them, rumination is the stuff of nightmares.

Until this reading you, like most of the planet, had never heard of it or knew it had a name.

The ruminator is not a monster. Yet, the ruminator feels like an outcast. Other than instilling a personal feeling of being a pariah-like recluse, rumination serves no real purpose to humans.

With the exception of extracting poison or drugs given in a hostage or terrorism situation, rumination serves no valuable human purpose. Most of us will never be poisoned or in captivity and therefore rumination serves no utility.

Most bulimics, who have this ability to regurgitate by just flexing their gut, secretly think they are sideshow freaks.

Since our thoughts become laws, for all intents and purposes, until the habit is controlled and stopped, this is true. To be fully vested in society one must not hide in closet practicing habits that they are embarrassed about.

Again, mankind is not meant to be isolated; any activity that by its nature must be practiced in secret or private is damaging to the individual and needs to be discontinued. Rumination just like its sister bulimia, is socially unacceptable.

Steve Starr "The Human Regurgitator" is not a ruminator. He is a performer doing a feat of entertainment. Any real ruminator can spot this, as the esophagus never flexes.

You might ask how I, your humble author Roger Bezanis, so intimately know so much about bulimia and rumination. The raison d'être that I am so versed is because I was bulimic for two years and before that anorexic. I am an authority as I have actually lived these two amazing (and life threatening) habits / lifestyles. I am also and always will be a skilled ruminator though I do not practice it.

I know / understand the motivations / psyche or emotions that comingle to create this aberration in humanity that exist in no other species on earth. Man has free will and that is good. It is in a toxic environment that our best intentions can go askew.

When I was in my late teens and early 20s, I was anorexic and bulimic. I dropped from 175 lbs to 125 lbs in a month and a week (anorexia). I became anorexic as I went off to college. I was wired on vitamins and orange flavored Jolly Rancher candy. Dropping weight, I looked like a sick 40-year-old man.

The final week of my anorexia involved not sleeping for a week. I couldn't sleep as my body was wired like a bomb. After 5 days of 24 hour a day consciousness, I finally fell asleep for 16 hours. When I awoke, it was time to finally eat. As mentioned before, I had dropped from 175 lbs down to 125 lbs.

Roger Bezanis

Roughly two weeks later, I discovered bulimia. Bulimia is simply the expelling or purging of food matter after eating.

What I did was not at all healthy. I could have done a controlled fast or adapted another healthy diet but without knowledge I starved myself.

A short time after giving up bulimia, I went from the frying pan to the fire so to speak.

Within one year of giving up anorexia, I became bulimic. Very soon, I was spending ridiculous amounts of money vomiting up food that I had just swallowed. I might as well have been flushing $20.00 bills down the toilet.

Just like I mentioned before, I felt I was:

Worthless

A leper, pariah, outsider or stranger to mankind

Cheating the food I was eating

Hiding

An idiot

Cheating life as I was changing the rules

I was flushing my self-respect right down the toilet

Food was controlling me versus the other way around

The signs and symptoms of Bulimia:

- **Closet eating, seldom eating in public**
- **Hiding food**
- **In the office, hiding food in a desk drawer**
- **Late night grocery shopping sprees**
- **Poor teeth (as stomach acid wears away at the enamel)**
- **Large amounts of money spent on dental work and caps**
- **Quick trips to the toilet immediately after eating**
- **Rinsing ones mouth after use of the restroom (rinsing acid from the mouth)**
- **Excessive spending on food**
- **Obsession about weight**

- Obsessive eating of junk food (or any food) but not gaining weight
- Undigested food (chewed) particles in the toilet after the suspected bulimics use
- Strange splattering on the walls of the bathroom the Bulimic frequent most often (food splatters)
- Eating for comfort when stress arises
- A bulimic may also be overly health conscious. Not necessarily in the business of health but practically an expert on the subject.
- They may also be obsessed with caloric intake and food content (sodium, salt sugar etc).
- Most bulimics are careful to clean the toilet after every use but occasionally make a mistake and leave food matter behind.
- In general bulimics tend to be perfectionists (this is not always true but it is very common).
- They tend to be very controlling individuals, as control equals safety. A bulimic must control everything they can so that they are in charge and can keep their secret, secret.

Be aware that anyone who is thrust into a job, which is dependent on looking good, may be stressed to extremes. Those that are affected most with bulimia and anorexia are actors, strippers, food servers and models. Yet anyone can be a bulimic. Keeping the secret is an all or nothing venture. They tend to believe that their habit is all that helps them hold onto their sanity. Bulimics are not necessarily lean yet they usually are not terribly overweight. It is very hard for even the most skilled bulimic to fully empty their stomach. Otherwise they would not still have bowel movements and they do.

Yet the strain from constant vomiting can damage the esophagus, stomach, lungs and more. What is always ignored is that once the body receives food, it goes into digestion mode and starts producing all the material it needs for the task.

This includes bile (from the gallbladder), which is vital to proper digestion. Some bulimics will vomit 8 to 10 times a day, although the average is closer to 4-5 times a day.

One of the main things keeping the bulimic in check is the cost of the habit. It is not cheap to always be hungry and constantly purchasing food. Just like cocaine it is not cheap to have this habit.

The dollar cost of being a bulimic is staggering; depending on how extravagant one's taste happens to be for this kind of gratification. Imagine flushing 25-70 dollars down the toilet every day. The 25-70 dollars does not include the food that the bulimic intends to "keep" and not vomit up. Bulimia is not as expensive as a cocaine habit but just as addicting.

Bulimia, like any addiction, requires the addict to believe he is helpless to do anything about their condition without the use of drugs or confinement / hospitalization. This is patently false.

This kind of frantic attitude toward food is accompanied by the belief that they are victims of something outside their control.

Gorging oneself to the point of physical illness is not a new problem. A popular belief was that all of Rome (circa 1800 A.D.) was using vomitoriums to expel unwanted ingested food for the sole purpose of ingesting more food, thus being more social.

This is a slight misunderstanding mixed with some truth.

The vomitorium was actually an access tunnel used at a stadium or theater for public or performer access during or after a show. In most theatres, these passageways are restricted to actors for entrance or egress from the stage. Some live theatres still have vomitoriums. Nonetheless, these passages are meant for ambulation, not in any way for human waste of any type.

As for the factual part of this misunderstanding, some Romans of the aristocracy were practicing upchucking of their meals on occasion. The practice appears to not be widespread but did occur. It was certainly not an accepted and or common practice among the Roman commoners. Eating enough to get sick is clearly not a new problem. It has existed as long as man has been eating. For early man, Mother Nature was the wild card affecting survival. Monsoon, drought, snow etc of course plays havoc on the food supply, creating major shortages. When food is scant the initial reaction is to gorge oneself when it is found. This over reaction can cause digestive upset and induce vomiting on contact. Too much sustenance introduced too quickly can even cause death depending on how emaciated the hungry man was.

Food must be introduced slowly to the starving individual.

Other factors that can influence how humans view food are:

Fear of mortality

Fear of hunger or no more food

Peer pressure to fit in and look a certain way (be skinny)

Fear of loss of control of one's body (getting fat)

Obsessive desire for unlimited pleasure

Distorted view on oneself (always think they are fat)

Fear of disease

Fear of bowel movements

Education or lack of it in the area of nutrition

Other

The purging of food from the body can be accomplished a number of ways:

Shoving a finger (or something) down the throat creating a gag reflex

Voluntary regurgitation (up chucking on command)

Laxatives used at extreme strength

The way I finally beat Bulimia

Breaking any habit, from biting ones nails to shooting heroin, starts with a personal choice. Sure a solution can be forced on someone, but unless "The Someone" decides to be the author of the choice, the change will not stick. Witness the revolving door of celebrities forced into rehab that revert to their pervious patterns.

When I decided that, once and for all, any food entering my mouth had to stay there, I was able to allow myself to reenter society. I knew I had to do something or I was going to die a lonely man with rotting teeth.

In order to kick this problem, I knew I had to tell someone (a large group) of people that I was bulimic. I attended a weekend retreat called the Wall offered on the San Juan Islands off the coast of Washington State. This event was a combination of intense activity and deep discussion. We did Tai Chi, ran walked two miles a day and ate a Spartan diet of rice with some protein.

This retreat was like a sort of boot camp yet had nothing to do with addictions or diseases. It was strictly for discovering what ones mental and physical limits were. Men and women had separate sleeping quarters in a military barracks like environment.

The weekend was all about completion. One did not have to run the two miles; they could walk it but had to complete it. Personal introspection was encouraged and no personal comments or self-realizations were ridiculed. Being so isolated and in such a safe environment made my decision to go public with my weakness easier, yet it was not easy at all.

Attendee after attendee stood to up to blather on about something or the other. I not only could not hear a word they were saying, my heart was beating over one hundred times a minute. I was terrified to stand out and spill my guts.

The after dinner sharing session droned on and on. Then I took center stage and through my fear, shame and embarrassment, I told the whole room of 45 people my dirty little secret. I was bulimic! I was finally honest about who I was. I felt so free and relieved; far more than I ever had before.

Roger Bezanis

I explained in detail how I did what I did. I promised the group for myself that I would never upchuck again.

It was alternately one of the most difficult and most rewarding things I had ever done. I was no longer a space alien. I had again re-entered the land of the living. I was no longer in a world of light and shadow. I was alive again. This was in February, 1982, I was 21 years old.

The rest of my quest was to recondition myself into new healthy habits. I recognized that as a bulimic I wanted to eat everything. But now to avoid being a bloated sick version of myself, I had to make adjustments or that would be my fate.

One enjoyable way I discovered that I could eat was to go to a restaurant and order 5-8 items on the menu and have a bite or two of each. I never allowed myself to take home leftovers, as that would be giving food power over me. Since I paid for the meal, it was mine to do whatever I wanted with it.

I taught myself to always leave food on my plate. I also made it a regular habit to never overeat during the holidays. My target was to lose a pound or two during every holiday seasons. This is a challenge, yet lots of fun.

The key to handling Bulimia:

- The Bulimic is not a social active person, as his habit must stay hidden.
- Understand that no bulimic really wants to be a bulimic.
- He or she feels alone and isolated and hungers to be normal.
- Every bulimic loves the taste of the food.
- Every bulimic feels ashamed and or embarrassed, while flushing their self-respect down the toilet.
- Do not make the bulimic wrong. No one can ever make the bulimic more wrong than he or she is making himself. Instead encourage him to look at his behavior to evaluate its survival versus contra survival potential.
- Support them in regaining their self-respect via education of nutrition and love.
- Help the bulimic get honest with society by announcing publicly to as many people as possible who and what he was. This may involve writing a letter but should be done in person as much as possible. The world is rooting for the bulimic to regain control of his or her life. The world loves a good success story.
- If necessary, give the bulimic a safe place to break their habit. A quiet place may mean a house or cottage to rest, sleep and focus on who they were and who they are becoming. Encourage him or her to document in written form what their life has been like. These

writings may one day help someone just like them.

- Follow these steps and the later points on the steps to beating addiction and you can help anyone.

Conquering/Controlling Bulimia

- Never grocery shop alone. This is another step to keeping honest about what you are eating. After a few months and much success, you may shop alone.

- As necessary, graze (nibble healthy treats, grapes, apples slices,etc.) throughout the day, never eating any one big meal. Keep fresh fruit handy for the quick nibble or for momentary grazing.

- Use a very small plate (if necessary) to control portions until you can naturally do it.

- If eating in a restaurant, get out of the habit of cleaning your plate. Restaurants do not understand you, your needs or your urges.

- Eat slowly. Eating is not a race. Savor every bite, as this is the last time you will ever taste it. In macrobiotics it is encouraged to chew food 100 times before swallowing.

- Always try to eat with a friend (not in isolation).

- Avoid fast food, (due to sugars, sodium, grease, etc.), as it would even make a non-bulimic vomit. So-called "fast foods," un-balance the body and ultimately leave the body open to infection and sickness.

- Avoid buffets as this encourages over eating.

- Keep remaking the choice to not be bulimic until it is no longer an issue.

- Own a scale and use it first the thing every morning to insure you are meeting your targets and goals for your body.

- Start and maintain an exercise program that contributes to your targets and goals.

- Make friends with a former bulimic and support each other.

- If so needed, get roommates who support you and your quest.

- Do a detox, using formulas or perhaps a sweat or sauna program to get your body free of the waste that it has been craving.

- Be good to yourself. No one can put you through the kind of hell that you can. No one will ever feel as ashamed as you will about your weakness. Know that your weaknesses are just this side of your strengths. You can get there. You just have to decide to do it.

Defeating urges is not a psychiatric problem, yet psychiatrists insist that it is. They assume that your moods and habits are due to a lack of medication. It is just the opposite. The amount of toxicity (from junk food) has overwhelmed your liver and made it very difficult to think straight.

Anything you do to help yourself should involve reactivating your liver and kidneys.

When they are working at their maximum, your urges are controllable. Have you noticed that your urges come almost the same time every day? This illustrates that your liver and kidneys need support at that moment and doing anything worthwhile to help them, will help you.

Do not let anyone tell you that to beat your condition you have to be hospitalized or drugged.

There is another well known eating/starving habit.

78 What is Anorexia?

Definition: Anorexia (pronounced—AN-UH-REX-E-UH) is the practice of not eating or starving oneself in an attempt to control our body image and weight. A person who is anorexic may be remarkably lean or skinny yet sees himself or herself as very rotund or overweight. The anorexic may be taking vitamins or supplements (tablets or capsules) for metabolism at a remarkable rate (8 to 12 times a day or more).

Note: Any one or two of these signs does not guarantee that anorexia is present. But when a number of these symptoms are present, then it is time to be interested. Up to 95% of those pronounced to have anorexia are women. But do not neglect the slow rise in men obsessed with their weight. It was believed the off spring (baby boomers) of the depression of 1929 and WWII families (who had to conserve food, etc.) were the most likely candidates for eating issues. Because parents enforced deviant eating habits on their children, a case can be made for manic control of food as the result.

It is even a joke to kid someone who leaves food on their plate, that "You should be ashamed of yourself not cleaning your plate; there are children who are starving right now in South Africa."

Some post WWII mothers even resorted to hiding food so that the food in question would "last longer." Now that is some odd computational thinking. For the child of the 1960s, it was a crime to not clean one's plate. Somehow making the plate the determiner of how hungry the child was makes no sense.

Even today there is a push to take leftovers home from restaurants. Sure it is food that is paid for, but a certain percentage of those who use doggy bags do it compulsively.

Oddly, the term doggy bag originally meant it was for the dog. It's only been since the 1990s that that term has completely fell out of vogue for the "To-go-bag."

Rationing was common in WWII households and these two eating abnormalities may very well still have their roots in this conflict. Add to that the push-pull of advertisers promoting fit bodies on one channel and a moment later another commercial is promoting the latest Pizza toppings and crust.

Regardless of the source of their motivation, an anorexic person craves control. Like the bulimic, controlling one's environment is just as paramount as controlling one's body. Interestingly, the higher the family economic stratum, the more likely an eating deviation will be present

Signs and Symptoms of Anorexia

- Perfectionism
- Constant fear of gaining weight
- Fear of food or eating
- Use of diet pills or stimulants
- Eats very little
- Exercise to extreme on stomach, hips thighs
- Reclusive
- Own more than one scale
- Always watching exercise tapes or DVDs
- Owns extreme amounts of exercise equipment
- Counting calories and weighing food before eating
- Extremely tight fitting clothes or extremely loose clothes
- Constantly weighing
- Mood swings
- Sunken eyes
- Hollow cheeks
- Colon cleansing junkie
- Detox (herbal or otherwise) junkie

Anorexia is just as devastating as Bulimia and features many of the same traits but not all. At its heart, Anorexia is a severe distortion of a person's body image. While the mirror reflects skinny, the person perceives that there is fat than needs to come off.

It has been said, "You can never be too skinny or have too much money." Perhaps the money aspect of that statement is true but the rest of it is pure folly.

Imagine the people held in concentration camps. Walking bags of bones, these people did not intend to lose weight at the rate they did. An Anorexic needs to lose weight, as they are always fat. Right up until their death.

Not all Anorexics starve themselves to death but small percentages have slipped through the cracks and have. Some of you older readers will remember "The Carpenters." They were a musical duo (Richard and Karen) that reached their pinnacle of fame during the mid1970s.

Karen never received the diagnoses of Anorexia, as in 1975 it was unknown. When she died in 1983 she was 80 pounds. She had been 140 lbs. in 1975 and quickly (via a water diet) dropped down to 120 and then 115 pounds.

Karen Carpenter routinely used prescription drugs for thyroid disorders and huge amounts of vitamins to help her feel better as she slowly wasted away. She sought out medical help and received drugs, which aided in her demise.

No one ever accepts help unless they want it. Anorexia is a cry of "Help me help myself; I want to gain control of my life." The person who is starving themselves for beauty or image needs to compare black to white. Literally the anorexic person, no matter how lean, sees himself or herself as fat.

Anorexia, at its base, is an aversion to eating based on a distortion of personal perception. The anorexic is literally starving, as they believe they are grotesquely overweight. One of the easiest ways to help them is via comparisons. I will explain this later.

Help them via comparison and education but not drugs or surgery. These sorts of attitudes about food and image come from very extreme points of view.

Eating aberrations are far more common than we think. One estimate indicates that 4 out of every 10 people have a distortion toward food that corresponds to a distorted view of their body.

The bulimic and anorexic use their secret habit for an emotional purpose. These emotional attachments skew the perceptions of the Bulimic and Anorexic, thus justifying their very extreme behavior.

A huge problem with anorexia and bulimia is that the participant has no real concept of how their body works. Most have no real understanding of what it takes to maintain their body via diet.

With so much misinformation on human health, the bulimic and anorexic must fully understand the complexities of their own body. The question that needs answering is what makes MY body tick?

Too often, the fear of gaining weight is alloyed with no real understanding of what the body needs to survive. It does not matter what works for others, it matters that the subject fully understand and appreciate their body and condition.

Beating Anorexia

Have the anorexic individual identify 3-5 celebrities who the anorexic agrees are not too fat and not too lean.

Get full body photos of these celebrities. Have the anorexic compare full body photos of their body to the body of the healthy celebrity previously identified. The purpose here is to have the person see the differences between a healthy body and an anorexic body.

Next it is very important to start to educate the anorexic on what food is and how the body uses it.

Finally, the pictures of the healthy celebrity should be blown up and placed around the mirrors of the anorexic so that a comparison is always possible.

Does the anorexic need drugs or surgery? No. The anorexic needs education and the ability to see and identify similarities and differences among themselves and others. He or she also needs proper nutrition that they are themselves participating in, either by food preparation or via shopping for the ingredients.

Anorexia and Bulimia as per medical "experts" is a nervous condition than can only be treated with drugs and surgery. I refuse to use this term, as this gives license to abuse to drug and give surgery to people who will be only be poisoned and made weak by these efforts.

All disease requires the acceptance that there is no personal responsibility for their condition. This is false and is a victim mentality.

The anorexic and the bulimic must make a moment-to-moment choice to participate in their slow demise. No one can make that choice for them. They may have lost sight of it, but it is a choice. They were not caught by a bug or attacked by something beyond their control.

Beating Any Addiction

- Deciding one can be cause over one's body and life.
- Deciding to be in charge of one's own life and body
- Admitting the problem (the larger the group the better) as a secret will remain a secret if it is not acknowledged
- Education on the subject and how it affects the body
- Education on proper nutrition
- Proper nutrition
- Continually deciding to be in charge of one's own life and body
- Use of as support group
- Avoiding isolation as isolation can lead to secrets such as bulimia or anorexia
- Continually deciding to be in charge of one's own life and body

In conclusion we chose who we are, what we do, how we live and our state of health. Anorexia, bulimia / rumination are choices that are made from moment to moment. Do not let anyone tell you otherwise. Drugs and surgery are not the answer. The answer lies within.

Each of us has the power to control what we do. Our society has taught us that this is not the case. Just because we are told that the sky is pink does not make it pink. Just because the so-called "authorities" say that this condition needs this kind of handling does not make it so.

What is true is true for you. You must be the one who decides that you want help. You do know what the truth is. You do know when you are being lied to. That is why you are reading this book.

You can identify truth and make your life healthy and happy.

Choose yourself, choose man and help me help the planet. The biggest helper you will ever have is you. I need you but the planet needs you more.

Final Notes on Addictive behavior

Who is the AMA or the APA (American Psychiatric Association)? These two organizations have a vested interest in convincing the American public that they are sick. One way or the other they want every American on one drug or another.

If you believe you are sick, you are a candidate for drugs and surgery, you immediately become a valuable resource for BIG PHARMACUITALS & INSURANCE. If you are not on the medical and insurance rolls you are useless.

79 Control = Cause

You have no doubt noticed that much of this book is taken directly from my life. This chapter is no different.

Much of my early trouble in life came from being in a hurry to do anything else other than what I supposed to be doing. In the 4th grade we were given an I.Q. test. Having zero interest in this examination, I hurried through it marking the questions randomly. All I wanted to do was play outside. As a result it was believed that I had the I.Q. of a rodent.

Rightly or wrongly, I was placed in "slow" groups for the next 5 years of my school life. The results of that I.Q. test would haunt me until I was in 10th grade in high school.

Back in the fourth grade, the first consequence of my flippant approach to evaluation was to be placed in the "slow" reading group. Every three days or so, our class divided into two groups all of those who could read and all of those who couldn't.

The good readers were given written assignments and the poor readers (five of us) were grouped together to read out loud. Ridden with stage fright, dyslexia and who knows what else, reading out loud was nearly impossible.

While reading out loud, I would stutter, stammer and improvise what I thought what was on the page. To hide my nervousness, I would go so far as to give my opinions on the book and the writer. I was unintentionally very funny, yet I was completely out of control.

Standing up to read, it would all start again.

First Mrs. Reel (my teacher) would warn the rest of the class, "Pay no attention, Roger is going to read." She might as well have told them to take copious notes on my performance.

Bumbling and fumbling, the class laughter would swell to a crescendo and then I would finally sit down, released from my torment.

Kids laughing, Mrs. Reel laughing, Me, I was dying.

Three different times teachers from adjoining classes barged in wanting to know what was so funny. There I stood the center of attention. Mrs. Reel, doubled over howling, sponging tears from her eyes, would cackled, "Its Roger, he's reading"!

Swaying back and forth did help me read better. Yet Mrs. Reel told me to stop and just read. Reading out loud felt like my skin was being peeled away.

Jumping ahead to the 10th grade, it was about to start all over again.

Roger Bezanis

I took an English "Elective" class on Greek Mythology; it sounded like a good idea. One of our first assignments was to create our own myth, and then read it out loud in front of the class. My good idea was not so good after all.

My myth was on the "God of Hamburgers."
(An interesting subject choice considering the content of the last chapter)

As I stood up to read, my entire previous trauma returned. I was in 4th grade all over again. But this was worse, these were my own words, and I still could not read them.

I was in terror as I started mumbling the "God of Hamburgers."

I lost my balance, stuttered, made faces; gave commentary on my reading and fell backwards over the table I was leaning on. I was Jim Carrey, Don Adams (Get Smart), Jerry Lewis and Woody Allen all wrapped up into one.

Kids were rolling on the floor with laughter. On guy told me he wet his pants he was laughing so hard.

With four lines left to go on my story, the bell rang signaling the end of class.

I was an unintentional riot. Mrs. Thomas (my teacher) told me that I should be on stage, and refused to give me my grade until the class heard the full myth again the next day. I was going to have to do it all again the next day!!!!

I was going to die.

Something happened for the first time. Kids told me, "You are so funny" etc., I was asked, "Did you mean to do that?" I did not know what to say. I said, "Yea, I meant to do that, it is all practiced and stuff, I do that all the time."

Now I was in big trouble. Because the kid asked me that question, I was going to have to do it all again and this time mean to be funny.

I went home and rehearsed fake nervousness for hours. I perfected the art of stuttering. This was mandatory, as my "funny reputation" was on the line. I turned my affliction into an act.

When I performed the next day I was funny, yet not as funny as the first day. Because I was rehearsed I was not nervous at all.

Standing in front of a crowd did not bother me! I was under control. My stage fright was gone. I could finally read all of the words on the page.

Jimmy Stewart, an actor from the 1940s to 1980s, was a terrible stutterer. Yet, in his films he did not stutter at all. On film he was rehearsed. In life he was the victim of a mechanism out of his control.

The reason my affliction was "released" was because that kid asked me, "Did you mean to do that"? This question might as well have been, "Roger, who is the source of your stuttering"? Or, even more simply "Who did it"?

By me saying, "Yea, I meant to do that, it is all practiced and stuff, I do that all the time." I became cause over my difficulty. I might as well have said, "I did it."

Being creator of my trouble meant that I could have or not have my reading / stage fright crisis at will. When I said, "I did it" the problem VANISHED.

This story may seem like an allegory for taking responsibility for one's life and it is. But this story is 100% true.

No quandary can remain a quandary once the source of it has been correctly identified. Bombs do not detonate around people who take responsibility for their creation.

I always thought someone or something else made me the way that I was. Nervousness must have come from my shoes or the center of the Earth. Surely I had nothing to do with it. And I did not, until I correctly said, "I am the source of my nerves."

Explaining exactly what I accidentally did has caused six stutterers to become former stutterers. Taking ownership, thus naming the correct source / cause of a problem it the first step to eliminating it. Again, six out of six have had the same results.

What are the limits of this or uses of this? I have no idea. Feel free to find out.

Remember the author of the story can write his characters anyway he or she wants. You are the author of your own life. You are the author or your own story.

Do not forget, control equals cause, equals zero affect.

Keys to mastering any habitual personal problem:

- Name the problem (I stutter, etc.)
- Answer the question: who is the source of the problem? The answer is always YOU!
- Practice the affliction until you are extremely good at it and can do it anytime on cue.

Crowds of as many as 1500 people cause me no fear whatsoever. Public speaking to 15 or 15,000 is welcome and fun.

Roger Bezanis

Where Do We Go Now?

Due to the controversial nature of my writings on Big Pharmaceuticals, soft drink makers, and other purveyors of death Oprah will probably not have me on her show, as she would lose advertisers. This means you have to talk this book up. Between us we can affect the lives of millions. I am speaking to everyone within earshot constantly. I am lecturing and teaching 13-20 weekends out of the year. The reason this book is making a difference is because of your efforts. People actually sit around and quote this book!

80 Success Stories

"By using the tools in my book, in only four months I repaired years of damage and lost 61 pounds. At 46, (2007) I have re-achieved my high school football playing weight."
- *Roger Bezanis - Author*

Dear Mr. Bezanis,

I have experienced tremendous benefits from utilizing the techniques learned from your book, Diagnostic Face Reading and Holistic Healing. By supporting the Liver, I have found relief from irritability (my husband is thrilled by this). I am now even, calm and better ability to deal with stressful situations. Through supporting my kidneys the way you recommended, I have discovered the most thrilling thing!! My ability to run has exponentially jumped! Even when I was a child I had difficulty running. I had no asthma or other "lung conditions" diagnosed, but I just couldn't run without becoming very short of breath. It felt feel like my lungs were going to explode. With your advice and information in your book, I have repaired my lungs, heart, and kidneys! I am now able to complete in 5K runs without stopping to walk! Now that is amazing! My endurance is far higher, my strength is noticeably better and my recovery time is really quick! I am shocked!! Thank you for this wonderful information and help!

L-
Kokomo, Indiana

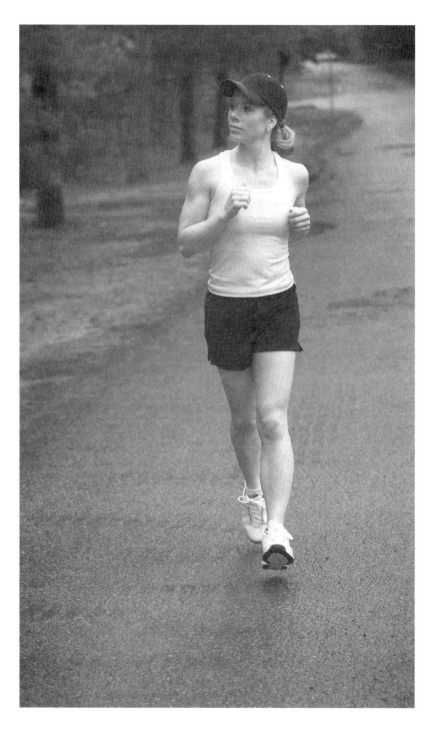

Roger Bezanis

Mr. Bezanis:

I am writing you back to tell you how much I appreciate you taking time out of your busy day to help me. Hope I can sufficiently articulate how thankful I am for your help.

These last two years have been very difficult without any alternative health practitioners to guide me in this healing process.

Cystic acne has ruined my life. I have tried many natural methods for healing acne, psoriasis and depression, but none of them ever really seemed to make much difference.

I have tried numerous supplements, and none of the creators of the formulas ever spoke to me about how to help my body heal itself.

This is why I was surprised and elated to talk to you.

Because of your kindness and remarkable book, these problems are completely fading from memory.

I now know I can live again.

The first Photo was taken around 2 months ago (August 24); "photo 2" was taken two days ago (Oct 22). I had no idea my face improved this much. The change has been far, far more than I had realized and in such a short time.

Thank you for your time and devotion in helping others get well. I'm sure many people are equally as grateful for your involvement in alternative health as I am.

Thank you again sir,
Michael

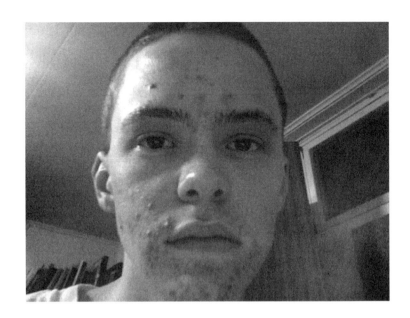

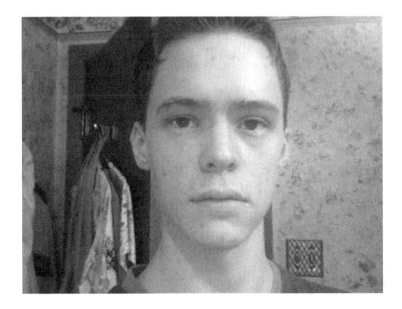

Roger Bezanis

Dear Roger!

I just want to let you know about my experiences with the Diagnostic Face Reading and the Energy Balancing.

As a Naturopathic Doctor, Iridologist, and Colon Hydrotherapist at Nature's Best Wellness Center, I work with clients in various states of dis-ease. It has always been a challenge to help them understand the connection between their health & their lifestyle choices. Since I began incorporating your Diagnostic Face Reading & Energy Balancing into our Wellness Center, the results have been phenomenal! With your book I can now show them, on their own face, body systems that may need support. By then knowing the right questions to ask (as you teach in your book) we can identify not only if they are in need of support, but what herbals that their body can use to help support and ease their state of dis-ease. When I help a patient feel noticeably better in one visit I always hear "How did you do that?" I point to the book because the answers are there. Your book has made healing an exciting experience for me and my clients. I actually have people coming in to see me who think that I am a healing magician all thanks to you and your amazing work.

Thank you again,
Laurie Ousley, N.D.

Nature's Best Wellness

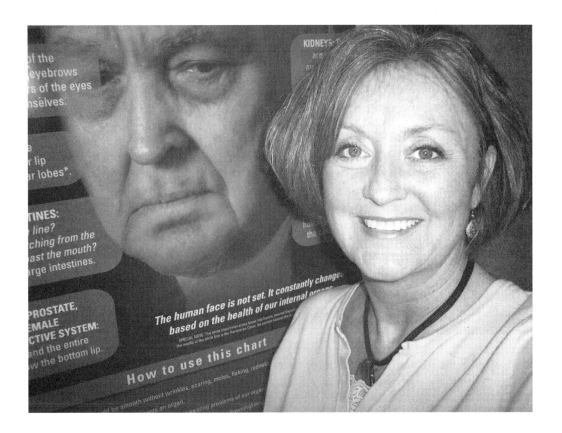

Roger Bezanis

SHOULD HAVE BEEN DEAD

I was given 5 years to live 5 years ago.

I was given notice that I have no hope of cure. My cholesterol was at around 3500. My triglycerides were at around 11000. Yes I should have been dead. This is very crazy. I was to the Mayo Clinic, UCLA and many others. I had the best studying my case. I was in the hospital all the time. My hospital stays were never ending. I had chronic pancreatitis, high blood pressure, blood sugar levels, depression and severe anxiety.

I was on more drugs than I could count.

I can't even remember them all. My hair had fallen out. I was always sick and hardly out of bed, I just wished for death. If I could die it would be all over. All of the pain of what I had lost would go away. My time with my horses was lost. So was the beach, school, hikes, quads, rodeo, gym, dancing and travel ALL gone. Just being my natural happy self was not possible. One day after I was released to go die, I was driving and I came to a red light. I looked over and saw a sign on a building for Natural Health and Wellness. I could not help it, I had to go in. My life changed that day. I went from drugs to herbs and from a crazy diet, I slowly learned how to eat minus all the bad stuff sugar, fast food, caffeine etc. I slowly got back in the gym and now I have everything back.

All of my numbers are normal again and my doctor (who I met that day) gets all of my referrals. All of my friends know who he is. Changing my life has saved my life.

CRAZY STORY HUH?
Thanks again

S-

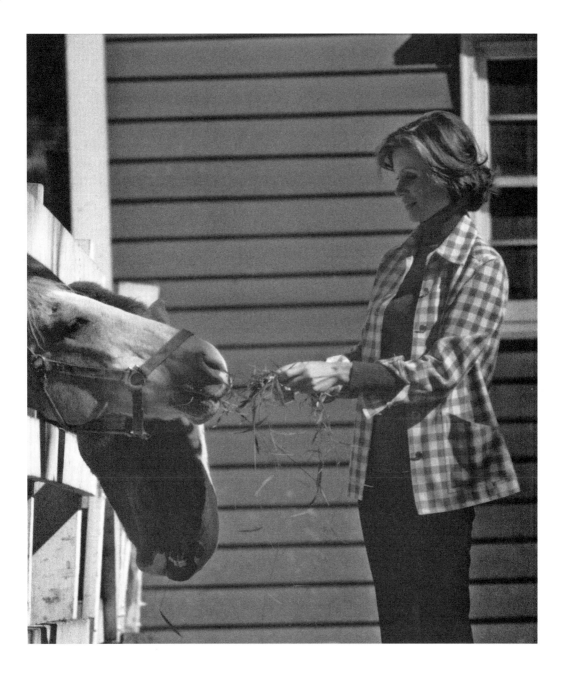

Roger Bezanis

WHAT A CHANGE!!!!

You Roger Bezanis are truly an inspiration! I used to drink 4 cups of black coffee a day understanding that it was good for concentration and energy. But I was always tired. I have often had trouble in that area.You do give great ideas! Now instead of the coffee I have a cup of hot water with half a lemon and Cayenne pepper. Now with your suggestion about eating citrus in the morning and evening (from your writings) I gave that a try too. My congestion is far better and with my lemon concoction that you suggested and I no longer desire coffee. I no longer need a nap by 2-3 PM and I now walk first thing in the morning (1/2) a mile and 2 miles in the evening when I would during my usual meal time. I am not hungry.

My family still eats dinner at the same time but I am out for a walk. I walk during dinner to avoid temptation and get some more exercise. But I am so full of energy I always feel like I could walk further. And I sleep a lot better.I remember reading that it is possible to improve skin by helping your liver. I thought that was funny because I was not going for better skin but it has improved so much, that I don't wear makeup anymore!!! These are very small changes but big changes over all. It's nice to get out and enjoy the Fall Season too, walking more and spending more time with nature. I am just so excited that you took so much time out to check in with me. That means a great deal to me you are grrrrrrrrrrrrrrreat! Now you know you are a true friend!!!

MUUUUUUUUUUUUUUUUUUUUUUUUUUUUUUUUUUUUUUA

Love

"E"

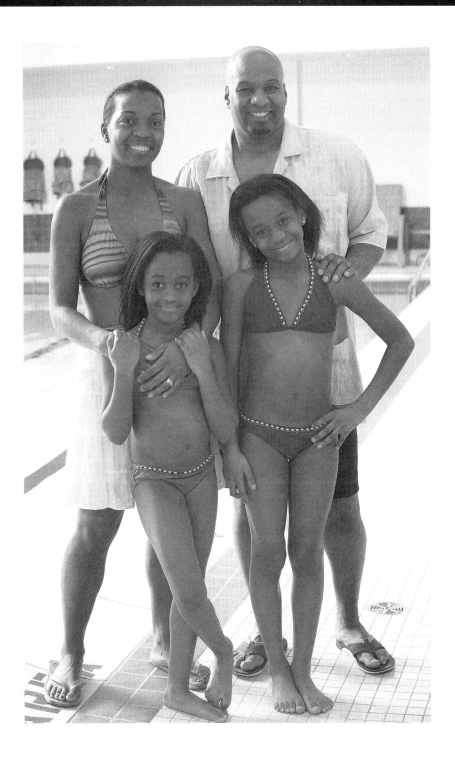

Roger Bezanis

My name is Elaine and I live in Aberdeen, Scotland. I take thyroxin for an under active thyroid. Other than that I am healthy at 5'2".

A few weeks ago my husband rooted me on as I took part in large marathon in Dublin (Southern Ireland). On race day my weight was 123 lbs. I felt great and was ready to go and take on the challenge that lay ahead.

Everything was great including the temperature, cool and crisp, perfect marathon weather!

Later running (around the 16 mile mark) I had to slow. Every part of my body felt pain. I felt puffy and bloated!! I looked at my hands and ankles and they were huge. Nothing like this happened during training.

I was determined none of this was going to beat me! But 12000 other entrants would, they were now all passing me!!

The next 10 miles were torturous. I've never felt such pain. I do not remember all of it, but I finished 6 hours and 21 minutes and 9278th place.Immediately after, returned to the hotel, soaked in a cold bath, (supposedly to help reduce inflammation).

After my bath I was feeling bloated so I weighed myself and I tipped the scales at 144 lbs!! I had gained a whopping 21lbs in just a few hours!!!!!

I was panicked but at the same time realized that it was probably inflammation and/or fluid retention, (I had drank a lot during the race!)

On my return home, whilst I was checking myspace for messages, I thought of Roger and whilst I appreciate he's real busy and may not of had time to help me I wrote to him anyway, almost instantly he replied with a message, mentioning my kidneys were probably in distress and that I should eat dark grapes and avoid bread, rice, pasta, cereal etc. These foods all would make me retain water.

Immediately after reading his words, I headed off to the shop to buy as many dark grapes as I could get my hands on, (I was getting real desperate!!).

I split the grapes up in to bunches, (about 15 grapes each bunch) and grazed all day and for the next few days too, not instantly but within hours of eating the grapes, I needed to pee and pee and pee!!

This went on for a few days; remember there were 21lbs of fluid that had attached itself to me!! The marathon was on the 27th of October and by the 3rd of November; I was feeling like myself again. Upon weighing myself I was so pleased!! I was a couple of pounds lighter than when I

DIAGNOSTIC Face Reading and Holistic Healing

started a delightful 121lbs!! All thanks to grapes and Roger!!

I cannot thank you enough for helping me out. It was so distressing and made me feel so lethargic. I had no idea that something as simple as grapes were so powerful.In my photos, you can see that I am not exactly big. But later after the race I was huge. My face, hands etc were all puffed up

This is remarkable.

Best Regards,
Elaine

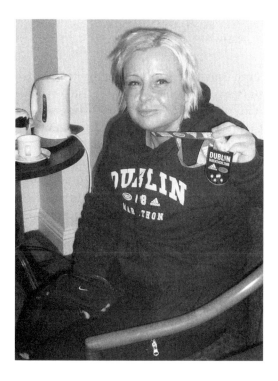
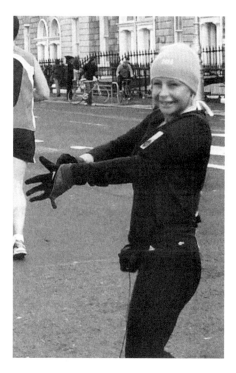

Dear Mr. Bezanis,

Your books have been a wealth of valuable information, thank you. You have helped me, my family and friends extensively. My mother and her sisters love your work. I have had a lot of experience with herbs and grew up familiar with them. Since I now am more aware of their effects, I take more now than ever before. Because of that, things have changed so much for me.

I was very self conscious of a spot on my right cheek not far from my ear. It had been there for about eight years. By following your recommendations, it is 95% gone! I had considered laser removal, but with my darker complexion there were chances the spot may get darker! I thought I was doomed. Thank goodness, I didn't waste any time or money on those procedures. Your simple approach has made all the difference in the world.

Also, I recently started going through menopause. I can honestly say that taking the herbs and using the diet you recommend has helped my hot flashes considerably. I still have half a cup of decaf a day. Yes, I am working on getting rid of it too. My moods are much more manageable. Insomnia has now kicked in but I have noticed that if I take in more of my herbs for the liver, plus exercise, I sleep like a baby. Speaking of exercise, if I take the herbs you speak about before a workout, I feel more energetic. It's great to know that it's so easy to decrease or eliminate my aches and pains after my workouts. Thank you again for helping me.

All the Best,
Sandy Pacheco

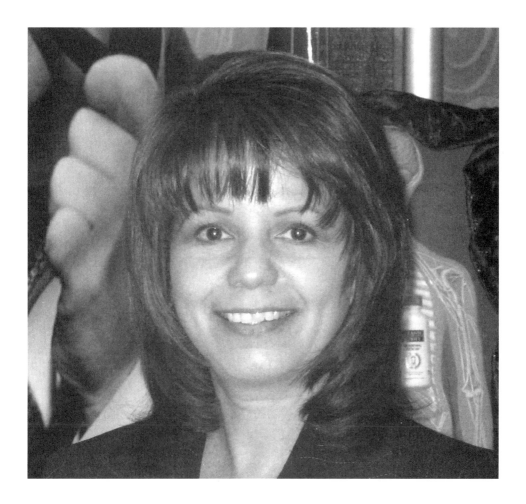

Roger Bezanis

Dear Mr. Roger

My sisters and I are all mature women. I am 71 but I feel 60! Two of my sisters listen to you and have read your book. They feel great too. The others might come around but until then, they are stuck with their aches, pains and problems.

When my daughter told me about what you did I was not sure what to make of it all. I only wish I had known about you years earlier. I can only imagine what it would have been like to live those years without all the aches and pains that I had. As you know I had ovarian cancer. When I went for my first chemo treatment the doctors thought they had the wrong examine information because they could not find the cancer anywhere. You said I would be surprised if I did what you said to do to handle for my cancer, and I was. So were the doctors. Just to be sure I still got the chemo but it was just for safety sake.

I always treat my liver just the way you say too and now my moods are never a problem. My bad back is a thing of the past. Now I am never sore from working around the house. I don't have acid reflux, high blood pressure or allergies either.

Thank you for being such a good friend. I don't know what I would do without you.

My name is Rachel Navarro and this is okay to print.

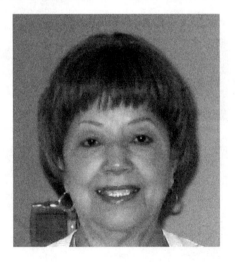

164 Pounds   225 Pounds

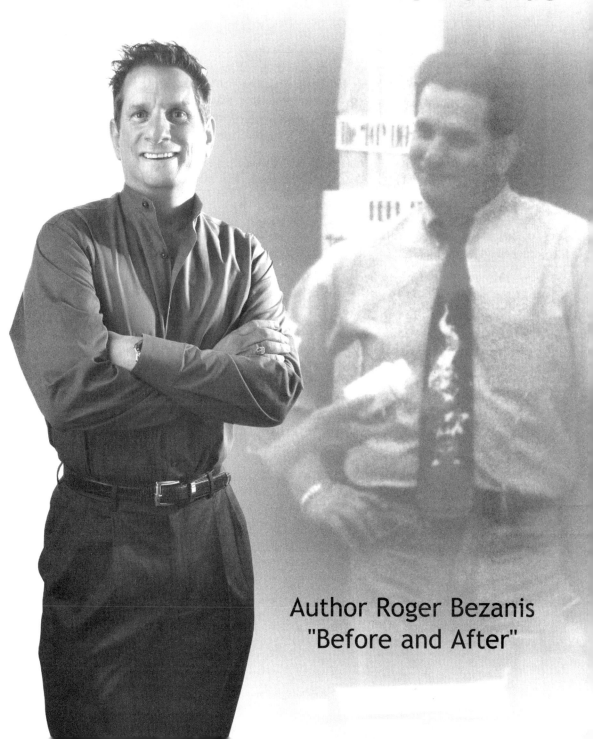

Author Roger Bezanis
"Before and After"

About the Author

*"Don't believe the lies from the AMA and FDA.
You can fix any problem of the body."*
— **Roger Bezanis**

Roger Bezanis has fervently worked in the field of health since 1991. He is the world's foremost expert on face reading and teaches Diagnostic Face Reading™ around the globe. An authority on detoxification of the human body, master formulator, educator, speaker and motivator for social and health change, he is constantly on the go. He is entirely self-trained and therefore not beholding to any group, social or medical dogma.

Debunking the brainwashing, deceptions & lies spewing from the Big Pharma, FDA, AMA & APA mega-criminals drives him. The self-regulating question that motivates all of his labors is "does it work"? Results are the beacon that illuminates the road to health.

Because of his miraculous vision and ability to make the complex simple, he has re-trained thousands of practitioners via his lectures and presentations. Rogers's ability to see and understand connections that heretofore have remained invisible is a marvel to medical science.

His presentations, classes, weekends and lectures are often standing room only. Seldom has a light so bright emitted from such a powerful speaker, transporting us home to health.

Find out where Roger is speaking next and bring your whole family.

How Roger has changed...

American Diet / Raw Food Diet
225 LBS — *164 LBS (his high school football playing weight)*
35-inch waist — *29-30 inch waist*
26 % body fat — *13-15 % body fat*

I eat a 98% raw food diet that features little or no protein (only the trace amounts found in fruit & veggies). This is a very old, yet cutting edge approach to health. It works.

Every morning I start with 12 to 36 ounces of fresh squeezed OJ or tangerine juice. Those who have employed my diet have dropped weight (as needed) and body fat. I live for Caesar salads (with no croutons or cheese), Pico de Gallo and anything fresh out of the ground.

Remember, if the worst thing that you eat is some dressing (that is out of a bottle), so be it. It is also better to shop at farmers markets and eat locally grown organic produce. Your body will be better grounded.

The most important aspects of life are circulation / energy / oxygen. With these points "in", the body can heal anything. It is never too late, until you stop breathing. This book bleeds with passion and is the focal part of my life. I am here to help mankind. That is the totality of my purpose. It is my mission to leave earth in better shape than when I found it.

You now have the full weight of my knowledge/understandings and awareness. Your journey is not over; it is beginning at this very moment. You now must be responsible for your new awakenings. You are fully conscious and obligated to push these truths forward, thus reversing the brainwashing administered to mankind.

Ignoring this responsibility is tantamount to turning your back on "who you really are." Please don't make me do this alone. Together we can change the future of our globe. We are engaged in a battle of epic proportions, the outcome of which will determine the future of this planet. It is a huge job.

Man needs your help. I am one person against a machine of untold power. Having finished reading this book it is NOW up to you to take it forward carrying on my words and work. The chapters in this manuscript are your friends. Use them often.

Stand up straight and enlighten everyone you care about with my message. Take this book to work and leave it on your desk. Keep a copy in your car and on your living room table. Unborn generations are counting on your efforts.

The future of earth is in the hands of our children. Because of that, get this book into the eager hands of every-pre-brainwashed-under-20-year-old you know. The world must at least become aware of the title of this book. The future of mankind is hinged on you taking responsibility for what you now know.

We all need your help. The choices you make henceforth will affect all of us.

Which side of the ledger will your name appear on? Will you sit back and do nothing? Will your name appear among the remarkable people who changed the world for the better? We must not fail or we move a little closer to the brink of oblivion for mankind. Do you want the blood of such a disaster on your hands?

What you do with this book is up to you. Perhaps you will put it down and never speak of it again. Could you forgive yourself if you did? The choice you make will shape the future of earth.

Welcome, I have been waiting for you.
Your Friend,
Roger Bezanis

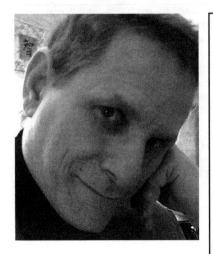

Do you have a Success Story that you would like to share with the world? "Do you have a great before and after picture that will shock people?"

If you do and you would like to submit one or both of them for use in my next book, just follow the instructions below:

Send them to:
Empirical Health Products
230 S. Olive St.
Ventura, Ca. 93001

Include the statement: "My pictures and success story are okay to print and use." Then sign it, date it and send it. They can also be sent by email to roger@pbiv.com